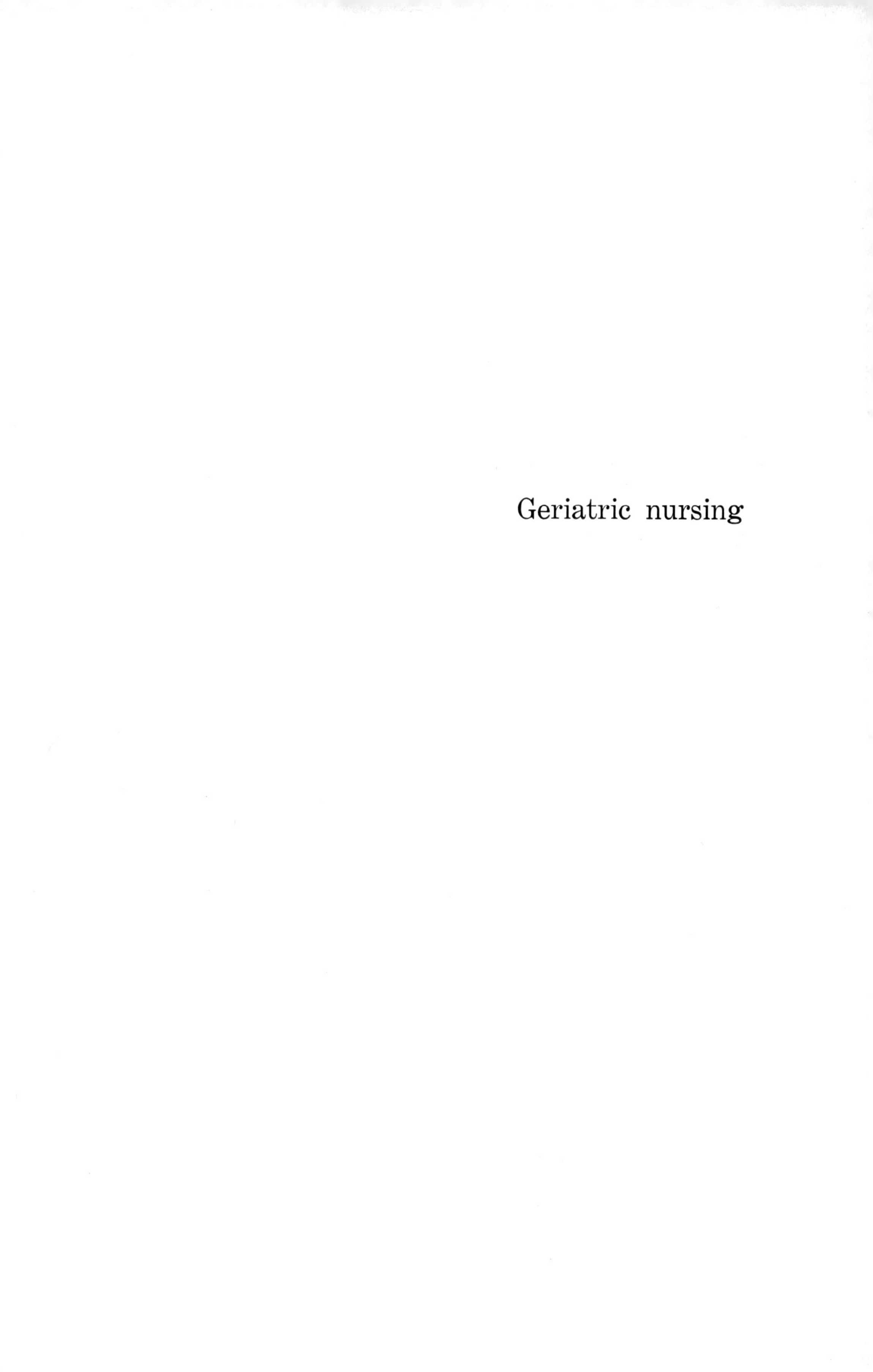

Geriatric nursing

Geriatric nursing

Kathleen Newton, R.N., M.A.

*Formerly Associate Professor in Out-Patient Nursing,
The Cornell University–New York Hospital School of Nursing,
New York, N. Y.; formerly Department Head, Out-Patient Nursing Service,
The Cornell University–New York Hospital Medical Center;
formerly Staff Nurse, The Visiting Nurse Association
of Plainfield and North Plainfield, N. J.*

Helen C. Anderson, R.N., P.T., M.N.

Associate Editor, American Journal of Nursing, *New York, N. Y.;
formerly Nurse Consultant, Vocational Rehabilitation Administration,
Washington, D. C.; formerly Nurse Consultant, Rehabilitation Education Service
Project, State Department of Health, Olympia, Wash.; formerly Assistant Professor,
School of Nursing, University of Washington, Seattle, Wash.;
formerly Instructor and Supervisor of Orthopedic Nursing, School of Nursing,
University of Washington, Seattle, Wash.*

Illustrated

Fourth edition

The C. V. Mosby Company

Saint Louis 1966

Fourth edition

Third printing

Previous editions copyrighted 1950, 1954, 1960

Printed in the United States of America

Standard Book Number 8016-3643-4

Library of Congress Catalog Card Number 66-13349

Distributed in Great Britain by Henry Kimpton, London

Preface

In this edition we have incorporated changes of the last decade that affect not only the responsibilities of the nursing profession for the health and welfare of the aging and aged in our population but also the nurse's competence in care of the elderly person who becomes ill.

The last few years have been marked by rapid social change, huge strides in scientific knowledge, and mastery of almost unbelievable technical procedures. In these years nursing has also become more fully aware of the contribution it should make to maintenance of health of the elderly and of how it may contribute effectively to the ever-expanding and increasingly complex galaxy of services needed to keep the aged well, to restore them to health, or to care for them if they cannot again become well.

It is our hope that joint authorship has helped to broaden the scope of the book yet preserve its practical usefulness for nurses working with older people in all areas of nursing practice. Although the basic format remains the same, chapters have been rearranged and altered and some have been largely rewritten. Material has been added on such conditions of the elderly as osteoporosis and emphysema, which are now being recognized much more frequently. A new chapter on the prevention of illness has been prepared. In addition, prevention is emphasized throughout the book since it is our belief that in this area lies one of the greatest challenges to nursing in care of the elderly.

Grateful appreciation is again due Miss Margaret R. Bonnell, librarian for the Muhlenberg Hospital, Plainfield, N. J., for her continued interest and helpfulness.

Kathleen Newton
Helen C. Anderson

Contents

Unit 1

General background and the aged

Chapter 1

Introduction

Our society appears to have awakened to the many needs of its older citizens and to be taking concrete action in their behalf. Perhaps the tremendous increase in the number of elderly persons in our population in recent years has translated a sentimental, but unproductive, concern into widespread activity toward their total welfare. In some older countries real regard for the aged has existed for years. In precommunist China, for example, the older person occupied a position of authority and respect. In the Scandinavian countries, provision is made for the security and contentment of the aged. More recently, England has begun to examine the needs and problems of its older generation and has taken action for their welfare.

Each year the chances of life extension improve. A Roman baby born 2,000 years ago had a life expectancy of 22 years. In 1959 in our country a baby boy had a life expectancy of 66.5 years, and his baby sister had one of 73 years.[5] It is obvious that we must do all we can to understand the nature of the needs of our aging population.

The last decade has seen tremendous growth in activity related to aging in all areas. Following the first National Conference on Aging held in Washington, D. C., in August, 1950, a Committee on Aging was created within the federal government. In that year the National Social Welfare Assembly, a large voluntary organization concerned with health and social betterment, formed a Committee on Aging. This committee was extremely active, particularly in the areas of employment, retirement, sheltered care, and the dissemination of information.

In 1961 the Committee became an independent organization, The National Council on the Aging.* Membership is available to workers in all the health professions, and to those in such other fields as industrial relations, labor, and general education. In 1956 the President of the United States created a Federal Council on Aging to coordinate efforts in behalf of aging persons in all the main branches of government and to broaden the range of federal activities. Recently an Office of Aging was created within the Division of Welfare Administration

*Headquarters: 49 West 45th St., New York, N. Y.

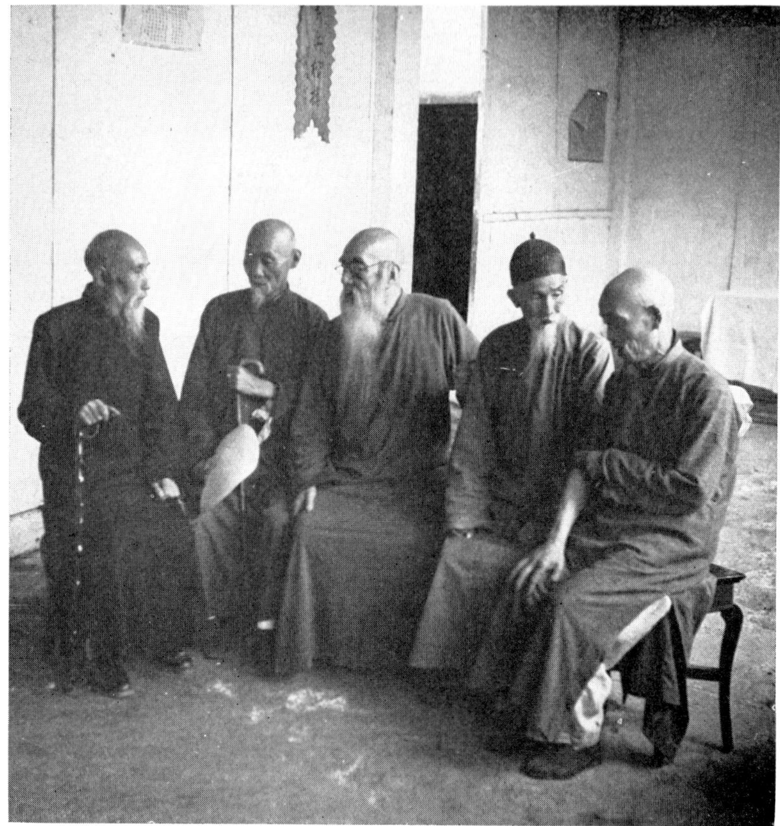

Figure. 1. In China the old person occupied a position of importance and participated in major family decisions. However, as elsewhere in the world, the role of the aged is being altered by rapid social changes. (Courtesy United Service to China, Inc.)

of the Department of Health, Education and Welfare. This Office publishes a monthly newsletter, *Aging*, which is available to all at a minimum cost; it also publishes reports on a variety of topics concerning our older population. In recent years the official and the voluntary agencies in this field have worked closely together.

There are now two scientific organizations devoted to the study and care of the aged. The American Geriatrics Society, started in 1942, is concerned primarily with the medical care of older persons and publishes *The Journal of the American Geriatrics Society*. Nurses may become associate members. The Gerontological Society, Inc., started in 1944, is concerned with all aspects of aging and publishes the *Journal of Gerontology*. Membership includes natural and social scientists, as well as social workers, nurses, and physicians.

Two organizations for institutions giving sheltered care to the elderly are the American Association of Homes for the Aged,* an organization of voluntary

*Headquarters: 49 West 45th St., New York, N. Y.

Table 1. Expectation of life and mortality at specified ages*
(By color and sex, industrial policyholders,† Metropolitan Life Insurance Company, 1962)

Age (years)	Expectation of life in years					Mortality rate per 1,000				
	Total persons	White		Colored		Total persons	White		Colored	
		Male	Female	Male	Female		Male	Female	Male	Female
5	67.9	63.9	71.1	61.9	66.5	0.4	0.4	0.3	0.5	0.5
10	63.0	59.0	66.2	57.0	61.7	.3	.4	.3	.4	.3
15	58.1	54.1	61.3	52.2	56.7	.5	.7	.3	.9	.4
20	53.3	49.3	56.4	47.5	51.9	.9	1.2	.4	1.6	.9
25	48.5	44.7	51.5	42.9	47.1	1.0	1.3	.6	2.2	1.1
30	43.8	39.9	46.7	38.4	42.4	1.3	1.5	.8	3.2	1.9
35	39.1	35.3	41.9	34.1	37.9	1.9	2.4	1.2	4.7	3.2
40	34.5	30.8	37.2	30.0	33.6	2.8	3.9	1.8	6.0	4.2
45	30.0	26.5	32.6	25.9	29.3	4.2	6.3	2.8	8.2	5.6
50	25.7	22.4	28.1	22.1	25.2	6.8	10.6	4.4	13.1	7.9
55	21.7	18.7	23.8	18.6	21.3	10.3	16.5	6.6	17.5	11.3
60	17.9	15.4	19.6	15.3	17.6	15.7	24.6	10.4	25.0	17.7
65	14.5	12.4	15.7	12.4	14.3	24.7	37.5	17.6	37.9	26.2

*Courtesy Metropolitan Life Insurance Co.
†Includes persons with premium-paying Ordinary policies for small amounts of insurance.

and nonprofit institutions that, for the most part, provide skilled nursing and medical services for elderly people. Its aims are to raise standards, to encourage professional training of personnel, and to provide a medium of communication among homes with similar aims. The American Nursing Home Association,* an organization of proprietors of nursing and convalescent homes, was set up to develop standards of care, to exchange information of mutual interest, to assist in the development of regulatory legislation, and to promote the welfare of its members. This organization publishes a monthly magazine, *Nursing Homes.*

Since 1955 the American Medical Association has had a Committee on Aging, and the majority of state medical associations now have corresponding committees whose main function is to foster more interest in the aged by members of the profession. Many other national organizations in the health and welfare field, such as the American Psychological Association and the American Public Welfare Association, have similar committees. The American Nurses' Association organized a Geriatric Nursing Section in 1962.

Most states now have definite activities in the field of aging. These may be governors' committees or commissions, legislative committees or the like. Their functions vary and include fact-finding aimed at changes in legislation, alteration of public attitudes, and cooperation with other states and with federal agencies.

Voluntary organizations for the aged are the Senior Citizens of America, founded in 1954, and the American Society for the Aged, Inc., founded in 1955.

The first university course in problems of the aged was offered by the University of Minnesota in 1933 as part of the program in human development. The

*Headquarters: 1346 Connecticut Ave., N.W., Washington, D.C.

teacher was the director of the Institute of Child Welfare. Since then, courses have been given for doctors, nurses, social workers, and others preparing to work with and care for older persons.

Some of our universities offer units of study and institutes for graduate nurses who desire additional knowledge and specific skills to qualify in the care of our aging population. In 1959 the American National Red Cross developed an eight-hour course, stressing preventive hygiene and preparation for later years. It is offered in many localities to interested persons over 40 years of age.

The word *geriatrics* is of Greek origin and means care of the aged. Geriatrics is, then, that branch of medical and nursing science that deals with the treatment and care of disease conditions in older people, including constructive health practice and prevention of disease. The word should be distinguished from *gerontology,* which is the study of the process of aging. Geriatrics is not a new word. It appeared in the *New York Medical Journal* in 1909 in an article by Dr. I. L. Nascher, who later used it in his textbook, published in 1914. This was the first textbook in this country to be concerned with the clinical care of elderly people.

The words *aging* and *aged* should be clarified. Aging is a process that begins with conception and ends with death, although in this book it has been used to designate the person who is past middle age. Aged means old. The aged exhibit the mental and physical characteristics that we recognize as the results of a long aging process, although tremendous variations exist. Some people are physically and mentally old at 35 years, whereas others are young at 65 years. In this book, however, 65 years has been more or less arbitrarily taken as the age at which the term *old* may be legitimately used. This is the age when retirement from active employment is generally expected, and Old Age and Survivors Insurance (Social Security) benefits are usually received, although benefits can be started at age 62 for both men and women.

The terms *young-old* to designate persons from 60 to 75 years of age and *old-old* to designate persons over 75 years of age are sometimes used. This is because of the enormous proportionate increase in the number of persons 75 years of age and older and because of the fact that this group has special characteristics, for example, a much higher incidence of chronic illness than persons under 75 years of age.

Senescence also denotes the interval of life at which changes characteristic of age have taken place. It is not incorrect to use the word *senile* to designate persons over 65 years of age, but common usage has branded it with the stigma of futility and deterioration. It is seldom used in reference to normal old age.

The number of older people among us is increasing rapidly, and indications are that there will be further lengthening of the cycle of life. In 1850, according to statistics of the Metropolitan Life Insurance Co., only 2.6 percent of our population reached 65 or more years of age. In 1962, this figure increased to 9.3 percent.[5] It is believed that by 1970 over 20,000,000 persons will be 65 years of age or older. The medical, social, and economic implications of this are enormous.

The increase in length of life is due largely to control of communicable diseases, lowered infant mortality, improved child care, and diminishing influx of young people from other countries. Actually, to life after 40 years, less than three years (2.3) for men and six years for women have been added since 1900. From the standpoint of medical research this is most interesting. The implication is that if the effort expended in controlling diseases of older people were to be made equal to that spent in controlling diseases of the young, there could be an even greater span of life.

Most improvement has occurred since World War II, with the advent of antibiotics, which have so successfully combated pneumonia and other infections, but relatively little progress has been made in the control and treatment of the chronic diseases occurring in old age. In our country the proportionate number of persons with degenerative diseases, such as heart disease, is higher than that in some economically less favored countries. It is believed that this may be linked with our high standard of living—nutritional patterns and general way of life.

Since medical science has contributed so much to lengthening the life-span, it is generally accepted by the medical profession that physicians must assume responsibility for the lives thus prolonged. As a companion science complementing medicine, nursing has a responsibility to help in making these later years healthful, happy, and economically productive.

One concept of geriatrics is basic. It is that old age can be satisfying and need not be a period of idle sitting and waiting for the inevitable, death. Medical science is working to bring the incapacitated person back to what is normal for his age. It is not a matter of making the old young again, but of maintaining the best health possible for each age level. The older person should be able to use his normal capacities, as at earlier intervals of life, to gain the satisfactions that ought to be and can be part of his later years. The phrase *the problem of the aged* should appear less often in our future writing and thinking as scientific and social progress continues.

REFERENCES AND RELATED BIBLIOGRAPHY

1. Chandler, Albert R.: The traditional Chinese attitude towards old age, J. Gerontol. **4**:239-244, 1949.
2. Harris, Dale B.: Maturity and aging; a course in the Institute of Child Welfare of the University of Minnesota, J. Gerontol. **3**:18-20, 1948.
3. Johnson, Wingate M. (editor): The older patient, New York, 1960, Paul B. Hoeber, Inc., Medical Book Department of Harper & Row, Publishers.
4. Mathiasen, Geneva: The aging. In Lurie, Harry L. (editor): The encyclopedia of social work, ed. 15, New York, 1965, National Association of Social Workers.
5. Metropolitan Life Insurance Company: Statistical bulletin, March, 1963.
6. Moore, Robert A.: The medical approach to the problem of aging, J. Gerontol. **4**:90-94, 1949.
7. Ravin, Louis S., and Tibbitts, Clark: Community programs and services. In Cowdry, E. V. (editor): The care of the geriatric patient, St. Louis, 1963, The C. V. Mosby Co.
8. Simmons, Leo W.: Social participation of the aged in different cultures, Ann. Amer Acad. Polit. and Soc. Sci. **279**:43-51, 1952.
9. Stieglitz, Edward J. (editor): Geriatric medicine, ed. 3, Philadelphia, 1954, J. B. Lippincott Co.
10. Thewlis, Malford W.: The care of the aged (geriatrics), ed. 5, St. Louis, 1946, The C. V. Mosby Co.
11. U. S. Department of Health, Education and Welfare: Nursing homes, related services and facilities, Washington, D. C., 1964, U. S. Government Printing Office.

Chapter 2

The nurse and the older person

Most young women enter the nursing profession because they are interested in others and wish to aid persons who are less fortunate than themselves. They are willing to study and are eager to participate in the realities of life. This interest will be well employed and deeply appreciated in geriatric nursing. No other field tests the nurse's maturity and sincerity of purpose more rigorously. No emotionally mature person expects nursing to consist only of interesting activities and contact with attractive patients who constantly express gratitude. Complete development demands that satisfaction be obtained from pursuing socially useful ends rather than from personal tribute. It is easy to be attentive to an attractive child; almost everyone responds to charm in others. It is harder to be as thoughtful of ill and overly emotional elderly patients. The nurse must be relatively mature before she can give effective nursing care to the elderly patient.

In the past nursing and the allied social professions have developed social conscience in many areas, but they have tended to avoid serious consideration of the problems of the elderly, largely because our society has been geared to youth, not age. In the nineteenth century elderly people were rare and were treasured; until very recently we have not, in our social planning, taken into account the fact that this group is increasing in numbers, and that their special needs must be considered. There are inescapable signs that the era of the older person is emerging.

ATTITUDES OF THE NURSE

Perhaps unconsciously, nurses have seemed to shun the aged. Some psychiatrists explain that in the homeless, friendless, and insecure we see a future image of ourselves. We shrink from the reminder that our hair will become gray, our joints knuckled, our voices cracked, and our place in society less valued. All around us in the social scheme we ourselves have built, we find that the aged are less wanted than the young. We may then identify ourselves with our elderly patient, and, rejecting this image of ourselves, we may reject the patient.

Fear is probably an important component of our reaction to the aged patient:

Some of our fear of age is based on the attitude we acquire in our culture, some of it comes from the kinds of persons we ourselves are, and some of it comes from the fact that younger people often do not really know or understand the aged. Whatever their bases, we should try to understand our own reactions so that we can control them better, even though we may not be able to change our attitudes immediately. Only time and marked changes in social attitude achieved by individuals working singly and together can guarantee to us personally a good measure of satisfaction in our own old age.

We should begin with the basic premise that the aged are no different from any age group except that they have lived more years. Some are attractive and responsive, whereas others are disagreeable and even repellent. Many extremely interesting persons are hidden by the mantle of anonymity that the term *old* places over them. An understanding of the process of aging, however, requires a tremendous amount of research in both the scientific and social fields. For example, why do some people live and work for years under an apparently deadly burden of physical illness, whereas others succumb so easily? Just how much of what we commonly think is characteristic of the aged is truly characteristic? Is some heart disease caused by forced retirement and the obvious discarding of the older person by his fellow men? We do not really know the effect of the mind on the physical condition of our aging people. We are all fearful

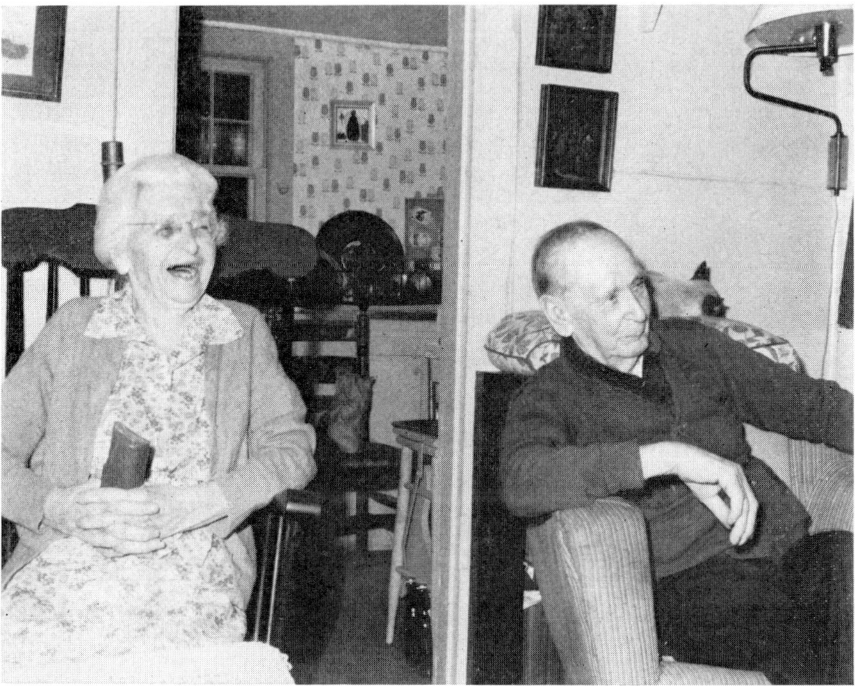

Figure 2. Television programs may stimulate a chuckle, a hearty laugh, or serious discussion by aged persons whose social contacts are limited.

of the day when our minds may fail, yet how much do we know about mental illness? How much of it may be the result of unavoidable pathology, and how much of functional disturbance born of boredom? Is the inattention of elderly persons caused by hearing loss and dulling of mental faculties, or is it sometimes merely lack of interest because the discussion holds no significant meaning for the older person? Many of these and other questions must be answered by science, but, until they are, the nurse should avoid making assumptions that are without scientific basis as she cares for older patients.

A nurse should think of an aged person as someone like herself at a certain stage in life, not as a member of a group apart. All human beings, old or young, have basic needs; when we are old, we shall still need recognition, novelty of experience, security, and love, though the ways of satisfying these needs must change. New interests should develop, and a great deal of satisfaction may still be in store for persons of advanced years.

REACTIONS OF THE OLDER PERSON

Older persons seldom regard themselves as old. We all witness the same experience: The high school student feels grown up. To the college student, the recent high school graduate seems painfully childish. To the student struggling for his doctorate, the college freshman seems very young. The interesting thing from a personal standpoint is that the individual does not get older. Other persons get younger! This simply means that the spirit is ageless, even though it must look out from slowly altering and aging physical features. Many a person at late maturity has been rudely confronted for the first time with the evidence of his own organic deterioration upon meeting an old friend. He looks at himself in the mirror and realizes that changes have taken place in himself also. He has not been aware of them. It is often a shock to an aging person to be suddenly called grandpa by a stranger. Perhaps he never had children, much less grandchildren. Nurses who thoughtlessly or even affectionately call a patient grandpa are losing sight of him as a personality.

Changes other than the physical ones take place with age. If the maturing process has been satisfactory, an individual should have attained a more balanced sense of values and developed a freedom from the excessive self-consciousness that plagues youth. There may have been progress toward wisdom—the quality that enables us to be at home at all times and in all places with tolerance and with the inquiring curiosity of a child. The nurse who takes the trouble to know her aged patient may often benefit from a philosophy of life that only the passing of years can bestow.

The elderly patient will respond as the kind of person he is. He must be treated as an individual. It must not be assumed that the patient is necessarily emotionally mature because he has lived many years and because his hair is white. Maturity is not a matter of years. There are many white-haired persons who are still children emotionally. It must be remembered that the patient brings to his illness the type of personality he already has—a personality that is the result of the interaction of heredity with a complex arrangement of environmental factors. One generalization that can be made about the older patient is that his personality reactions are often based on the mores of another era. He may have been very liberal and tolerant for his own era, and though it may appear, by contemporary standards, that his reactions have become fixed into a set pattern, in reality the changes he has been able to make could only reflect a relatively large amount of flexibility.

PERSONAL QUALITIES OF THE NURSE

What qualities enable the nurse to give good care to geriatric patients? The competent nurse needs a sympathetic kindliness and thoughtfulness without pity. She needs a sense of humor, that quality which serves so well in every aspect of living. She needs tolerance, but not the tongue-in-cheek tolerance that amusedly accedes to the patient's wishes. Tolerance must be based upon the value of every life, regardless of its endowment by nature or of the effect that environmental forces have had upon it. The nurse needs patience and tact, for the aged do become garrulous at times and occasionally appear somewhat unreasonable. The nurse needs flexibility, since older people may appear fixed in their ways, and

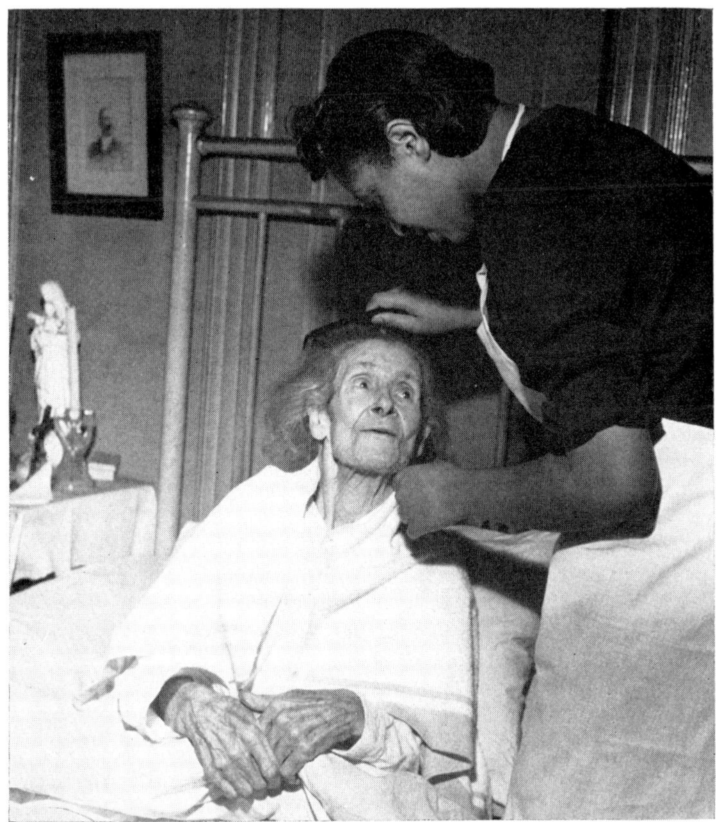

Figure 3. Almost every patient responds to expert and sympathetic nursing. (Courtesy Visiting Nurse Service of New York; photograph by Hazel Kingsbury.)

needless adherence to procedure achieves nothing and makes them unhappy. She needs friendliness, warmth, and genuine interest in people because the aged are often lonely and alone. She needs persuasiveness, for she may need to manage the patient without appearing to manage him. She needs teaching ability, and she needs physical energy and the knowledge of how to use it wisely.

The nurse should be particularly observant of the emotional needs and the emotional reactions of the geriatric patient. Signs of worry must be noted. The need for explanations is particularly obvious during the first few days of clinic or hospital care, when numerous alarming tests may be in progress. Worry and fear often may be allayed by careful explanation, by reassurance, or by just letting the patient talk and express his fears. He may be thinking in terms of old-fashioned folklore about treatment and care of illness, or about treatments that were accepted as medically sound in his youth. The nurse should listen to the patient and use records and other available sources of information to acquaint herself with his home background and usual environment, since it will enable her to support him more effectively in any uprooting that his age or illness may entail. The nurse should notice the need for assistance and consideration in details of personal care so that the patient is spared the embarrassment of requesting help.

The need for privacy should not be overlooked. The older patient may be shy. He may have lived alone or with one other person for years. He may have had his own room. That room, no matter how poor, still ensured a precious prerogative, privacy. The elderly person may be painfully conscious of the physical infirmities that have caused him to lose out in competition with those around him. If he has been forced by illness, unemployment, and subsequent poverty to accept a situation entirely different from that to which he is accustomed, he may be inordinately grateful for even the smallest attention to the niceties that are sometimes difficult to provide in a large ward of a general hospital or related facility. An individual room when initial adjustment is being made, a screen carefully placed, a door carefully closed for assurance of privacy when a bedpan or commode is being used, an extra towel placed in the water to respect modesty when assistance is needed in getting out of the bathtub—these are but a few of the small things that can be done to make care during illness or infirmity less painful.

The nurse should adapt herself to the particular needs of each patient. Not all older people are deaf; the common habit of shouting at them on the assumption that they are is deplorable. It is well, however, to realize that many elderly patients have some hearing limitations. The nurse should make an effort to speak slowly and distinctly. She should face the patient as she speaks and should stand in a good light in case he is dependent upon lipreading. Whispering or mumbling to others in the room on the assumption that the patient will not hear is inexcusably rude and is demoralizing to the patient. Asking questions of family members in the presence of the patient when he can speak for himself is equally demeaning.

Understanding the need of each patient for personal independence is essential in good geriatric nursing. It may seem easier and less time consuming to help the patient out of bed, put on his shoes, and wait upon him in many ways, rather than permit him to care for himself. It must be remembered that the ability to do for oneself is tremendously important in human happiness. It is good nursing to arrange the schedule so that morning preparation for breakfast will begin earlier than usual and be completed in time to save disruption of meal schedules. The elderly person will then be spared the feeling of inadequacy that results when he is hurried.

Optimism is essential in caring for all elderly people. Sometimes, considering the multiplicity of their ills, the impression is that the situation seems hopeless. This is seldom the case. Many older persons adjust to their chronic ills and get along very well for years. Many can be benefited by the medical and surgical procedures that are now available. There are very few who cannot be improved by supportive medical treatment and by thoughtful and kindly nursing.

Judgment is needed in answering the questions of aged patients, in referring questions to the physician when necessary, and in making certain that answers are explicit and easily understood. The elderly person who is ill, clutching at the hope of recovery and self-sufficiency, may misinterpret statements by the doctor or the nurse. If misunderstandings occur, full and simple explanations should be repeated.

Careful observation should be made to detect signs of new chronic disease, and pertinent information relating to illness should be noted. The patient may forget to include some significant incident or may think that certain symptoms are not sufficiently important to mention when the physician takes the history. He may, however, mention them later to the nurse. Older people often suffer from a number of ills. They present extremely complex diagnostic problems in contrast to younger persons, who may have an acute illness but whose body systems are otherwise functioning well. For example, an elderly person may suffer from congestive heart failure, pneumonia, generalized arteriosclerosis, diabetes, osteoporosis, tumor, and cataracts. Chronic diseases differ from acute ones in having a much more insidious onset. Early signs may not be noticed by the patient, or he may not recall their time of onset accurately. Complications of any chronic ailment can appear, and obviously the nurse must be keenly aware of their possibility and have definite knowledge of their early signs. It is equally important that the nurse be constantly alert for signs and symptoms of acute illness. For example, chronic symptoms of cough, nasal congestion, or headache may mask signs of incipient upper respiratory infection or pneumonia.

Teaching ability

The nurse should use patience, clarity of expression, and be discriminating in what she teaches. Along with the essentials, she must be able to assist the patient, or persons responsible for his care, in learning what seems to them important; she should remember that what she tells them is useful only insofar as it is directed toward the patient's own felt needs, but she can assist by recalling questions that have been on the patient's mind or in teaching in relation to needs that he finds difficult to express.

Teaching should not be delayed, since the patient may need repeated explanation; each visit of the public health nurse should contribute to essential learning. In the hospital, dismissal is sometimes quite abrupt and gives little op-

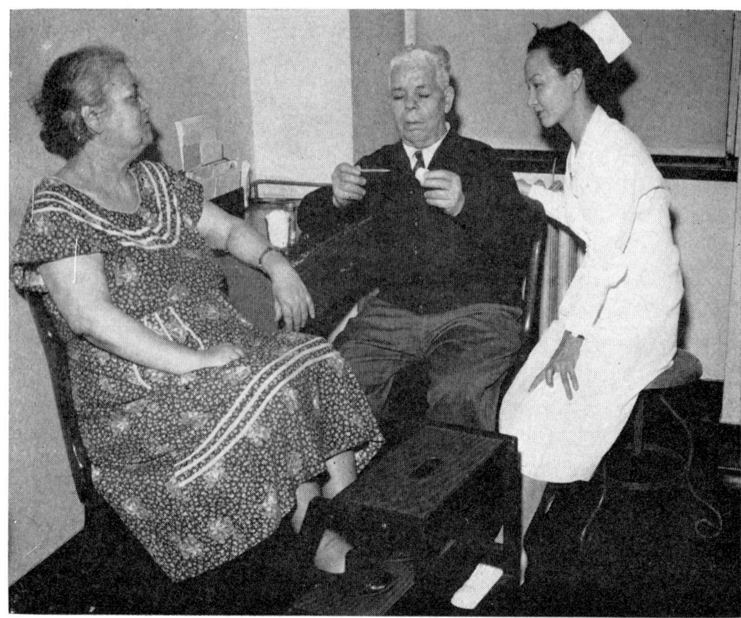

Figure 4. This elderly lady, who is almost totally blind and has several other ailments, was able to leave a hospital for the chronically ill when the nurses in the clinic devoted time to teaching her husband the procedures necessary for her care.

portunity for answering final questions. Often, in their excitement, patients and their relatives fail to understand instructions. When they reach home, or after the nurse leaves, many questions arise to worry them. If written instructions are used, they should be brief and clear and should contain only the key points of material that has been discussed with the patient or his family. For example, uncertainty is caused by such simple details as whether the patient should be permitted out of bed. Sometimes the elderly patient is being cared for by others who are also old and who are unfamiliar with recent medical thinking in regard to ambulation. They may feel, despite having been told otherwise, that allowing the patient out of bed may be dangerous. Written instructions often give reassurance to the patient and his family and assist them in carrying out instructions effectively.

In the haste and confusion of the doctor's visit or their visit to the doctor's office or the clinic, the patient and his family may forget to ask some questions that have caused them concern. It is well to advise that they write their questions before seeing the doctor.

The shortage of nurses and all other professional health workers, now and in the foreseeable future, makes it apparent that more and more nursing of chronically ill aged persons and, in fact, of ill persons of any age will be done by family members. It will become the responsibility of the nurse in the home, the clinic, or the hospital ward to teach safe and adequate nursing techniques to family members and to adapt this teaching to each individual situation (Chapter 10, Care in the Patient's Own Home).

CONTINUITY OF CARE

In the aged, recovery from disease is often slow and may be incomplete. Progress should not be interrupted because of lack of planning for care in the transition from hospital to home or institution. The nurse must know the resources of her community and should not hesitate to initiate plans for continuity of nursing that will be in operation by the time the patient is able to go home. Family members may need to come to the hospital to learn certain aspects of care. Additional bedside nursing and instruction may be required at home. Local health departments frequently assume responsibility for this nursing, especially in areas in which no visiting nurse agency exists. Service is available to rich and poor.

Referrals to public health nurses must be thoughtfully written by the nurse in the hospital. Medical orders must be signed by the doctor, and other professional workers may make valuable additions to the form. The nurse in the hospital should try to imagine herself to be the public health nurse and to anticipate the information that would be most helpful to her were she meeting the patient for the first time.

Referral forms must also be carefully completed by the nurse who visits the patient. Her report will give the nurse in the hospital some idea of how effective the hospital care and instruction have been. It will also enable the nurse in the hospital to reevaluate her own impression of the patient as she saw him in his unfamiliar hospital environment, and it will tell her whether the information she gave was pertinent and helpful.

Completed forms should become part of the patient's permanent record in the hospital. If the patient returns to the clinic or the hospital, they are helpful to the nurse who cares for him. When patients have received nursing care or supervision at home before entering the hospital, a written referral to the hospital is a valuable aid in speeding effective nursing care and treatment. Unfortunately, this procedure is not yet widely used.

REFERENCES AND RELATED BIBLIOGRAPHY

1. Arnstein, Margaret: Balance in nursing, Am. J. Nurs. **58**:1690-1692, 1958.
2. Charles, Don C.: Outstanding characteristics of older patients, Am. J. Nurs. **6**:80-83, 1961.
3. Goldfarb, Alvin I.: Responsibilities to our aged, Am. J. Nurs. **64**:78-82, 1964.
4. Hall, Bernard H.: The mental health of senior citizens, Nurs. Outlook **4**:206-208, 1956.
5. Henderson, Cynthia K.: Nursing aspects. In Cowdry, E. V. (editor): The care of the geriatric patient, ed. 2, St. Louis, 1963, The C. V. Mosby Co.
6. Hulicka, Irene M.: Fostering self-respect in aged patients, Am. J. Nurs. **64**:84-89, 1964.
7. Randall, Ollie A., and others: The problem of extended illness and old age, Am. J. Nurs. **54**:1220-1225, 1954.
8. Schwartz, Doris, Henley, Barbara, and Zeitz, Leonard: The elderly ambulatory patient; nursing and psychological needs, New York, 1964, The Macmillan Company.
9. Shafer, Kathleen Newton, and others: Medical-surgical nursing, ed. 3, St. Louis, 1964, The C. V. Mosby Co.
10. Thompson, Prescott W.: Let's take a good look at the aging, Am. J. Nurs. **61**:76-79, 1961.
11. Tibbitts, Clark: Social change, aging and public health nursing, Nurs. Outlook **6**:144-147, 1958.
12. Tibbitts, Clark (editor): Handbook of social gerontology, Chicago, 1960, University of Chicago Press.

Chapter 3

Basic sociopsychologic needs

Basic sociopsychologic needs of older people are those of human beings of any age living anywhere. The aged do not suddenly change when a certain number of years have been lived; just as they have been throughout their lives, they remain flexible or rigid, penurious or generous, cheerful or gloomy in facing the world and their own problems. They are individuals who attend to things promptly or who procrastinate indefinitely; they think things through and plan ahead or they act impulsively with little thought of the future. By sociopsychologic needs are meant those requirements over and above the basic creature comforts or legally termed necessities. They include the need to love and to be loved and to secure companionship, recognition, participation, and personal achievement. They must be met if a feeling of personal worth is to be maintained and if true happiness is to be achieved.

The ability of any individual to find means to meet his basic personality needs within the circumstances in which he lives has not been found to be related to age to any appreciable extent. The best prescription for happiness in old age appears to be happiness and contentment in middle age. One study showed that persons eighty years of age and older were as happy as those who were sixty-five.[6] There was little relationship between socioeconomic status and happiness. Health, although more important than actual age or socioeconomic status, was less important than might be expected. The closest relationship occurred between the ability to keep active, to the extent that activity had been part of the pattern of earlier life, and continued social approval, which is so important.

Basic needs for the aged have been succinctly defined by a member of the Society of Friends as "the need for somewhere to live, something to do, someone to care."[16] This description may seem oversimplified since basic needs are interrelated. It brings out fully, however, the need for "belongingness": belonging in a home and in a community, belonging to a job or occupation, or belonging to another person and to the social group in which one lives. "Somewhere to live" and "something to do" means having some economic security and some activity that wins approval from others as work worthy of accomplishment. "Someone to care" implies not only the personal recognition, but also the social recognition of one's worth as a human being. To this list some writers would add other needs, implied but not stated, such as the need for freedom of movement and of decision. In addition, many feel that there must be some stimulation and some novelty of experience to add interest to the older person's days. If there is to be true happiness and contentment, there should be equilibrium between two conflicting drives in human nature, the one demanding security and routine and the other clamoring for novelty and adventure. The need to worship is also basic and is closely allied to the need to love and to be loved.

Economic security has been cited as being less important than emotional security for happiness in older persons, and few would argue that wealth alone can ensure happiness. Economic security, however, does become more important as the years go by. Old age is not a period of making new friends who may fill emotional needs, but rather a period of losing them as, one by one, friends and relatives scatter and die. A feeling of desolation and panic often besets the older person who faces economic insecurity in addition to becoming aware of his aloneness.

Chapter 4 deals with the economic implications of unemployment of the aged. Many are not economically self-sufficient, and the attitude of the working world toward them not only robs them of economic security, but also strips them of a feeling of adequacy and personal value. This is true not only of persons over 65 years of age. The insidious social influence of discrimination against the older worker, which causes insecurity, frustration, and unhappiness, begins with middle-aged persons, those between 40 and 65 years of age. It is during these years that people need desperately the opportunity to achieve and to accumulate worthwhile working experiences.

The need for approval through personal achievement, sometimes called public recognition, persists throughout life, though in age the emphasis is focused on past accomplishments. The older person, denied satisfying experiences in the present, resorts to preoccupation with the past. This makes it doubly important that worthwhile accomplishment take place in the more active years and that intellectual interests be developed that will sustain the individual, so that in old age he will not have to lead a merely vegetative existence.

WHY BASIC NEEDS ARE NOT MET IN OUR SOCIETY

Security for each individual within his group depends upon the extent to which he shares in the common culture. He needs to know what others expect of him and what to expect of others. He needs to have developed a definite concept of his role within the group. The position of the elderly as a group within our society is not clear; we have mixed and conflicting attitudes that are, naturally, shared by the older people themselves. For example, we cut off older people from gainful employment, yet we expect them to care for themselves. We speak of them with deference and respect, yet we restrict their social participation and avoid their business counsel. We acknowledge their experience and wisdom, yet we decide to "do for them" and fail to secure, at times, their participation in plans for themselves. Because we deal with older people as a group instead of as individuals, we may impose a sense of values upon them that is not in accord with their own values and life experiences.

There are several reasons why the satisfaction of achievement for older people is difficult to obtain in our society. Our rapid industrialization has been an important factor, for with it came urbanization. Government aid, social interest, or participation from interested welfare groups probably cannot compensate older people for what our trend away from rural living has cost them in loss of participation in basic worthwhile human experiences.

In most primitive cultures each member was part of the tribe; he survived or perished with the family and the tribe; he contributed the best he had according to his ability; he was an individual, and, as he grew old, he still deserved and was accorded active participation in the group. In the agricultural period of our life as a nation the same principles prevailed. As members grew older, they gradually relinquished some of their authority; they turned over the management of the farm, home, or business to younger family members. They still had ownership in the home. They did not have to feel that they were dependent upon their children. Odd jobs about the house and grounds kept them occupied and gave them the feeling that they were still needed and useful. Old women were busy teaching the girls of the family how to make candles, how to make soap, how to cool the butter in warm weather, and perhaps how to weave materials and make clothing. Now the light switch, the box of soap flakes, the electric refrigerator, and the dress shop take care of these necessities. Now the young people work each day to earn money to pay for them, and the old ones are left sitting. Our urban-technologic society has made us renters of apartments instead of owners of homes. It has made us wage earners who work a regular number of hours in order to buy a living. Sons no longer learn a trade from their fathers and carry on the firm's name from one generation to another. Sons have moved to the city, learned a trade, and question the parents' knowledge. Many elderly people are thus made to feel that they know nothing about what is going on nowadays, that they are far behind the times.

The family home often must be given up since children can no longer contribute to its maintenance. Older persons find themselves in crowded city apartments living with strangers. The trend toward urbanization has uprooted the aged person and has placed him far from friends and the scenes of his active, happy youth at the time when his need of emotional response from this source is the greatest. For example, a rural couple may have a son who goes to work in a distant city or a daughter who marries a man working in a city. After the father dies, the mother finds that she cannot do the work of keeping up the house alone in the country. She is reluctant to sell the home in which she has lived for so long, but taxes accumulate, and eventually the home is sold for a small amount and the woman goes to live with her daughter. The apartment may be small. She stays for a while and then goes to visit her son.

In the city dwelling of her children, the older person often feels that she has no function and is at loose ends. The way people live in the city is strange to her. There is no garden to putter in. The old friends with whom she has visited occasionally since girlhood are too far away to visit. She is lonely and unhappy.

Often her children cannot understand why. Sometimes in their effort to provide well, they rob her of the last vestige of independence by overprotection and by not letting her do the small things she could still do to make her feel needed and useful. Urbanization has changed family relationships; for instance, in the past daughters-in-law and sons-in-law were usually local people known to everyone in the community. Now they are often strangers to the parents, who know nothing of their background and by whom the parents are in turn misunderstood. The elderly people sit about bewildered and unwanted or shunted between various sons and daughters, and they finally may arrive in an institution for the aged.

The unmarried aged person faces a similar situation. Illness, inability to work, and other circumstances may make it necessary to leave familiar friends and surroundings and live in a distant city with little-known relatives where welcome is uncertain and adjustment is difficult.

The younger people, caught in the meshes of our rapid industrialization, cannot be held entirely to blame for the plight of their elders. Many families are laboring under terrific pressure to meet high city rents, keep up accepted standards, pay taxes, and educate children. It is no wonder in this pattern of life that the older people appear as a burden to the young. In rural living people dwelt in roomier quarters; homes were handed down from one generation to another, several generations often sharing the home. In the farm or family establishment there was room for the grandparents, room for the magazines, the comfortable chairs, the pipes, and the knitting needles. Many of the personality conflicts arising in close family living were avoided. One of the nearest things in city life to this family unit of the past is the small grocery or vegetable market where successive generations of the family are employed. Grandparents may spend a few hours each day in work that is suited to their physical capacities and have a share in the ownership of the business. They may be deprived of some important components of a healthful day—moderate exercise in fresh air and sunshine—but they are often happy, for they at least are active, useful members of the family.

Another reason why the aged suffer from lack of feeling of personal worth is that essentially we are a nation of modernized foreigners. The desire of many of the people who came to this country was to become Americanized as quickly as possible, and in their haste they have turned from everything that was foreign. Children have been reluctant to admit that their parents speak with a foreign accent. Rejecting their foreign origin, children have become alienated from their parents. The authority of the elders has been challenged, and their opinions and judgments have been tossed aside as belonging to a past era or a foreign society that could not possibly have any relation to contemporary values. Marriages between persons of entirely different cultural backgrounds have further increased the misunderstandings. Church ties have become more tenuous, and lack of religious teaching in the home has decreased the prestige of parents.

The need for belief in personal worth includes the capacity to love and to be loved. Each individual must feel that there is at least one person in the world to whom he is extremely important. No individual of any age in any society can

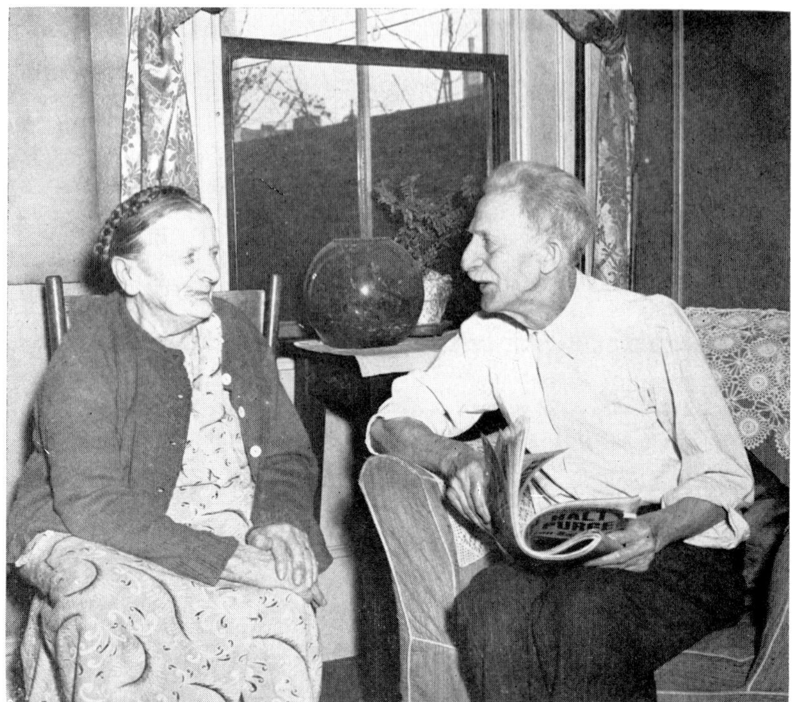

Figure 5. The aged couple living together is a unit of our society that we should strive to preserve. (Photograph by Anne M. Goodrich.)

be happy or content unless he firmly believes that he is capable of being loved by others. The method of demonstrating this need differs at each age level. Babies and small children demand an all-embracing love for themselves and they may respond with tantrums, enuresis, or other marked reactions if love is denied them. In old age the demonstration of this need may be a turning to religious fanaticism or an intense preoccupation with a particular cause or movement. To many people the assurance of God's love is gratifying and gives peace of mind when the need for love is not met by human beings.

In adolescence and young maturity, sex plays a primary role in the demand to love and to be loved. Man reaches the highly competitive stage of his existence. Competition to secure a mate becomes a primary drive and is closely followed by the effort to excel in the life work that has been chosen. Men must feel that they are able to win and to hold the love of women and that they are indispensable in their work. Women must feel that they are attractive to men and that they possess the qualifications needed to make good wives and to be good mothers. To some extent these needs are constant throughout life, and the longer the aging person can retain the qualities that are distinctly masculine or feminine, the better his adjustment in later life will be. A moderate number of failures in love and in other personal relationships will not necessarily demoralize a person in his maturity, since he is not faced with the physical helplessness that the infant and small child feel and that the aged person dreads. His reaction to his failures will be determined by his emotional maturity and his own ability to face obstacles and to profit by overcoming them, or else to rationalize them to the satisfaction of his own ego. In middle age the person may feel that much is yet ahead for him. The older person does not have this alternative. His gratifications must be in the present, and thus his personal failures in securing satisfaction of his needs are felt more keenly.

Happy and satisfactory sexual life may continue many years after the possibility of procreation ceases. Age plays mental tricks on human beings. To the self-conscious adolescent it seems barely possible that sex could still be of interest to persons of 40 years of age. The adolescent may be greatly embarrassed if a new brother or sister arrives in his home. This demonstrates that the way people feel at certain stages in life and the way others think they feel may be entirely different. The older person often does not feel old. He feels no different until he is suddenly faced with the fact that persons around him consider him old. Sexual activity in marriage should continue as long as it meets a need for the persons concerned.

As age progresses, it is true that sexual activity as a means of obtaining the assurance of love and acceptance gradually gives place to other means. The need

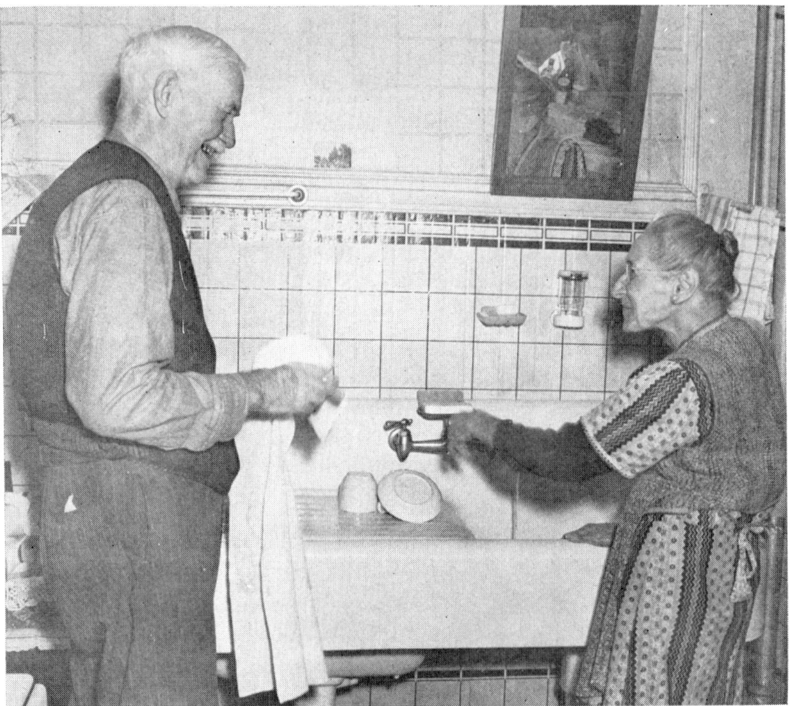

Figure 6. Old couples come more and more to depend almost entirely on each other for company, tending in many ways to return to the early days of marriage. (Photograph by Anne M. Goodrich.)

for love is still met by tenderness and affection. Sexual activity is only one method of expression of love, and because it decreases with the years is no sign that love is at an end, provided real love exists. Well-adjusted couples find many other mutual interests that serve to further the bonds of affection. It has been found that not only do children emancipate themselves from parents, but also that parents whose children are grown tend to return in many ways to the early days of marriage, before the demands of the children for love and attention may have limited that given to the marriage partner. Many aged couples come to rely more and more upon each other for companionship, sometimes feeling almost no need for outside friends. One member comes to identify himself so closely with the other that the loss of a spouse represents almost truly the loss of part of oneself. The Chinese principle of the yang and yin demonstrates the relationship of the two members of a harmonious couple. The two sections of the circle are formed in such a way that one completes the other to form the perfect circle, and if either of the sections is missing, there is scarcely a semblance of a circle. This relationship should not exclude old friends and the making of new ones of all ages, for they add pleasurable breadth and depth to living. Friends are also a reservoir of comfort and help during illness or when one of the couple dies. When a mate dies, substitutes must be found in other persons, in creative activity of some kind, in interest in others. It is at this time that the aged person turns hopefully to sons and daughters and to friends and familiar surroundings in his loneliness. He is at a distinct disadvantage as compared to a younger person in that he makes friends less easily, and his chances of finding or wishing to find a solution in another marriage are limited.

For some people, the need for love is never filled in a sexual fashion. Many people do not marry. To them a favorite nephew or niece or some special friend may supply an emotional need. This is quite satisfactory insofar as it does not either become an excessively domineering influence or result in too great a dependence, resulting in a burden upon the recipient of such affection. The single person who faces old age may have less difficulty in filling his personal need for affection than the person who has married and whose husband or wife has died. The single person may have developed substitutes through the years that can tide him over the old-age period. There are, of course, a few persons whose bitterness in failing to attain normal fulfillment of this need increases with age.

Our widespread policy of forced retirement and our reluctance to reestablish aging persons in steady employment have deprived them of the satisfaction and security of routine that is essential in the lives of all. The man who has caught a certain bus and worked in the same office for twenty years cannot suddenly stop this practice without a feeling of loss. The daily routine plus the stimulus and novelty of working and of going back and forth to work are badly missed. Since there are no longer any details of news to bring home, no new acquaintances to be made at work, and no definite work to be done, one day drags endlessly into the next. The wife at home misses the routine of her husband's working schedule and the breaks in monotony that his excursions into the outside world contributed to her day. Sometimes the presence of a retired husband in the home creates a real crisis. Even if the couple's adjustment has not been too harmonious, both members may have worked out satisfactory patterns for the hours they were together. These often cannot be sustained in the constant togetherness of retirement. Many retired men seek recreation and other pursuits outside the home to occupy the hours previously spent at work.

Lack of income and of health often may preclude the possibility of a vacation that would at least bring a change of scene for the elderly. The busy younger world has little time for them, so that the aged are driven to association almost entirely with people of their own age. Here conversation may range from refreshing reminiscences with contemporaries to morbid preoccupation with physical and mental changes in themselves and in those around them.

Oliver Wendell Holmes wrote a tribute to the single woman of his day, much of which might apply to the aged person in ours.

> The great mystery of God's providence is the permitted crushing out of flowering instincts. Life is maintained by the respiration of oxygen and of sentiments. In the long catalogue of scientific cruelties, there is hardly anything quite so painful to think of as that experiment of putting an animal under the bell of an airpump and exhausting the air from it. . . . There comes a time when the souls of human beings, women, perhaps more even than men, begin to faint for the atmosphere of the affections they were made to breathe. Then it is that society places its transparent bell-glass over the young woman who is to be the subject of one of its fatal experiments. The element by which only the heart lives is sucked out of her crystalline prison. Watch her through its transparent walls;—her bosom is heaving, but it is a vacuum. Death is no riddle compared to this. . . . How many have withered and wasted under as slow a torment in the walls of that larger Inquisition which we call Civilization!
>
> For that great procession of the unloved, who not only wear the crown of thorns, but must hide it under the locks of brown or gray,—under the snowy cap, under the chilling turban,—hide it even from themselves,—perhaps never know they wear it, though it kills them,—. Somewhere,—somewhere,—love is in store for them,—the universe must not be allowed to fool them so cruelly. What infinite pathos in the small, half-unconscious artifices by which the unattractive young persons seek to recommend themselves to the favor of those to whom our dear sisters, the unloved, like the rest, are impelled by their God-given instincts![8]

A FUTURE FOR US

Finally, when the sins of commission and omission that lead to the plight of the aged have been laid at the feet of society, what can each thoughtful individual in that society do about it? What can each mature person do toward seeing that his own basic needs will be met in that future society in which he will spend his own old age? It should be remembered that society is simply a large aggregate of individuals. Our personal attitudes and responses will affect society as a whole in time if we really seek to make them known. It might be well for all of us—for we must anticipate that some day we, too, will be old—to consider our assets and our liabilities, to analyze our resources in terms of our needs. Are we doing work of which we shall be proud when we are old? Are we obtaining a promise of economic security? Are we cultivating new friends? Are we developing a variety of interests, especially those that can be carried on or cultivated with advancing years? Some would call this preparing for old age, but it might be also called living fully in the present, with only a small look to the future. Often we shall find that, if we concern ourselves with meeting basic needs in an organized fashion in maturity, our old age will take care of itself—at least insofar as it can be directed by us.

REFERENCES AND RELATED BIBLIOGRAPHY

1. Anderson, John E. (editor): Psychological aspects of aging, Washington, D. C., 1956, American Psychological Association, Inc.
2. Birren, James E. (editor): Handbook of aging and the individual, Chicago, 1960, University of Chicago Press.
3. Charles, Don C.: Outstanding characteristics of older patients, Am. J. Nurs. **61**:80-83, 1961.
4. Gitelson, Maxwell: The emotional problems of elderly people, Geriatrics **3**:135-150, 1948.
5. Hall, Bernard H.: The mental health of senior citizens, Nurs. Outlook **4**:206-208, 1956.
6. Havighurst, Robert J., and Albrecht, Ruth: Older people, New York, 1953, Longmans, Green & Co., Inc.
7. Havighurst, Robert J. (editor): Aging in western societies, Chicago, 1960, University of Chicago Press.
8. Holmes, Oliver Wendell: The autocrat of the breakfast table, New York, 1955, Heritage Press.
9. Hunter, Woodrow W., and Maurice, Helen: Old people tell their story, Ann Arbor, 1953, The University of Michigan Press.
10. Kutner, Bernard, and others: Five hundred over sixty-five, New York, 1956, Russell Sage Foundation.
11. Linden, Maurice E.: Emotional problems in aging, Jewish Service Quarterly **31**:80-89, 1954.
12. Mathiasen, Geneva: The aging. In Lurie, Harry (editor): Encyclopedia of social work, ed. 15, New York, 1965, National Association of Social Workers.
13. The nation and its older people; a report of the White House conference on aging, 1961, Washington, D. C., 1961, U. S. Government Printing Office.
14. Schwartz, Doris, Henley, Barbara, and Zeitz, Leonard: The elderly ambulatory patient; nursing and psychological needs, New York, 1964, The Macmillan Company.
15. Simmons, Leo W.: Social participation of the aged in different cultures, Ann. Amer. Acad. Polit. Soc. Sci. **279**:43-51, 1952.
16. Stern, Leon T.: After sixty-five, Philadelphia, 1945, Social Service Committee of Philadelphia Yearly Meeting of Friends.
17. Tibbitts, Clark (editor): Handbook of social gerontology, Chicago, 1960, University of Chicago Press.

Chapter 4

Employment and economic security

Employment regulations and practices and the economic status of persons who are 65 years of age and older constitute pressing problems and are receiving attention from both official and voluntary agencies. Although many employers are reluctant to hire older persons, there are a significant number who are willing to retain old employees and who take a more liberal view about allowing them to work after the set retirement age. The average employer, however, does not want the person who is growing old. Unemployment, even for individuals in their forties and fifties, has disturbing implications. With each succeeding year of life the chances of finding secure and satisfying new employment are cut down, and not enough effort has been made to fit the older person into work that will be suited to his lessened physical resources yet keep him employed and self-supporting.

When any person cannot work, cannot find employment, and has inadequate personal resources, he becomes dependent. The number of aged persons in our population is increasing and because of their difficulty in finding and keeping employment, the implications of the consequent economic stress are far reaching.

Nowhere else in the world and at no previous time in history has there been such an increase in the older age group as in the United States today. We have had an unusually high percentage of young people in our society, and even today half of our population is under 30 years of age; this is in contrast to some of the older settled countries of Europe. It is a result of the fertility of our people, the large influx of young people from European countries, and success in controlling diseases that destroy young people. In 1900 persons over 65 years of age constituted 4.1 percent of the total population. In 1962 the percentage had risen to 9.3 percent, and by 1975 it is estimated that the percentage will be approximately 9.6 percent, or more than 20 million people over 65 years of age. This means that approximately one person in every ten will be 65 years old or more.

EMPLOYMENT OF OLDER PEOPLE

In 1900 63.2 percent of the men 65 years of age and older were working, whereas in June, 1958, only 26 percent had some income from employment.[5] Although the percentage of elderly men in the labor force continues to decline, the percentage of women working after age 65 has increased.[6] In 1900 a man might expect 2.8 years of life in retirement; today he expects about 13 years, and this will increase after he reaches 65 years of age if present employment policies continue and the life-span continues to lengthen.

The ratio of persons 65 years of age and older to persons in the productive years has increased from 9 percent in 1850 to 20 percent in 1964. It is anticipated that the trend toward a smaller number of employed persons over 65 years of age will continue, despite present efforts to reverse it. One reason for this statistic, however, is the proportionate increase in the number of persons who are 70 years of age and older. In 1960 persons 75 years of age and over numbered 5,359,338 out of a total of 179,325,675; their number has increased by 29 percent since 1950. This age group is designated the *old-old*.[13] Another reason is the huge number of young people born soon after the end of World War II who are now beginning to join the labor force.

Even at high employment levels during the war, only one third of the persons over 65 years of age (men and women) were employed. Recent figures show that only about one fourth of the men are employed, and this percentage is perhaps declining. Many older persons are working in agriculture or individual business. With a few notable exceptions, large industrial plants do not employ older workers. Insufficient provision is made in our society for the gainful employment of older women, and women constitute much more than half the number of persons living beyond 60 years of age. In 1964, 10 percent of all women over 65 years of age were in the labor force. The projected figures to 1975 show only a slight increase. This trend may be altered as a result of the recent federal civil rights legislation that provides for equal employment opportunities for women and of the efforts of citizens' groups to eliminate discrimination on the basis of sex. The federal government has removed age barriers to employment, and it is hoped that private business will do the same. Fifteen states have now passed laws to help prevent discrimination in employment because of age, and a number of others are considering such laws.

It would seem that our society has perhaps awakened just in time to the financial danger for our aged persons of the future. During the last few years rapid progress has been made toward hastening the development of voluntary retirement plans. There are indications that social security, which represents compulsory insurance, will continue and will become a greater source of economic security. Unemployment of our aged and our failure to have provided any form of country-wide old age insurance that covers all of our citizens have placed a large financial burden on the earning capacity of this generation. If we continue to shelve our older workers, if the high cost of living and high income tax eliminate the possibility of adequate personal savings during the earning period, and if inflation continues to reduce retirement income, the wage earner of the future will be sadly burdened. Though the trend is toward more than one wage earner per family, in the majority of instances the average family unit of three and one half has only one wage earner. It is during their active years of employment that workers should be contributing to their own retirement so that they will not in their own later years become dependent upon others.

Employment should not be terminated merely because of age. Much more attention must be paid to finding suitable employment for the older person, and retirement should be delayed for those who want and are able to continue in productive work. A number of state employment service offices affiliated with the United States Department of Labor provide special job counseling and placement for persons 45 years of age and over; they annually place one and one quarter million in employment. The Department of Labor and other government agencies, industrial managements, and labor unions are conducting research to determine the extent and nature of discrimination, and to acquire facts about the capabilities and characteristics of the aging and older workers. In spite of progress, much pressure and creative assistance is still needed from citizens' groups to encourage job development and employment for the elderly.[14] This is a much more important objective than plans for the economic support of aged people who are idle; though some, of course, cannot work, and social planning for their care is necessary.

Consequences of unemployment. We might turn for a moment from the economic implications to other influences of our present unemployment situation on the aged. Most people like to work and to be self-sufficient and self-supporting. This is true except for those persons in whom, for a variety of reasons, the will to achieve has been blunted or destroyed. The unhappiness and frustration suffered by unemployed older people cannot be measured in dollars and cents. Idleness and retirement are not conducive to man's happiness. Older people must be productively employed in the present, since they cannot speculate upon plans for a future that may not be theirs. Forced retirement at the peak of productivity may produce frustration and insecurity, may make the remaining years futile and unhappy, and may even shorten life. Older people cannot adjust to new situations as readily as they could in youth, and the working habits of forty years cannot be suddenly interrupted without profound feelings of desolation and loss. The retired individual may wander about, unhappy and bewildered. Mental confusion may finally rescue him from reality, and he may dwell upon a happier time—his youth—or else he may be plunged into a truly devastating anxiety state.

Charles Lamb in his essay, "The Superannuated Man," expresses the plight of the man used to a schedule of work and suddenly cut adrift with an abundance of leisure:

> I could scarce trust myself with myself. It was like passing out of Time into Eternity—for it is a sort of Eternity for a man to have his Time all to himself. It seemed to me that I had more time on my hands than I could ever manage. From a poor man, poor in Time, I was suddenly lifted up into a vast revenue;

> I could see no end of my possessions: I wanted some steward, or judicious bailiff, to manage my estates in Time for me. And here let me caution persons grown old in active business, not lightly, nor without weighing their own resources, to forego their customary employment all at once, for there may be danger in it.*

WHY OLDER PEOPLE ARE NOT EMPLOYED

It is the duty of all of us, as nurses and as citizens of our communities, to think seriously of the implications of the shift in age of our population. Leadership in a humane and realistic approach to the situation must probably come from altruistic professions, including nursing. One cannot study the group behavior of man without feeling that he is truly shortsighted. Our conduct toward our aged members represents one of the glaring inconsistencies of our time. While our left hand has been busy ensuring life in infancy and combating infection and preserving life, our right hand has been equally busy curtailing the usefulness of the older person. Thus, paradoxically, while we preserve the life of the person, we kill him socially.

Why, we might ask, have we, the leading democratic nation of the world, with our professed emphasis on the personal worth of the individual, allowed this situation to occur? There are many reasons. In fairness to persons who are struggling with the problem, it must be said that we have no precedent to follow, for never before in the history of the world has there been proportionately so large a number of older individuals in one nation's population.

One reason for our rejection of the aged in employment circles is an attitude of mind that characterizes Western thinking. Anthropologists have described our society as one that places the highest value on youth and beauty and upon the ability to achieve physically in highly competitive enterprises. This seems to have become a definite cultural trait. The movies have fostered the myth that youth and beauty alone can surmount all obstacles. This attitude of mind is quite foreign to the Oriental world, in which prestige, pride, and satisfaction come with age. For example, in nationalist China it is a compliment to assume a person to be older than he is. In this country the judgment of age is a serious affair: Underestimates become a compliment and overestimates a social blunder.

Another reason for difficulty in employment among older people is our newness as a nation. Persons coming to our shores were young, energetic, and aggressive. They set to work developing and industrializing our vast resources. In this period of great expansion and growth, an inordinate value that persists to this day was placed on speed and efficiency. In our eagerness to produce and to sell, we did not stop to consider the real worth of our endeavors beyond their commercial importance. Thus, the values we thought worthwhile demanded the time and effort of the young and energetic and relegated the more mature persons to the sidelines. Our culture is geared to the life of the young. One sees this everywhere. Our traffic rules, our recreational facilities, and our housing are but a few examples. Nowhere is this more apparent than in industry. In our eagerness for speed and efficiency, we have created a situation in which a

*From Lamb, Charles: The Superannuated Man. In The Last Essays of Elia, London, 1952, Macdonald & Co.

25-year-old promoter of a brand of deodorant or a convincing writer of television jingles may receive a higher salary than a college president.

The loss incurred by eliminating services of the older worker who has had time to develop a social vision and a philosophy is inestimable. This is difficult to evaluate in an industrial-technologic society. When one compares the painting, the sculpture, and the architectural achievement of artists at various age levels (for example, the paintings of Renoir), one cannot help but conclude that development of the inner man and depth of character may often come with age and living. This we might all wish to see reflected in the culture we bequeath to the next generation.

Individual capacities are not given sufficient attention in regard to employment. After World War II, when numerous workers returned to their jobs, there was little room for the older person. Little effort was made to suit employment to his decreasing physical abilities, and almost none was made to utilize his special capacities. The inflexibility of retirement rules bears grim evidence of the lack of consideration for individual capabilities. Some men are old at 30 years, while pages could be written about men 65 years of age and more who have contributed immeasurably to human enjoyment and progress.

Workmen's compensation laws have contributed to curtailment of the employment of older workers. These laws, which provide financially for certain workers injured in hazardous employment, exist with variations in all states. Workmen's compensation laws militate against the employment of older workers, even when individuals are willing and anxious to waive all compensation rights if they may only be employed. The pressure of public opinion among the aging populace may force the revision of workmen's compensation laws in the individual states in the future. Many labor contracts now have clauses stating that a certain proportion of workers must be in the older age group.

Employing agencies are inclined to employ the younger person who is a better risk, since they themselves have to contribute to the insurance of their workers. There are indications, however, that the older person properly placed is not a great work risk. Changes in policy may be slow in coming partly because of our centralization of industry. Many large companies have pension plans and accident and illness insurance which, they believe, make the hiring of older persons almost impossible.

Industry has only begun to consider the contribution that older people can make if they are given suitable part-time work. Deeply entrenched in the minds of many industrial employers, and often in the minds of the individuals themselves, is the conviction that a worker cannot make work adjustments after he is 40 years of age or thereabouts. This works a particular hardship upon the unskilled workers, that large segment of our population who have the larger families, whose connection with their place of employment is more tenuous, and who cannot save for a rainy day. The older employee has a better chance of being retained if he is an executive or a so-called white-collar worker. A study of top business executives revealed that 44 percent were over 60 years of age. However, an executive over 40 years of age who leaves his employment often feels that it is too late to make a new start. This has resulted in the formation of a club in which unemployed executives who are over 40 years of age can discuss their mutual interests. The man who secures employment is automatically disqualified for continued membership. He then assists other members to secure employment.

Needless unemployment of older people should be corrected by education. Thoughtful analysis of the worker's productivity in a few situations has revealed that the older worker does have certain limitations. However, what he may lack in both physical and mental speed, he may make up in dependability and judgment. During the war years when every hand was needed, the older worker demonstrated his ability to compete with any age group as a steady, reliable, loyal, and happy worker. Many preferred to work rather than avail themselves of the social security benefits to which they were entitled, and the list of persons receiving old-age assistance fell far below predicted levels. Some, for the first time in years, were enjoying the satisfaction of working in a situation in which they felt essential.

The older worker is often an asset. If alterations in work situations, such as shortening the number of working hours, are made, and if attention is paid to individual assets and liabilities, there is no reason why many older persons may not be employed indefinitely, with benefit to industry and business, to themselves, and to the rest of society. All fields of human endeavor need both age groups among their workers. The speed of learning and accomplishment, the imagination, and eagerness to take risks in the young must be tempered by the stability, experience, and mature judgment of the older person.

The argument has been presented that we must retire the older person in order to make room for the younger. This is simply another way of saying that there are not enough jobs for everyone. We might pause for a moment to speculate upon the fallacy of insufficient work for the people of all ages in our country who want to work, when at the same time there are jobs for which workers cannot be found. Domestic help, for example, is completely unavailable to the elderly or to middle-income persons at a price they can afford, yet often this would enable chronically ill and elderly persons to remain out of institutions. So much attention has been focused upon status as it relates to various forms of work and upon the low status of many kinds of physical work that, at present, needed services are not available to many who can purchase them while, ironically, there is unemployment.

Retirement. The generally high standard of living in this affluent society, with technologic progress making for less time needed to earn the necessities and the luxuries, has led to the genuine conviction on the part of many that retirement is a privilege in such a fortunate society and that it should be accorded to everyone and should be enjoyed. It is quite possible that early retirement will be the rule in the future. It is equally possible that this may indeed be a relatively happy period of life for the majority of people, if plans for a secure economic future can be assured and creative and satisfying interests aside from work can be developed.

Ideally, preparation for retirement should begin while one is in the thirties and forties. Employees should take responsibility for group and individual preretirement conferences and counseling. Gradual reduction of work or partial retirement over a period of five to ten years has been recommended and tried. Such an arrangement is still far from widespread, but some encouraging developments have taken place recently, even though this plan presupposes a long time in the same place of employment, which is often not the case.

Employment and chronic illness. Some people cannot be employed because of chronic illness. When we were a young nation with a preponderance of young people, we turned our attention to the control of the diseases of childhood. This preoccupation with diseases of the young left little time for study of the diseases of age, while at the same time it added immeasurably to the preservation of life in the young and indirectly to the marked swing toward a much larger number of old people. Though the contribution of the early leaders in public health should not be minimized, it now seems necessary that more attention be paid to research in diseases of older people.

Many of the chronic illnesses of older people cannot be cured. Many can be controlled in part, and, what is more important, the person can be taught to live with his disease and can often be relocated in the working market so that his chronic illness will not lessen his earning capacity too greatly. Sometimes this may mean that a new skill must be learned, and our attitudes about this learning must be revised. Many are inclined to think that the older person cannot learn a new trade, that he is not worth training. In some state vocational training programs, the tendency in the past has been to accept fewer candidates over 50 years of age on the grounds that funds and resources were limited and attention must go to those who give promise of the longest number of productive years in the new vocation. This concept is changing rapidly, and truly remarkable success in the rehabilitation of older people is being accomplished.

ECONOMIC RESOURCES OTHER THAN EMPLOYMENT

Providing security for aged citizens, should they of necessity be idle in their later years, is equally as important as measures to ensure a longer life of useful employment. Several plans now operate to provide some economic security, and, though improvements are being made constantly, none of them at the present time seems wholly satisfactory. Personal savings and personal insurance are helpful, but even before the present high taxation and inflation, it was found that a very small part of the population was able to accumulate enough in savings and insurance to guarantee economic security in old age.

In contrast to the situation twenty or even ten years ago, the majority of elderly persons now have a small income from one or more sources. It is impossible to determine exactly how many persons receive benefits, since sources overlap. In March, 1963, about 10,000,000 persons 62 years of age and over received income from Old Age, Survivors and Disability Insurance (social security), and 4,645,000 wives and other dependents of retired and deceased workers also received income from this source. In 1962 the average monthly payment to a retired single male worker was $81.70; that to a single female retired worker was $62.40; that to the retired worker and aged wife was $127.10; and that to the aged widow was $65.40.

In 1956, old-age assistance from various sources was given to 2,500,000 persons: 1,000,000 received pensions for public service, 500,000 received railroad pensions, and 500,000 received private pension benefits.[14] The number of recipients of old-age assistance has been declining steadily since 1950, apparently in part because of the increasing numbers of persons receiving Old Age and Survivors Insurance and income from other types of benefits. In March, 1963, it was 2,214,000. Public service and railroad pensions decreased in 1960, whereas the number of private pension plan recipients rose to 1,780,000.[6]

Total income is extremely low for the age group as a whole, especially when it is realized that only one third of the total number of members and only one fifth of those who are retired have insurance to cover medical care or hospitalization in event of illness.[13] In 1956, the median income for families with a head of family 65 years of age or older was $2,500, compared to a median of $4,783 when the head of family was 55 to 64 years of age.[5] The average income for elderly persons living alone or with relatives was $796 a year. Of all elderly family units, 24 percent had savings of less than $1,000, and only 19 percent had as much as $2,500 in savings. There has been little change in these figures during the past ten years, although the upper 30 percent now have savings of $10,000 or more. In 1963 less than 30 percent of the nonmarried persons had savings of $5,000 or more; over half had less than $1,000. From these known figures it is obvious that the elderly as a group have a low standard of living. Persons with income largely from established pensions, which do not increase with increased living costs, have great difficulty.

Voluntary insurance. A plan of voluntary old-age and retirement insurance to which the worker and the employer contribute throughout the time of employment is one way of ensuring financial security in old age. It is in this type of insurance that many social and economic leaders feel the greatest hope for future security lies. The details for transfer of policy in event of change of employment have not been sufficiently well worked out, though progress is being made. In this type of plan retirement can usually begin before a stipulated maximum age if the worker wishes. The benefits are commensurate with the age of the worker when he started paying and the time he has been employed, as well as with the amount of his salary. This type of insurance seems to have value in that it represents voluntary savings supplemented by the employer and does not interfere with the recipient's feeling of independence. Also, in this plan the individual's contribution goes to his heirs if he dies before retirement. In the past, employers were reluctant to initiate this type of insurance policy for their workers. Since it is voluntary and since the employer contributes a percentage equal to that of the worker, he may feel no moral or personal obligation to participate in such a plan. As a result of union pressure, a tremendous increase in the number of industrial pensions has occurred in recent years.

Government plans. In 1935 Congress passed the Federal Old Age and Survivors Insurance Law under the Social Security Act, which provides payments to certain aged persons and their families. Amendments passed by Congress in 1950, 1952, 1954, 1956, 1958, and 1962 have made changes in the law. This insurance again represents the earned income of the individual as well as the contribution of the employer and is in no sense charity. Payment is dependent upon what the worker earned as computed from a record of his earnings, which is kept by the Social Security Board. The worker and the employer contribute equally toward this government insurance, each paying 3⅝ percent (as of January, 1963) of the earnings of the worker in covered employment up to $4,800 a year. This will go to a maximum (with present legislation) of 4⅝ percent in 1968. Successive amendments have extended coverage to more persons, so that by 1956, 92 percent of all employed workers were covered; money collected by the federal government is set aside to cover payments and the cost of the program. There are some limitations to the plan. Full benefits cannot be collected until the worker is 65 years of age or over, although payments and benefits may begin at reduced rates for both men and women at age 62. In this we are behind some countries of Europe who begin their benefits at 60 years of age. Denmark was the first European country to do this. The Social Security Act provides payment for workers who reach the age of 62 years and, in the event of their death, for their wives if they are over 62 years of age. Widows who have dependent children, unmarried children under 18 years of age, and other dependent persons are provided for. The amendment of 1956 provided income beginning at age 50 for eligible persons who become totally disabled and are unable to work.

Social security is essentially an insurance, not a savings, plan. Nothing reverts to the worker or to his beneficiaries if he does not receive all that he has contributed. All of his contribution, however, remains in the federal fund and is used to cover payments to others covered by the total plan.

The amount contributed to social security, although now relatively large and matched equally by the employer, does not provide a premium that will give enough insurance for comfortable living, even if emergencies are barred. Benefits are based on the average monthly earnings during the time spent in work covered by the Social Security Act. If the average yearly earnings were $3,000, the monthly benefit would be $95. If and when a dependent husband or wife reaches 62 or 65 years of age, an additional amount of $35.70 or $47.50 is provided.

When the Social Security Law was first passed, payments could not be made to persons under 75 years of age if they earned $15 or more per month. Successive amendments have altered this ruling to keep pace with inflation and to permit greater flexibility in administration of benefits. As of January, 1962, the covered person who is 65 years of age or older may receive regular monthly payments if he makes no more than $1,200 a year (including income from self-employment); if he earns more, he forfeits one dollar for every two he earns between $1,200 and $1,700 each year.

Another plan providing income for needy older people is federal-state aid (OAA). In this plan the federal government assists the state, providing the state meets certain criteria. The state may then add to the federal allotment as much as it wishes. If the state does not have the funds to meet the federal amounts, the maximum payment may fall below the amount that could be given by the federal government alone if it were matched by the state. The amount given to the individual depends upon the funds available and the policies of the state. Some states have very generous policies and allotments to individuals, whereas others consider many factors such as the ability of relatives to contribute, and all other sources of possible income. Average payment for all the states was $77.85 per month in 1962. In all states, law demands that the individual be 65 years of age or older. In most states, he must prove that he has been a resident of the state for a specified length of time, which varies from a short period to a maximum of five years. The federal act did not require the older person to be a citizen of the country to be eligible for assistance, but about one half of the states have citizenship requirements for eligibility. Old-age assistance is secured through application to the department of welfare in the city, county, or state, and for many aged persons this constitutes a painful method of securing economic support.

The Medical Assistance for the Aged (MAA Kerr-Mills) program passed in 1960 under the Social Security system provides some economic reimbursement for elderly persons who qualify. This may vary from 50 to 80 percent of the cost of services as designated by the state. As of November, 1963, however, only twenty-eight states were participating in the plan.[10]

The amendments to the Social Security Act signed by the President on July 30, 1965, not only established a program of health insurance for the aged, but also expanded the Kerr-Mills program.

The health insurance program, popularly known as Medicare, provides two kinds of insurance: hospital insurance, which is financed by special contributions paid by the employee and employer, and medical insurance to assist persons over 65 years of age to pay for doctors' services and other medical items and services not covered under the hospital insurance program. The medical insurance program is voluntary. Subscribers will pay $3.00 a month, which sum will be matched by the federal government.

Unemployment insurance, which is also provided for under the Social Security Act, is intended for persons who are employable but who are temporarily out of work. Theoretically, the aged person who is still able to work should be eligible for this insurance, but actually when retirement is forced upon him, he is considered as too old to be employable and is directed to the old-age assistance program unless he can qualify for disability benefits.

Nongovernment aid. Fraternal orders, such as the Masons and Elks, lay aside funds for aid to needy members and their families. Some of them maintain homes for their aged members. Religious organizations provide some financial assistance for the old. Private philanthropic services that secure assistance for the aged are numerous, and the good that they do is enormous. Nothing, however, can take the place of plans of his own making to ensure economic independence for the aged person.

REFERENCES AND RELATED BIBLIOGRAPHY

1. Ball, Robert M.: Social insurance and private pensions. In Lurie, Harry L. (editor): Encyclopedia of social work, ed. 15, New York, 1965, National Association of Social Workers.

2. Burgess, Ernest W. (editor): Aging in western societies, Chicago, 1960, University of Chicago Press.
3. Donohue, Wilma T. (compiler): Education for later maturity, New York, 1955, Whiteside, Inc.
4. Dublin, Louis I.: Problems of an aging population, Am. J. Pub. Health **37**:152-155, 1947.
5. Mathiasen, Geneva: The aging. In Kurtz, Russell H. (editor): Social work year book, ed. 14, New York, 1960, National Association of Social Workers.
6. Mathiasen, Geneva: The aging. In Lurie, Harry L. (editor): Encyclopedia of social work, ed. 15, New York, 1965, National Association of Social Workers.
7. Mathiasen, Geneva: The continued employment of older workers, Geriatrics **10**:137-140, 1955.
8. Mumford, Lewis: City development; studies in disintegration and renewal, New York, 1945, Harcourt, Brace & World, Inc.
9. Randall, Ollie A.: The aging, the aged, Public Health Nurs. **40**:61-65, 1948.
10. Rogers, Edward S.: Medical care. In Lurie, Harry L. (editor): Encyclopedia of social work, ed. 15, New York, 1965, National Association of Social Workers.
11. Scheid, Phil N.: Training the average employee for retirement, J.A.M.A. **147**:1323-1324, 1951.
12. Shock, Nathan W. (editor): Problems of aging; transactions of the fourteenth conference, New York, 1951, Josiah Macy, Jr., Foundation.
13. Tibbitts, Clark: The Aging. In Kurtz, Russell H. (editor): Social work year book, 1957, issue 13, New York, 1958, National Association of Social Workers.
14. U. S. Department of Health, Education and Welfare: The nation and its older people; report of the White House Conference on Aging, Washington, D. C., 1961, U. S. Government Printing Office.

Chapter 5

Housing in health

Much thought is being given to where older people should live in health and during illness. It is the belief of persons who have studied their needs, as well as the needs of the total society, that aged people should live as long as possible in their own homes and own communities. When they are extremely feeble and alone, even though well, they should have special housing facilities. When they are chronically ill, elderly persons may do well at home with some assistance from family, public health nurses, and housekeeping and shopping services. When they are acutely ill, they should be in a general hospital. If they are chronically ill and have no relatives on whom they can depend for care, some elderly persons should live in hospitals for chronic illness or in nursing homes that, preferably, are close to and associated with general hospitals and that take into consideration their individual and special needs. Living arrangements should be as varied as the individuals themselves, and each individual should help to decide where he should or may live.

Effort is being made to keep the elderly person in his own community and away from the old folks' home. Denmark is a leader among the nations making this effort. We have passed through a period in which we strived to "put the aged person away" in some quiet spot in the country where he was removed from everyday living and was no bother to anyone. No bother, at least, to anyone but himself, for most older people are not happy out of their familiar surroundings. The older person does not want to be put far away from his relatives and neighbors. True, in our present society, some older people escape to homes for the aged because they prefer them to the social and economic insecurities in our present way of living. They dislike being a burden to the younger people of the family. But the old folks' home would seldom be their choice had the circumstances of their living been different. They suffer from loneliness and the feeling that no one cares. They adjust poorly to frequent changes to new homes. Their personalities starve for lack of the daily give-and-take experiences that are part of community living and that are the satisfying result of cooperative efforts. They miss the church, the school, and the local politics. Even the aged city dweller misses the few remaining local relationships that urban renewal, city planning, and superhighway building have left him.

Benjamin Franklin wrote:

> When they [the aged] have long lived in a house, it becomes natural to them; they are almost as closely connected with it as a tortoise with his shell; they die, if you tear them out of it; old folks and old trees, if you remove them, 'tis ten to one that you kill them.*

The reasons for this are quite obvious. As physical limitations increase, there is even greater need for daily contacts with friendly neighbors. The aged, like all of us, are interested in news about friends and neighbors. Their happiest memories are associated with experiences that combine familiar persons and familiar things. These in a sense become part of them in that they are so much a part of their thinking. A familiar view, a particular road or tree, a piece of cherished china or linen—these should surround them in old age. After visiting the older people in a small town, one observer felt that there was need for a paid visitor to call upon persons who are confined to their homes and bring them up to date regularly on the local happenings of the town.

Older people need a few cronies of their own age with whom to discuss the good old days, the political situation, and "what the world's coming to." But they tire of association exclusively with other older people. They need, also, the refreshing stimulation of contact with children and with young adults. They need the company of people of both sexes and of all ages.

We have passed through the rural and agricultural periods of living in the United States and the first impact of the industrial period that resulted in mass movement from rural to urban areas. Our industrial society made little effort to fit housing to the needs and natural desires of the individual. Instead, housing was fitted to the needs of industry. Living situations thus created placed limitations upon the possibility for happiness and satisfying experiences for everyone involved. As industrialization brought many workers to live in small urban apartments, a choice was forced upon the older persons if their young people had moved to the city. The older ones had to decide whether to live in their old surroundings, if they were financially able to do so, or to live in the city with or near sons or daughters. Urban housing arrangements were not always conducive to the harmonious living together of several generations. Although it was possible for some older people to have a place of their own in or near the city and thus to be near family members, this arrangement was satisfactory only as long as both members of the aged couple were able to care for themselves or for each other. When illness or infirmity finally made it impossible for them to carry on the necessary activities of daily living alone, families were faced with problems of care and housing outside of the home for the first time in our country's history.

The recent mass movement of more affluent city dwellers to the suburbs has further complicated the problem. Although many suburban homes are large enough to house an older relative, families are larger and the way of living has often changed from the one to which the elderly are accustomed. Although shop-

---

*From Van Doren, Carl: The Autobiography of Benjamin Franklin, New York, 1940, Pocket Books, Inc. (Courtesy Mr. Van Doren.)

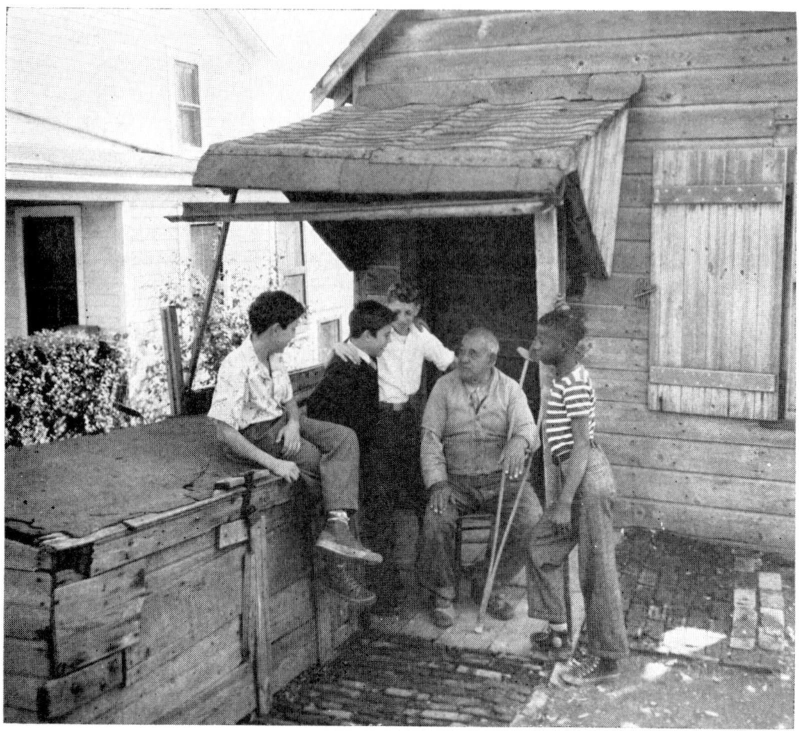

Figure 7. The older person needs association with persons of all ages. (Courtesy the Ulster County Health Department; Lipgar Studio.)

ping centers make shopping convenient for most housewives with automobiles, public transportation that means freedom to many elderly people is often inconvenient. Buses may schedule trips to the city, twenty or thirty miles away, but not to the local church or center shops. Because the elderly usually are dependent upon someone for transportation, their freedom is greatly restricted.

For those elderly persons who wish to live near but not with their children in the suburbs, there is almost no housing to be rented nearer than the city. Too, many of the elderly of today have been the city dwellers of the earlier industrial period. Having become used to the easy accessibility of shopping, services, and entertainment in the city, they often feel isolated in the suburbs.

There is true beauty in the aged couple who have faced life's problems and joys together and have been granted companionship in their old age. Every effort should be made to keep them together as a unit of our society. One of the greatest needs today is for housekeeping service for such couples. Sometimes all that is needed is someone to clean house, to do the shopping, or to help prepare a meal each day. Yet this service is almost impossible to obtain. The result is that the old couple will undoubtedly be separated if one or another of them becomes ill or infirm. One member may be sent to a nursing home, the other to a home for the elderly. Most large departments of welfare provide some

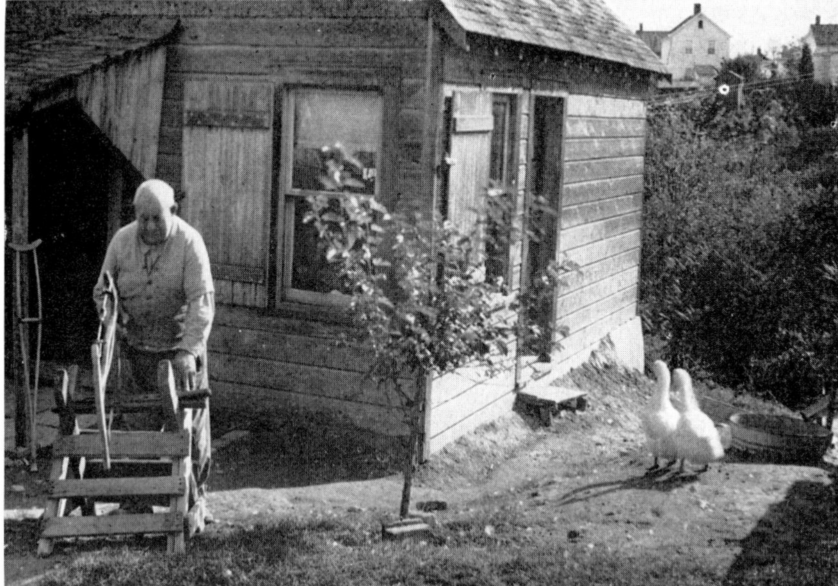

Fig. 8

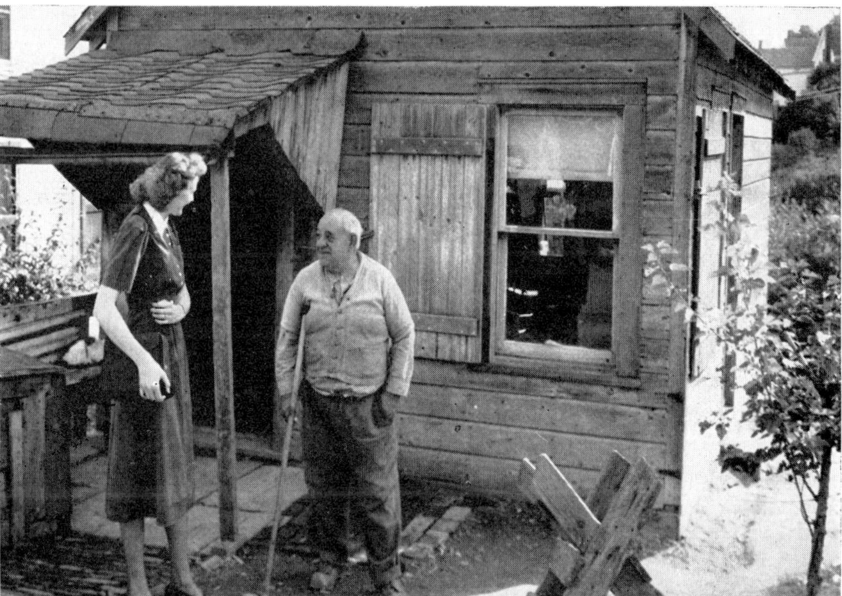

Fig. 9

Figures 8 and 9. This patient, who has arteriosclerosis, arthritis, and diabetes, is able to remain in his own home through regular visits from the nurse. He enjoys his community relationships, raises ducks for a hobby, and keeps busy with small chores about the place. (Courtesy the Ulster County Health Department; Lipgar Studio.)

funds for housekeeping service for deserving persons of all ages. But the funds available are most inadequate to meet the need. Though social agencies and social workers recognize the needs of the healthy aged couple or of the aged person living alone, they are almost always at the bottom of the list of persons who receive help. Preference is usually given to situations in which children are involved with next preference given to the chronically ill and disabled aged. Homemaker services are now being sponsored by visiting nurse agencies and other official and voluntary agencies. Fees for service vary with the kind of agency sponsorship. There are approximately 425 homemaker services today, or more than twice the number in 1961. There is a great need for more education of the taxpaying public and additional support for this kind of service, which contributes so much in happiness and self-sufficiency to aged people.

After a husband or wife dies many older people prefer to live alone, rather than with relatives or in any kind of group housing arrangement. To them the ability to maintain their own establishment represents a precious freedom and independence, regardless of how poor they may be or how great the hardships. In England, for example, it has been found that old men often do their own housekeeping, including cooking, cleaning, and laundry. They are in familiar surroundings and report that time goes fast, and they are relatively happy and content. They are often unhappy when participating in some form of communal living where they may sit for hours and days among strangers, with nothing to do.

England adopted the practice of *meals on wheels* for its shut-in elderly persons several years ago and has reported excellent success with this service. Meals on wheels has been only slowly adopted in this country. (See Chapter 7, Nutrition.) Another plan that is being considered is the use of school cafeterias to prepare and serve a hot evening meal daily for persons who can leave their homes for a meal yet cannot prepare meals satisfactorily and cannot afford the cost of suitable restaurant food. Elderly men living in rooming houses might benefit greatly from such a program.

RECREATION

Many older people are completely removed from relatives and old friends. Studies in gerontology point to the crying need for recreation resources for our aged. Many lonely older people sit in parks for hours; they haunt the rooms of the public libraries; in smaller communities they visit the corner cigar store or saloon. Some literally do not speak to anyone for days, even though they may live in a crowded city. Provision to meet persons of their own age who have interests and problems similar to theirs and whose physical capacities are relatively the same often adds greatly to their happiness and contentment. The need for this kind of service is greatest in large cities where community relationships are more tenuous, and some large cities are progressing rapidly in the development of recreation centers for the aged. Recreation centers should provide opportunities for the mingling and meeting of both sexes. They can offer lectures, discussions, movies, and exhibits embracing any subject from art to exploration and natural history. Group enterprises such as picnics, sewing projects, competitive writing projects, and art exhibits and social activities such as dancing and cardplaying are appreciated, as they are not otherwise provided for in daily living. Many elderly people are interested in learning, and some recreation centers develop a close association with universities and adult education classes. They may also have camps that will make suitable vacations possible. Vigorous efforts to develop effective recreation facilities for the aged are being made not only in most cities but also in many rural communities. In New York City, the Hodson Community Center was an early progressive development in this field. Susan Kubie and Gertrude Landau have described the work at the Hodson Center in their book, *Group Work with the Aged.*[10] An important feature of the program at this center is that the elderly people plan and help to conduct their own activities program.

The growing number of organizations of aging persons, such as senior citizens' clubs, indicates the initiative and interest of this age group in meeting their own needs and directing their own lives. Many persons prefer such social groups to the more highly organized day recreation centers where professional workers direct many of the activities.

COMBINED CENTERS

Some leaders in gerontology and geriatrics, such as Dr. R. T. Monroe in Boston, believe that we need centers that offer a wide variety of programs for elderly persons and that are patterned somewhat after the program of the Young Men's Christian Association. These centers would have rest rooms, recreation rooms, reading rooms, a cafeteria, and perhaps temporary sleeping quarters. They would include a general medical clinic, department of physical therapy, and the service of a podiatrist. The centers would also offer guidance, counseling, and social case work assistance. Adult education classes and planned recreation programs would be offered. The elderly in the community would have a say in preparing the programs and making any changes.

SPECIAL HOUSING FOR THE AGED

Definition and some existing arrangements

The term *infirm aged* usually designates the old person who is neither acutely nor chronically ill, but who suffers from general debility of age and often has one or more relatively mild chronic ailments. He can care for his personal needs and light household tasks but requires assistance with activities that are physically demanding. Some form of communal living may be necessary for this person, and unfortunately, he may have to go to a hospital-type facility because no suitable home is available.

The need for suitable housing for older people of different levels of economic and physical self-sufficiency has received consistently increasing attention. In 1949 the national goal of a decent home and a suitable living environment for every American family was written into the Preamble of the Housing Act. Under successive modifications of the Comprehensive Housing Act of 1954 many types of aid are now available through the Federal Housing Administration to meet the housing needs of the elderly. These include public low-rental housing projects, liberalized financing methods for home purchase and remodeling, mortgage insurance for both profit and nonprofit rental housing, and direct loans at low interest rates on a long-term basis.

Legislation administered through the Federal Housing Administration has made possible housing developments of many kinds. They include individual living units such as apartments, houses, or trailers that may be owned or rented by elderly persons who are capable of managing their own affairs. For those who need semi-independent living arrangements there are facilities that provide rooms, suites, or cottages. These may be in hotels, residence clubs, or motel-like developments that provide centralized dining rooms and housekeeping and other nonpersonal services. Multifunction facilities not unlike these have developed in response to the growing need of assurance of continued care in the event of illness; they include infirmary care, and more recently many have added a nursing home annex or unit for long-term care.

Retirement towns have also developed. These are self-contained communities, some of which provide for all essential services, including social assistance, health care, and recreation opportunities.

Some religious and fraternal orders maintain homes for aged members who have paid dues toward their future home. Some require large payments on admission or demand that all property be signed over to the home, the church, or the order. Waiting lists are long, and in most of these homes the increasing cost of living makes it difficult to keep up high standards of care. Almost all homes now privately operated accept persons who pay regularly and who can retain control of their own resources. Most states permit elderly persons living in such homes to receive old-age assistance if they are otherwise eligible. Some voluntary institutions require that the resident sign over his old-age assistance benefits, and out of this income each resident is given a small uniform monthly allowance.

Some elderly persons enter a home when they are still able and really anxious to carry on by themselves. They fear that their health may suddenly fail at a time when the protection of a home is not available to them. During the last few years some homes have developed plans whereby individuals become members of the home's family, yet continue to live in their own homes as long as possible. The Peabody Home and the Home for Aged and Infirm Hebrews, both in New York City, have experimented with this plan and believe it may be one answer to the pressing problem of long waiting lists in almost every good home for the elderly in this country. Elderly people are visited regularly by a social case worker from the home, and they are given assurance that there will be a place for them in the home when the need arises. It has been found that when they are relieved of the worry and fear of being alone and without protection, many older people carry on very happily and independently.

In 1961 the American Association of Homes for the Aged was organized under the sponsorship of the The National Council on the Aging, with a grant from the Ford Foundation. Its membership includes nonprofit voluntary and government homes for the aged. It has published a directory of nonprofit homes for the elderly that nurses who work with the elderly should find helpful.*

*The American Association of Homes for the Aged, 49 West 45th Street, New York 36, N. Y.

Foster home placement is meeting the housing needs of some infirm elderly people. By taking an elderly person into their own homes, some middle-aged women are finding a partial answer to how to fill the gap left in their lives by marriage of children and early widowhood. Careful selection of a suitable home must be made by the welfare agency involved, and wishes of the client and his family must also be considered. Follow-up at regular intervals is also advisable. The public health nurse can be helpful to the foster homemaker in preventing accidents and in maintaining optimum health both for herself and for her elderly paying guest. Older people may be happier in a foster home than in the home of relatives with whom they have had little in common throughout the years. Although the trend is toward greater use of foster homes, there are no accurate statistics available showing the number of old persons who are now living in them.

Many homes for the aged merge in form and management with infirmaries or nursing homes that provide care during illness. All three types of care are sometimes available in different parts of the same establishment. A discussion of the regulations governing these establishments and the problems of their management is included in Chapter 9, Housing During Illness. Useful guides for persons interested in housing arrangements are now available.[2, 14] A few essential criteria may be of interest to nurses.

Location. It is now generally felt that any establishment that houses the aged should be located either in or near a medical center where the best of clinical and diagnostic facilities are readily available when needed. They should be located where grounds are adequate, and where a court and view are possible. Their location should in no way restrict visitors or limit the residents from sharing in the everyday experiences of daily community living as long as this is permitted by their physical and mental condition.

Safety. An important feature in establishments for the aged is that they be safe. Many elderly people have been housed in old structures that are fire hazards. The newspapers in the winter of 1945-1946 reported grim evidence of this, for in that winter there were four serious fires in homes for the aged. Forty-four persons lost their lives and forty-nine were seriously injured,[21] and in 1952, the serious fire in a home in Florida reemphasized the problem. It must be remembered that older people cannot get about quickly, and safety precautions must be taken with this in mind. Smoking in bed by the residents must be forbidden. Main furnaces or other heating units must be inspected regularly, as must lighting, wiring fixtures, and gas cooking and heating equipment if it is being used. Brick or fireproof construction is best for the buildings, and it is well to avoid old buildings with several flights of stairs since it is so difficult to get older people up and down stairs. Recommendations have been made[2] that any building with over two flights have elevators and that those with more than fifty occupants have at least two elevators. Even if there are elevators, they are not always usable in the event of fire, and it is almost impossible to have elevator service that can quickly accommodate the number of persons in wheelchairs in some homes.

Attention to innumerable small details adds up to safety in homes where older people live. Lighting throughout should be adequate. Thresholds in doorways should be eliminated. Halls and stairways should be well lighted. A small night-light at every bedside would help to prevent stumbling when older persons get up at night. Bathrooms adjoining bedrooms prevent residents from unsafe wandering about at night. Entrances to the buildings should have ramps, and doorways throughout the building should be wide enough to permit the passage of wheelchairs. Rails along ramps and stairways and hallways give necessary assistance to feeble elderly persons. Small benches placed in elevators, at the ends of hallways, and on each flight of stairs help to prevent the aged from falling from excessive fatigue. Fire extinguishers should be set into the wall so that residents who are not attending carefully will not injure themselves. Electric irons in pressing rooms should be automatic so that forgetting to turn them off will not result in overheating. Beds should be normal height, and no throw rugs should be used.

General facilities. All homes for the aged should have recreation facilities or provision for participation in them in the area in which the home is located. Recreation should include passive participation with others such as watching an outside entertainment, activities like knitting or reading that can be done alone, and group activity, planned and arranged for by the residents themselves. Group discussions and dancing are examples of suitable group activities. A department of occupational or recreational therapy and the full- or part-time services of an occupational therapist or recreational therapist are most helpful. Such professionally trained persons may be able to train volunteers who can be extremely helpful in recreation programs.

Medical and dental facilities should be available, and most homes with fifty or more residents should have an infirmary with competent nursing service and a department of physical therapy. Other services that should be available are those provided by a beauty operator, a chiropodist, and a barber, unless all residents are able to leave the home and make their own provisions for these services. There is a trend toward the operation of clinics in some homes for the aged and in many public housing projects accommodating large numbers of elderly persons. These may be sponsored by the housing authority, the local department of public health, the local visiting nurse service, local voluntary community organizations, or a combination of these. The purpose of the clinic is to supplement the hospital clinic and private medical practice[3] by providing diagnostic services, screening for conditions such as glaucoma, preventive health education, and similar services.

Nutrition. Principles of nutrition for the older person in the home would follow those for the aged anywhere. It is obviously impossible to please every member at every meal. But the better institutions employ a skilled dietitian interested in older people, and budget a good part of their money for food. In the smaller homes it is possible to obtain from each resident some of the recipes and menus of which he is fond and to feature some of these occasionally; the response to this in the appetite of individuals and in general interest is often remarkable.

Meals in any home should be as far removed from institutional cooking as possible. Some progressive homes have spent much thought and expense on their dining rooms, with excellent results. Small tables rather than long ones make the dining hall seem more like a dining room in one's house. They also enable persons wishing to sit together to do so, yet permit others to eat alone. Many older people living in groups after being alone for years are annoyed by the table manners, conversation, or mannerisms of others, and in turn they often irritate others with their own peculiarities. Meal hours should be as close to normal as possible; most congregate living establishments tend to serve the evening meal too early.

Many homes demand that all residents appear for meals if they are physically able to do so. This serves to get withdrawn members into the group for short intervals. When a resident is extremely feeble, it is often best, if a cafeteria system is in use, to provide a porter system in which he can select his own food and have his tray carried to the table. The family-style way of serving is being replaced in many homes by the cafeteria system since food tastes differ so greatly. Water should be provided on the tables since many aged people do not take sufficient fluids and drink little between meals. The dietary requirements of old people are discussed in detail in Chapter 7, Nutrition. Some of the more progressive residences provide facilities for light cooking—breakfast or a snack—in apartments, and on each floor a more extensive kitchen to be used when entertaining guests. Residents in most homes are expected to eat at least one meal (dinner) in the dining room.

General policies. It is considered best that homes for the aged admit both men and women, even if women predominate. Married couples should be admitted and should have rooms so that they can be together. It has been the experience of most homes for the aged housing both sexes that romances flourish, and rarely a year passes without a marriage taking place.

Some regulations are necessary in all congregate living, but rules should be flexible. Residents should be free to come and go as they please, provided they have medical approval and carry some identification. Some homes have committees or councils made up of elected members of the home population who help to make the rules by which the group shall live and who are helpful in conveying to the home management the attitudes and feelings of the residents.

Residents should be encouraged to bring some of their favorite pieces of furniture and other marks of personal identity and individuality such as family portraits and knicknacks. Some residences permit automobiles and provide garage or parking space for them.

Visitors should be encouraged and hours of visiting should not be restricted. Every effort should be made to make family members feel that their visits are welcome and appreciated. Visits from family and friends are one of the most important means of a person's keeping a feeling of personal identity and worth.

REFERENCES AND RELATED BIBLIOGRAPHY

1. Abbott, Ruth D.: Public health nursing service in housing projects, Nurs. Outlook **12:** 41-42, 1964.
2. Alt, Edith (project director): Standards of care for older people in institutions, section ii, New York, 1953, The National Committee on the Aging, National Social Welfare Assembly.

3. Blanchard, Bradford M.: Geriatric care in the public housing area, Geriatrics **19**:302-308, 1964.
4. Bozian, Marguerite W.: Nursing in a geriatric day center, Am. J. Nurs. **64**:93-95, 1964.
5. Cryan, Eleanor: Foster home care for older people, Am. J. Nurs. **54**:954-956, 1954.
6. Glober, Lee J.: The high rise apartment as housing for the elderly, Geriatrics **17**:147-150, 1962.
7. Goldfarb, Alvin I.: Responsibilities to our aged, Am. J. Nurs. **64**:78-82, 1964.
8. Home-delivered meals for the ill, handicapped and elderly, Report of National Council on the Aging Committee on Guidelines for Home-Delivered Meals, New York, 1965, National Committee on the Aging.
9. Kleemier, Robert W.: Attitudes toward special settings for the aged. In Williams, Richard H., and others (editors): Processes of aging, vol. II, New York, 1963, Atherton Press.
10. Kubie, Susan H., and Landau, Gertrude: Group work with the aged, New York, 1953, International Universities Press, Inc.
11. Lawton, George: Aging successfully, New York, 1946, Columbia University Press.
12. Linden, Maurice E.: The aging and the community, Geriatrics **18**:404-410, 1963.
13. Mathiasen, Geneva: The aging. In Lurie, Harry L. (editor): Encyclopedia of social work, ed. 15, New York, 1965, National Association of Social Workers.
14. Maxwell, Jean M.: Centers for older people; a guide for programs and facilities, New York, 1964, National Council on the Aging.
15. Mumford, Lewis: City development; studies in disintegration and renewal, New York, 1945, Harcourt, Brace & World, Inc.
16. Posner, William: A foster home program for older persons, New York, 1952, National Council on the Aging (mimeographed).
17. Scott, Miller: Housing and welfare planning. In Lurie, Harry L. (editor): Encyclopedia of social work, ed. 15, New York, 1965, National Association of Social Workers.
18. Smith, Emily M.: Health services in selected housing projects and day centers for the aging, Paper presented at the Annual Convention of the American Public Health Association, October 6, 1964.
19. Tartler, Rudolf: The older person in family, community, and society. In Williams, Richard H., and others (editors): Process of aging, vol. II, New York, 1963, Atherton Press.
20. Van Doren, Carl: The autobiography of Benjamin Franklin, New York, 1940, Pocket Books, Inc.
21. Zeman, Frederic D.: Accident hazards of old age; the physician's role in a program of prevention, Geriatrics **3**:15-25, 1948.

Unit 2

Maintenance of health and prevention of illness

Chapter 6

General hygiene

General hygiene for the aged differs somewhat from that for younger persons. Many of the adjustments necessary are small in themselves, but for the aged person they may mean the difference between comfort and well-being and persistent discomfort or even predisposition to disease. Principles of good hygiene apply to all elderly persons, including those who become ill.

REGARD FOR THE PERSON

An older person should have as much personal freedom as is consistent with his safety. Untold discontent and unhappiness come to old people because relatives, friends, and others try to take charge of them in the belief that they are incapable of caring for themselves. One geriatrician goes so far as to say that older people need only two things for happiness and contentment—economic security and freedom to do as they please.

Attention to the details of hygiene is essential when illness occurs, and the nurse must take responsibility for many details left at other times to the individual. Care must be given, however, without seeming to manage the aged person or forcing unnecessary adjustments upon him. Old people dislike change, and their routine should be disturbed as little as possible.

The nurse should employ her good judgment to distinguish harmless activity from that which may be injurious to the patient or to others. She should know, for example, that the aged patient who persists in smoking in bed during the night is endangering others besides himself unless he lives alone. She must make him realize the seriousness of this and make him cease the night smoking, particularly for the time he is in the hospital or living with others. But the patient who wears two pairs of socks and a sweater when he sleeps is harming no one and should be permitted this self-indulgence. There is no place in professional nursing today for the inflexible nurse who fails to see her patient beyond the narrow confines of his starched white bed. Unfortunately, it must be admitted that a few nurses in the past have insisted, for example, that all hospital shades be pulled to exactly the same level even though one patient might complain of sunlight in his eyes or another believe he is denied the protection from draft that the drawn blind affords. How many aged patients have been made miserable in the hospital by such trivial rules as having to take showers instead of tub baths and to take them in the morning instead of at night. Perhaps for fifty years the patient's routine has been to take a tub bath just before retiring. Such unimportant rulings often make him unhappy and resistive to important hospital procedures. Evidence of such inflexibility on the part of nurses is fortunately quite rare today.

PHYSICAL CARE

Bathing and skin care. Many older people dislike daily baths and feel that they are not necessary. They show good judgment in their disinclination to bathe so frequently. As the skin atrophies, less oil is produced and perspiration decreases; drying of the skin occurs and there is less waste secretion on its surface. Frequent bathing is less necessary to remove dead skin and excess secretions and may cause drying and itching of the skin. Too frequent bathing may lead to an annoying skin condition called bath itch, which usually begins as dry, reddened, and itching spots of pinpoint size over the shin bones and may spread to other parts of the body. Specialists in geriatrics feel that bathing once or twice a week is usually sufficient for the older person. Extra bathing may be necessary in such a specific illness as uremia, when additional waste products may be found on the skin. Many bed patients should have baths, supplemented by sponging of the back, face, and hands if this seems necessary. Superfatted soaps, containing fat additional to that combined with the alkali constituent of the soap, can safely be used for older people. The newer neutral detergents are usually harmless to the elderly person's skin, but occasionally a sensitivity reaction to them occurs. Preparations containing silicone are now prescribed occasionally for elderly persons who are incontinent. They must be used with care since they are most irritating if inadvertently rubbed into the eyes.

Bathing the bedridden, helpless aged person is a difficult nursing function. One fairly satisfactory method is to move the patient from a bed or a wheelchair to a commercial bath or commode chair or to a wooden armchair that can be moved under the shower, so that a spray shower can be used. When a tub is located so as to be practical and workable for the nurse or family members, tub baths are generally the best means of getting the patient really clean, improving circulation, and making him more comfortable. The tub bath also offers the opportunity for the person to move his joints more freely than might otherwise be possible. Almost any patient, even when extremely old and completely disabled, will automatically assist with washing himself when placed in the tub.

Back rubs and general body massage are good for the skin of most bed patients. The geriatric patient who is unable to move about freely should have any skin surfaces on which weight is borne massaged every hour. Stimulation of circulation is one of the greatest benefits of massage, but it must be remembered that aged skin is thin and easily traumatized, and therefore massage should not be too vigorous. Witch hazel, mineral oil, and various emulsions and lanolin creams should be used on dry skin areas. Alcohol is drying to the skin and should not be used. Bony prominences may be protected from pressure by a piece of

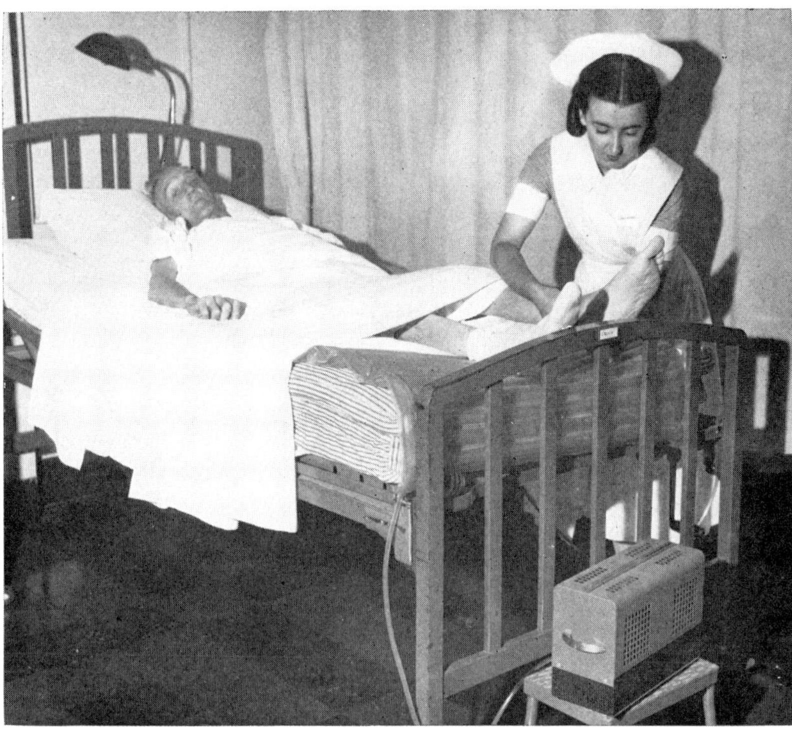

Figure 10. This electrically operated machine alternately inflates and deflates sections of the plastic overmattress. Massage and warm socks are helpful when circulation in the feet is poor.

rubber sponge, chamois skin, unshorn sheepskin, or new commercial sheepskin-like products. All of these may be washed in mild soap solution when necessary.

The feet usually show changes of age early since they may be the first part of the body to be affected by diminished peripheral circulation. The heels should be massaged thoroughly. The nails undergo changes that first may be considered normal but that may lead to disease. They become brittle and thickened, and normal cutting of them may eventually be impossible. Placing a wisp of dry cotton under the lateral edge of a nail that tends to curl inward against the flesh may encourage it to grow straight. The cotton should be inserted most carefully to avoid trauma; the broad end of a wooden toothpick can be used. The cotton should be removed before bathing. Well-fitting shoes that do not exert pressure on the toes help to ensure adequate circulation and more normal nail growth. Massage to the toes to stimulate circulation and specific toe exercises that increase circulation to the nail beds are sometimes helpful. Warm oil poultices should be used on horny, irregular toenails before cutting is attempted. The older person should not cut his own toenails if they are thus involved; if necessary, the services of a podiatrist should be secured. Castor oil is one of the best oils for softening and improving the texture of the nails. A large variety of suitable creams, many of which contain lanolin, are available for helping to keep the skin and the cuticle in good condition. Hand creams should be used generously by elderly persons and careful attention should be given to the fingernails. One dermatologist cautions against the elderly person visiting the beauty parlor for manicures for fear of infection to the cuticle. The use of rubber gloves for washing dishes or doing other work about the house helps to preserve what little lubricant is being secreted by the skin. If the hands become excessively dry, a lanolin cream may be applied at night and white cotton gloves may be worn to prevent soiling the linen.

Many dermatologists suggest that cosmetics be used by the elderly woman, provided they contain no irritating substances. Cosmetics can be protective, as, for example, the cream used as a base for lipstick and eyebrow pencil. Cream and powder applied to the skin of the face help to protect it from exposure to sun, wind, and dirt.

The hair becomes thin, dry, and colorless as the tissues age and blood circulation diminishes. Massage to the scalp and daily brushing help to preserve the hair. Lanolin cream in small amounts may be used for the massage, and oil treatments before shampooing are often beneficial. The hair should be kept clean, but too frequent washing should be avoided. Every three to four weeks is sufficient for the average older person. A mild soap dissolved for a shampoo is best for general use; special shampoos should be prescribed by a physician. The older person should be discouraged from experimenting with new shampoos since many preparations contain alcohol and other drying agents. Men often wash their hair several times each week; this procedure dries the hair excessively and may produce an annoying pruritus of the scalp. Occasionally, elderly men do not wash their heads often enough and develop a crust on the scalp. This can be removed by using pHisoderm or 3 percent hexachlorophene in a soap solution (pHisoHex), followed by a mild shampoo.

Whether he is in good health or chronically ill, the older person should be encouraged to care for the hair as carefully as in earlier years. In the hospital the older woman patient gets a real psychologic lift from having her hair brushed and arranged attractively. Permanent waving is often recommended. The patient should be encouraged to care for her own hair. The physician or the nurse who remarks about the attractive appearance of an older woman's hair is applying sound principles of mental hygiene.

Many women (and a fairly large number of men also) dye their hair. The need to have natural-colored hair is one that must be recognized in our society, where such a premium is placed upon youth. The tendency toward early graying of the hair is inherited, but graying may be hastened by illness, poor nutrition, worry, and emotional strain. There are no miraculous drugs that can restore natural color to the hair. The vegetable dyes and rinses, except for causing dryness, are harmless, and physical danger is encountered only when aniline dyes and dyes made from heavy metals are used. Once it is begun, use of dye must be continued if an acceptable appearance is to be maintained, and this requires time and may be costly. One of the nurse's most valued services in caring for a patient with a chronic illness may be in assisting the patient with the use of harmless hair dye. A woman patient may have hidden (or believe she has hidden) her graying hair from her husband for years. Continuing this innocent subterfuge during the last months of a terminal illness may add immeasurably to her happiness and peace of mind.

With age, the distribution and quality of hair changes. Hair in the axilla and pubic areas becomes finer and scanty, whereas that of the eyebrows becomes coarse and bristly. Hair on the face of women is often one of the most trying aspects of growing old. As one aging lady bluntly put it, "When we get old, we get hairy and we get horny." When the patient is ill for long periods or is unable to care for herself, the nurse may assist her in the removal of superfluous hair from the face. The only safe and permanent method of removing hair is by means of an electric needle. This procedure must be done only by persons who are qualified. Shaving or the use of pumice stone followed by the application of cream to prevent drying is fairly satisfactory, except on close inspection. Plucking of stray hairs from the face is often sufficient. The nurse who offers assistance to the extremely ill or helpless patient will find that her services are greatly appreciated and will contribute to improvement of the patient's morale. Hairs should not be plucked from moles but may be snipped close to the surface with small scissors; one should be careful not to cut or otherwise traumatize the mole. Stray hairs on the face may be made less conspicuous by daily bleaching with a weak solution of hydrogen peroxide and ammonia, provided that this does not irritate the skin.

Because of poorer neuromuscular coordination in the hands and decreased tissue tone with loss of subcutaneous fat on the face, many elderly men who use safety or straight razors frequently nick the skin when shaving. Although it is not easy to change the shaving habits of many years, many elderly men can be helped to accept the use of a good electric razor. The rotary blade type seems to be the most durable and efficient and can be used equally well by women who must shave hair from the face frequently. Elderly men should be encouraged to arrange equipment in the bathroom so that they can sit while shaving. Usually a stool and a small mirror that can be hung or propped just above the washbowl is all the change that is necessary.

Sleep. Old people may doze at intervals most of the day, although total sleeping hours may not increase. They sleep lightly and intermittently, and strangely enough, in most instances this does not seem to disturb them. Less sleeping may be done at night. It is not unusual to find aged individuals reading, getting up, wandering about the house, even preparing and eating a meal during the night, with little consciousness that such behavior may appear peculiar to others. The nurse should not expect her older patient to sleep as soundly as children on the pediatric ward or young adults. She should note whether he is awake constantly or intermittently. Little success is achieved in trying to alter the sleeping habits of aged patients, though the time-worn useful aids such as a warm drink, a back massage, and quiet surroundings may help to get their night of sleep off to a good start. Interesting activities to keep them awake during the day may result in better sleep at night.

Ventilation. Fresh air is important. The diminished chest expansion of most older people resulting from inelasticity of the rib cage makes it necessary that the air breathed have a normal amount of oxygen if enough is to be supplied to the body. The older person usually does not like very much fresh air; what most younger people consider good ventilation he may think is too much. Indirect ventilation is usually best for the older person since he is extremely susceptible to drafts, and, contrary to popular belief, this is not a notion but a physical reality. Many older people suffer from fibrositis, which produces vague muscle pains that are aggravated by chilling and drafts. Adipose protective tissue is decreased, and the volume of circulating blood may be less. Decreased activity lessens circulatory function, and the result is lowering of skin temperature and susceptibility to chilling from lowered external temperature and drafts.

Rest and relaxation. Older people need less food, less work, more rest, and more relaxation. They should avoid haste, particularly in the morning hours. Geriatric specialists instruct their men patients to take twice the time to shave that they took in earlier years, to dress slowly, and to avoid hurry of any kind. Some doctors believe that haste and hurry are injurious to the well-being of the aged person, regardless of the status of the heart, blood vessels, or other body systems.

The morning routine of the average busy hospital makes this need for a slower pace difficult to achieve. The ceaseless early morning round of collections of blood and urine specimens, basal metabolism tests, test meals, and visits to the x-ray department, to say nothing of the rush so often apparent on operating days, are not consistent with good geriatric care. Some of the routines and some of the pressures are necessary and cannot be avoided. The thoughtful nurse, however, who realizes the needs of her geriatric patient will make some effort to arrange routine procedures to suit his individual needs.

Noise is a further disturbing element to any ill person, but particularly to the older one who is finding hospital adjustment difficult and who may have a hearing loss. Partial deafness may set the patient on edge and make him alert to every sound. This interferes with the capacity to relax. Even though ability to hear conversation may be limited, the sound of a distant radio, shrill voices, or rattling equipment may be most disconcerting.

To ensure relaxation and at least partial peace of mind, every person who is ill in a hospital needs to feel that there is one specific person to whom he is assigned and to whom his needs are well known. The case method of assignment of patients to nurses helps to make the patient feel understood and secure in the hospital.

Rest is essential for the aged. The ability to relax completely for short satisfying periods is most helpful when old age has been reached. All elderly people should be encouraged to rest for at least ten to twenty minutes once or twice a day in the prone (face-lying) position. This helps to prevent flexion contractures at the hips and the kyphosis so commonly seen involving the dorsal spine.

Too much rest can be dangerous. It is important that the nurse who is caring for a patient in the home instruct the family of this fact. The nurse is seldom in the home long enough to see that the patient is out of bed as much as is desirable. She depends upon the understanding and cooperation of the patient

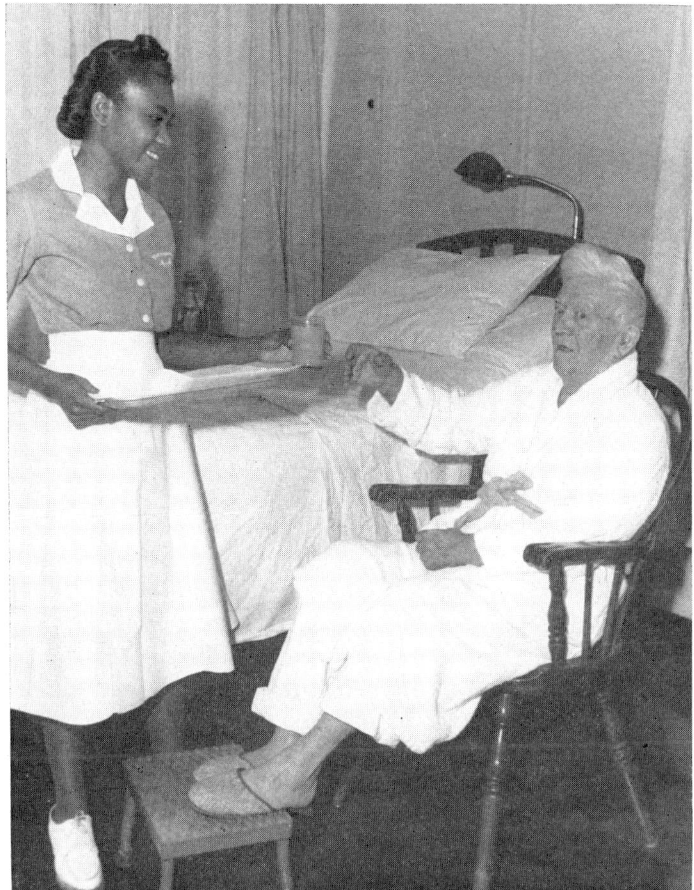

Figure 11. A footstool and a chair with arms add to comfort and safety. (Photograph by Robert Waldeck.)

and his family. The family should know that oversolicitous care and too much waiting on the older person may be damaging to him both physically and emotionally.

Most older people want to be out of bed, particularly if they can be up without feeling that they are a burden to their families. To most of them who are ill, permission to be up represents the doctor's faith in their recovery. The value of early mobilization to circulatory, respiratory, and other physiologic processes in all age groups is now accepted quite readily. In caring for the aged, one must remember that physical changes make the need for frequent moving even more urgent. Except for patients suffering from such conditions as acute coronary thrombosis, pulmonary embolism, and acute pneumonia, it is felt that every older person should be out of bed at least once each day.

Sitting in a chair each day adds to the patient's interest in his surroundings. The environment can be altered. He may be taken in a wheelchair to visit another patient, to look out the window, or to sit on a porch. He is much happier, and often the restless apprehension that so easily comes to an older patient is avoided. It must be remembered that no matter how great the age, life is still precious as long as the capacity to learn and to participate in mutual social experiences remains. To foster in elderly patients the desire to live and to learn and to maintain interest in their surroundings is an important responsibility of the nurse.

Every elderly person should have at least one chair that is the right size, shape, and construction for his safe use. The chair should be the right height so that his feet rest squarely on the floor, without uncomfortable bending of the knee or dangling of the feet. The chair seat should not be so deep as to press against the popliteal spaces and retard circulation. It should have arms so that arm leverage can assist him in rising from the chair, and there should be space under the front chair legs so that the patient can place one foot backward to increase his base of support and help to prevent his falling as he rises from the chair. Elevation of the lower extremities by using a low footstool helps to prevent pressure on popliteal blood vessels and thereby improves circulation in the legs and feet. A rocking chair is excellent in that it provides gentle and safe yet varied exercise for the lower extremities and to a lesser extent for the arms and the trunk also.

Posture and exercise. In age, muscular activity becomes less automatic, and a slumped posture may result in a sagging abdomen, rounded spine, and drooping of the chest and shoulders. Stiffened ligaments, tendons, and muscles often permanently fix these changes. Attention to posture and exercise is essential to well-being and helps to postpone physical infirmities. Exercises must, however, be carefully regulated by the physician. A great deal of harm has been done by an older person's trying to keep up the rigorous exercise routine that was maintained in youth. Thewlis believes that routine exercises should never be done by the older person immediately upon arising. If a routine of formal exercises is desired by the person or ordered by the physician, it is usually carried out in the afternoon or evening. As the number of aged in our population increases, commercial companies will supply recreation equipment appropriate to the needs of this growing number of mature customers. For example, the market for tennis rackets might remain constant, whereas the demand for golf clubs may be greater.

Exercises to improve posture are helpful for the aged, even though bony structures may be so altered that really good posture is impossible. Any improvement in posture will enable the body to use its remaining resources to better advantage. Improvement of posture and muscle tone has produced amazing results in fatigue states accompanied by low blood pressure. Breathing exercises are often helpful to the patient who is suffering from asthma. Marked increase of blood pressure and mitigation of symptoms have followed the strengthening of the abdominal musculature to give better support of the viscera in the correct position. Specific exercises must be prescribed by the physician and must be directed by a physical therapist, but teaching good posture and deep breathing is part of the daily nursing care of the patient.

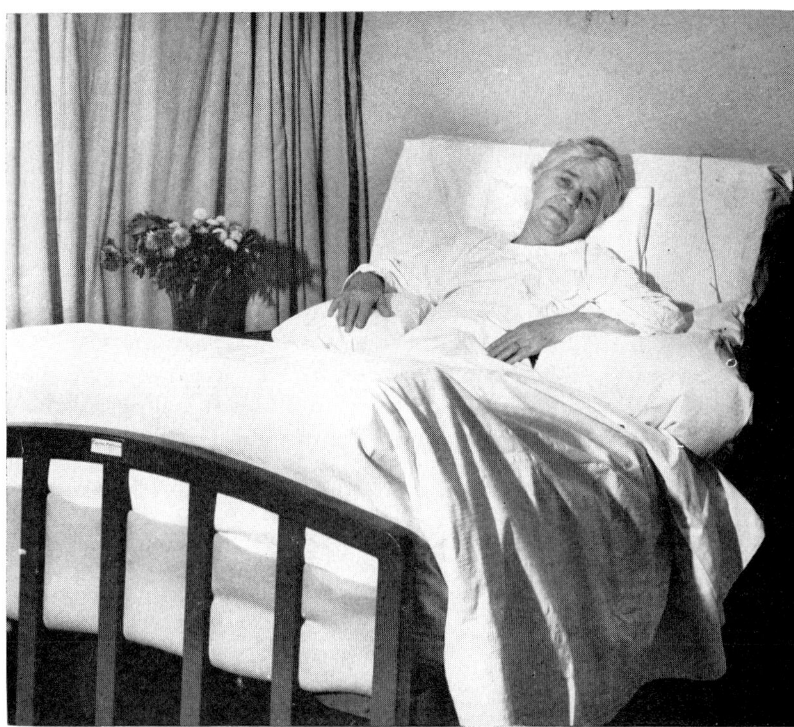

Figure 12. Pillows provide comfort for this patient. The head pillow placed lengthwise brings the chest forward and permits good chest expansion, and support of the arms prevents strain on the shoulders. The foot block gives support and provides something firm against which she can press her feet.

Unless there is some particular contraindication, nonspecific exercises or active arm and leg exercises and exercises to keep abdominal and gluteal muscles active and to strengthen the extensor muscles of the spine should be performed several times each day by every bed patient. These exercises may be learned by nurses from the physical therapist if instruction was not included in the nurse's own preparation. Supervision of daily exercises of a nonspecific nature is the responsibility of the nurse, and regular performance of them will help to prevent the loss of muscle tone that occurs in all bed patients unless activity is continued.

The older person should sleep on a firm bed since he is a ready candidate for postural deformity. Fortunate is the person who becomes accustomed to a firm bed in youth since such a bed is very likely to be prescribed in age, particularly if hypertrophic or osteoporotic changes are occurring in the spine. Actually, many people prefer a firm bed, and some patients report that they are unable to sleep in the hospital because of the soft bed. The nurse should be certain that this is reported and that a fracture board is placed under the mattress if needed. Bedcovers should be light and warm and should be tucked loosely to give the patient sufficient room to move about in bed.

Clothing. Clothing should be that to which the older person is accustomed and in which he is comfortable. There are few more distressing sights in the hospital than that of the lonely older patient sitting uncomfortably in his recently donned hospital garments while an attendant stuffs his clothes, symbols of his personal identity, into a white bag and disappears with them. Many hospitals are altering their previous policy and allowing the patient to keep some clothing at his bedside. If at all feasible, lockers for clothing should be provided on all wards. Too often the patient stays in bed because he finds hospital bathrobes and slippers cold and uncomfortable or not available when they are needed.

In chronic care facilities permitting and encouraging a person to wear his own clothing is an incentive to activity; it helps to encourage good bowel and bladder control and aids in socialization with others. The older person at home after hospitalization or illness should be encouraged to return to normal patterns of daytime dress. If an elderly woman, however, has been accustomed to spending the morning or much of the day in a bathrobe or housecoat it is unlikely that this practice can be changed.

Dermatologists recommend that wool not be worn next to the old person's skin because it may increase pruritus. Many aged persons believe that woolen underwear is essential for health and comfort, and, here again, hospital routine should yield to individual preference of the patient. There is nothing to be gained from forcing the patient into an ill-fitting hospital shirt when he may have worn flannel pajamas all his life—provided that his own belongings are clean and he can assume responsibility for them. It is imperative that the patient's shoes be kept at his bedside to be worn when he gets up. Even a few days in bed may cause loss of muscle tone, and foot troubles may follow the wearing of soft slippers that offer no support to the feet.

Eyes. Most people over 65 years of age need glasses, at least for reading. The nurse must be careful that glasses are not lost or knocked from a cluttered bedside table. When mail arrives, she should make certain that the patient has his glasses and that they are clean; the difficulty in seeing that suggests eye trouble is often caused by soiled glasses. Glasses should be put away carefully when not in use; loss of glasses has caused aged patients untold hours of anxiety in the hospital. The nurse must remember that older people dislike appearing helpless, and she must do everything possible to enable them to carry on with a minimum of assistance. Poor lighting can cause eye discomfort, so light over the bed should be adjusted to make reading without eyestrain possible. Reading is often a source of great comfort and relaxation to the elderly patient. If he has a room of his own, most physicians feel that there is no harm in his turning on the light and reading at intervals during the night if he is wakeful.

Irritation of the eye may follow a decrease in conjunctival secretions. Sometimes the lower lid droops (ectropion), and the necessary lubricating fluid of the eye is lost. Irritation and tearing may produce further annoyance. Secretions at the inner canthus of the eye may accumulate, particularly overnight, and may be uncomfortable and unsightly. The alert nurse is mindful of care that will make her patient more acceptable to persons around him. A sterile cotton sponge moistened with boric solution or physiologic solution of sodium chloride can be used to cleanse the eyes. Great care must be taken not to press on the eyeball or to irritate any exposed conjunctiva.

Smoke is irritating to the eyes, particularly to the elderly person's eyes. The elderly nonsmoker will sometimes have to be protected from persons around him who smoke excessively, but there are few complaints from the patient who enjoys smoking.

Teeth. The majority of people (three fourths of those 70 years of age and older) have lost all their own teeth by their seventieth year. Much could be done during the younger and middle years of life to prevent this loss. After the age of 34 years for men and 39 years for women, periodontal disease is the first cause of loss of teeth, though most people think of dental caries as the greatest danger. Defective bite from malocclusion results in absorption of bone surrounding the roots of teeth so that they loosen and are lost. When the deposits that form on teeth are not removed, they may progress under the gum margins and destroy the delicate fibers holding the teeth to their inner sockets. This often is the reason for the loss of teeth that may be entirely without cavities.

His teeth, or his lack of them, present a painful problem complicating the elderly patient's happy adjustment to hospital life and to the impositions of illness. At home he had his own secret container for his bridge or his artificial teeth. In the hospital he must ask the nurse for the necessary equipment, unless she is thoughtful enough to provide for his needs in this respect.

Effort should be made to motivate the patient to give adequate care to his teeth and mouth. Free hydrochloric acid may be lacking in the stomach, which may predispose to impaired digestion and poor oral health. Gum tissues become less elastic and less vascular, and the gums may recede from any remaining teeth, leaving an area of tooth not covered with enamel. This area is sensitive to trauma from brushes and coarse dentifrices. Popular dentifrices do not have sufficient abrasive property to wear through the enamel of the teeth but can injure the exposed tooth roots (cementum). Many aged individuals who do not wear dentures have decayed, broken, or missing teeth, which result in poor mastication of food and the avoidance of foods that cause discomfort when eaten. The effect of mouth health upon nutrition is marked. Surprising improvement in appetite has followed correction of unhealthy conditions in the mouth.

Any lesion in the mouth should be promptly reported to a physician. Cancer of the buccal mucosa, the tongue, and the lips is relatively common in elderly persons and sometimes follows pressure from a dental plate or irritation from jagged or broken teeth.

For psychologic reasons, if for no other, all elderly people who have lost their natural teeth should have dentures and should use them. Adjustment to dentures is often difficult, and the patient needs a great deal of encouragement. He should visit his dentist if dentures cause irritation or do not seem to fit properly. Many elderly persons have worn dentures for years and are reluctant to have them replaced if they become worn and ill fitting. Often they reason that the cost is too great, that they will probably not live long enough to make expenditure of money for a new set worthwhile, or they are afraid that a new set may not fit properly. Sometimes the dentist is able to avoid replacing dentures by lining old ones so that they fit better and are more efficient.

Diet. Diet for the elderly should consist of foods that are easily masticated, easily digested, and adequate in protein and vitamins. The older person changes food habits with reluctance. A balanced, regular diet is essential to general well-being, but it is useless to try to force new and unfamiliar foods upon the older person simply because they are good for him. Patient and persistent explanation of dietary needs is helpful, but much deliberate effort is necessary to make the food attractive.

Obesity, an enemy of long life, must be avoided. Obesity is rather rare in the very old since it is often not compatible with long life. Many obese persons die in their forties and fifties.

Elimination. Older people are inclined to worry about bowel function. They often become concerned if they have decreased bowel elimination. They may forget that they are not working as hard and are not eating as much, and therefore the output of waste products is naturally lessened. Gainful and attractive occupations that will detract interest from bodily systems and their functions are often helpful in decreasing concern over elimination. Any marked change in bowel habits, however, and any unusual reactions to normal doses of laxatives should be reported, since malignancies of the lower bowel are fairly common.

Many otherwise normal elderly persons have itching and discomfort about the rectum. This may be caused by lack of cleanliness, by dryness of the skin, or by lessened secretion of mucus from the membrane of the lower rectum. Many persons of all ages have small external hemorrhoids and skin tags, and the elderly are inclined also to have a slight tendency to prolapse of rectal mucosa, which may sustain trauma during defecation or from coarse toilet tissues. Geriatricians recommend that elderly persons be advised to cleanse the anal area gently with soap and water after each defecation. Soft toilet tissue moistened with warm water is quite adequate for this.[17] At the conclusion of this procedure any tendency toward prolapse should be corrected.

Regularity in going to the lavatory is important since it provides stimulus to evacuate the bowel. Motor activity of the intestinal musculature decreases with age, and supportive structures in the intestinal walls become weakened. It is believed, however, that muscle tone, motility, and contractile power of the gastrointestinal tract remain adequate into advanced age. Digestive residue reaches the sigmoid about 24 hours after ingestion. The accumulation of feces in the lower sigmoid and rectum stimulates the process of evacuation. Since the gastrocolic reflex reinforces this stimulus, the after-breakfast interval usually is a good one for bowel evacuation.

Sense perception is less acute in age so that the signal for bowel elimination may be missed, and constipation may occur, resulting in impactions. There is a tendency with aging toward incomplete emptying of the rectum at one "sitting." Frequently it is observed that immediately or a few moments after standing up, the stimulus to defecate will be felt again. If heeded, the person may then have a second defecation. Nurses often disregard this, especially with very elderly and somewhat confused patients, and they may even become irritated when the patient says he needs to return to the bathroom. The nurse should understand what is occurring and the patient should always be encouraged to heed this stimulus.

Difficulties in regular bowel elimination can often be overcome by alteration in diet and fluids. The diet should contain plenty of fruits and vegetables unless there are definite contraindications for this, and one of the most satisfactory ways of assuring improvement in elimination is having the patient eat six to eight cooked prunes for breakfast.[5] Usually it is recommended that the older person who complains of constipation take two to three liters of fluid per day. Many elderly persons do not consume this amount.

Some form of laxative may be ordered when bowel elimination is not satisfactorily improved by conservative measures. Glycerin suppositories or soap suppositories are sometimes all that is needed. Recently bisacodyl (Dulcolax) suppositories have been used widely for the very old person who must have some regular stimulus to evacuation or who is incontinent. Smaller doses of laxative are usually required in age than in the more active period of life. Many old people develop diarrhea easily. Mineral oil is not desirable for habitual use because vitamin A is soluble in the oil and is probably excreted without being utilized by the body. Saline cathartics are seldom used because of their drastic action and because they may cause dehydration. Milk of magnesia is seldom ordered because many elderly people have diminished hydrochloric acid in the stomach and because its excessive use also causes dehydration. The mild bulk laxatives such as agar-agar or karaya and psylla seed are most often selected by the physiciain for the elderly patient. Enemas may be needed, particularly if it is believed that laxatives cause digestive upsets. A pint of warm water with ½ tsp. of salt or 10 ml. of glycerin may be recommended.

Many elderly persons are troubled with flatulence, and escape of flatus from the rectum may become so pronounced that it interferes with their social activities. Reasons for this may include irregular bowel evacuation, constipation, and poor neuromuscular control of the anal sphincter muscles. The person who has this difficulty should be advised to discuss it with his doctor. Some physicians prescribe activated charcoal, which has been reported to produce remarkable improvement in many instances.[10]

Another annoyance that may plague the older person is frequency of micturition. One of the first signs of diminishing or failing kidney function is night frequency. The normal average adult kidneys secrete about two ounces of urine per hour during the day and, due to their ability to concentrate urine during sleep, about one ounce per hour during the night. This ability of the kidneys to concentrate urine may be gradually lost with age. In addition, decreased muscle tone in the bladder, with lessened emptying ability, may result in residual urine in the bladder and subsequent mild infection. Frequency and slight burning on urination are symptoms of which the patient may complain. Older women often experience the added difficulty of relaxation of perineal structures and older men difficulties associated with hypertrophy of the prostate.

Unless there is a definite contraindication, the nurse should urge her elderly patient to take sufficient fluids to dilute urine and decrease its irritating properties. Fluids may be limited in the evening, however, if nocturia is troublesome. If the patient is likely to be up and about at night, the nurse must be certain that his light is convenient at his bedside and that his surroundings are not such that he is likely to stumble or fall. If the patient is quite feeble, it is well to suggest that a urinal or bedpan be used during the night. Prompt response to a light signal is necessary if the patient with frequency is confined to bed. If complete incontinence occurs, bathing frequently is necessary to keep the skin clean and in good condition. Care of the incontinent patient is discussed further in Chapter 17, Nursing in Psychiatric Illness.

Genitourinary disorders. Hypertrophy of the prostate is extremely common in elderly men. Early signs are frequency of urination and difficulty in initiating urinary flow. People with these signs should be urged to seek medical advice before the condition progresses and causes kidney damage. Many older men who are receiving medical care for some other condition have some prostatic difficulty. The nurse must be sure that a urinal is kept at the bedside and that any new difficulties are reported accurately.

Some older women are troubled with a vaginal discharge. After the menopause, involutional changes of the genital structures occur, with partial atrophy and decreased activity of the cells lining the vagina, which in normal maturity secrete a fluid sufficiently high in acid to inhibit bacterial growth. When an insufficient amount of acid secretion is produced, vaginitis may occur and cause an irritating discharge. Occasional douches with a mild antiseptic or vinegar solution are often helpful, and frequent tub baths when permitted will make the patient more comfortable. Any unusual discharge should be reported to the physician.

Many elderly men and women are likely to have a problem with an unpleasant odor that may go unrecognized by themselves but that may be objectionable to others. This is the result in part of lessened acuteness of the senses of sight and touch and smell so that clothing is worn long after it should have been laundered or sent to the cleaners. Elderly men and particularly those who have hypertrophy of the prostate are inclined to dribble on their clothing at the conclusion of voiding with little awareness that this is occurring. Urging them to stand for a few seconds at the conclusion of voiding before rearranging their clothing may help to correct this difficulty. Elderly women should know that although bathing of the total body is not necessary each day, local cleansing is perhaps more important than when they were younger.

Accidents. Older people often do not see well, they may not hear clearly, and they may not move with ease. It has been found that neuromuscular coordination about the hips is impaired, and the ability to regain physiologic balance is diminished.[8] Vertical perception becomes less effective, and this interferes with establishing normal balance if it has been lost. This problem is further aggravated by poor lighting and particularly in going from a well-lighted to a poorly lighted room.

Many accidents could be prevented if elderly people had better medical care. Wider use of hearing aids and glasses, for example, would prevent many accidents. While the personal independence of aged individuals is respected, it is necessary to take precautions for their safety. Curbs, buses with high steps, and street crossings are a few of the most common hazards. The confusion of our busy cities with their heavy traffic, their noise, and the nervous preoccupation of their people contributes to the incidence of accidents. Public education as to the benefit from wearing hearing aids would help to prevent many traffic accidents. Older persons would be less likely to slip or stumble if they wore shoes with rubber heels both indoors and outdoors. The nurse may take part as an active citizen in her community in accident prevention. Better street lighting, control of speeding, increased time intervals for lights at controlled crossings, and sloping curbs at street corners are examples of items that might occupy her interest.

Falls rank next to traffic accidents as a cause of accidental death in the aged. Approximately 3,500,000 persons 65 years of age and older suffer accidental injuries each year,[12] and a large number of these occur indoors. Scatter rugs should not be used in the home in which an old person lives. Floors should be kept clean and dry and lightly waxed. Lighting should be adequate, particularly in halls and stairways. One thoughtful owner of a delightful home for the elderly considers that his most important rule is that the hall lights be on at all times. He knows that the residents will go to the bathrooms during the night and wishes to lessen the danger of their falling in the dark. Painting the lower step yellow may prevent accidents on stairways; yellow has a higher visibility than white. A small night-light by the bedside is helpful if it does not interfere with sleep. Low-voltage lights near baseboards in bathrooms and stairs can be left on during the night, with small expenditure of electricity.

Excess furniture and equipment such as boxes and stools should not be left in an older person's room. Children's toys must not clutter rooms or hallways, and furniture should not be rearranged without the older person's knowledge. Even if his vision is good, it is unwise to do much rearranging of furniture since an elderly person is likely to forget and depends on long-established habit in moving about in his room. Accidents may follow the sudden change when the older person is taken to the new environment of a hospital where physical surroundings are unfamiliar, particularly if his vision is impaired.

Accidents in the bathtub are frequent. The elderly must be cautioned to have the bathtub filled and to test the water before getting into the tub. Many severe and even fatal burns have resulted from a person suffering a heart attack, cerebral accident, or fainting spell while lying in a bathtub with the hot water running or from stepping into a tub of very hot water that had not been tested. A rubber mat in the tub lessens the danger of slipping. A railing around the tub provides a firm support to grasp when one gets in and out of the tub. It is tiring to stand in the tub, and there is danger of slipping. A stool should be placed by the tub so that the older person may sit while drying himself.

All drugs in the home in which an elderly person lives must be clearly labeled in large print. No poisonous drugs should be kept in the medicine cupboard where an absent-minded older person or one with failing vision may rummage during the day or night.

If the older person is inclined to get up and wander about the house during the night, it is well to lock the doors securely to prevent his wandering out of the house and perhaps falling or otherwise injuring himself. Basements and cellars are a particular hazard and should, in most cases, be kept locked during both day and night hours.

Many accidents occur in kitchens. Many people still persist in using kerosene to start wood fires. Many light the kitchen stove or the gas when wearing kimonas with dangling sleeves. Others leave boiling pans too near the edge of the stove or fall sleep when food is cooking, thus allowing liquids to boil over and extinguish the gas flame. Older people are sometimes inclined to turn on the gas and forget to light it. If gas is used and there is an elderly night prowler in the house, it is often well to lock the kitchen door so that gas cannot be turned on accidentally.

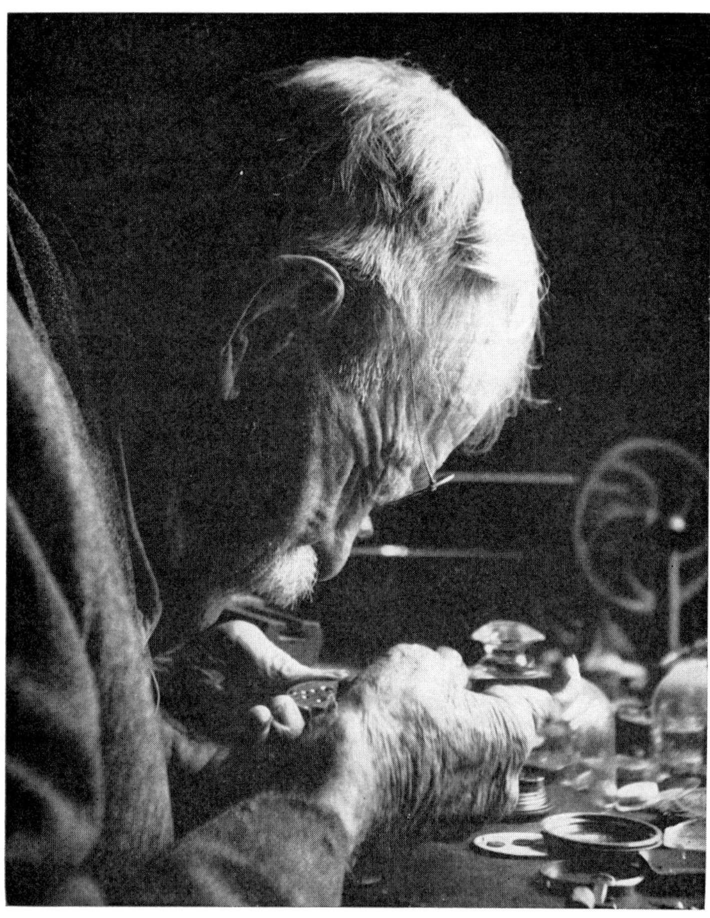

Figure 13. This old gentleman was fortunate in having good eyesight. He continued his lucrative hobby of repairing watches until his death at 94 years of age.

MENTAL HYGIENE

No one, young or old, can keep mentally healthy without stimulating activities and associations with others of both sexes. Keeping the patient happy and content when he is confined by illness is difficult in his own home. But here, at least, he is surrounded by familiar faces. Keeping him happy and content in the unaccustomed surroundings of the hospital often taxes the ingenuity of the nurse. Fortunately, the trend is toward relaxation of the "antivisitor legislation" all too common in hospitals in the past. The patient today can be a little more sure of seeing his loved ones when he needs them most—when he is ill. Dear to the hearts of all of us, especially to older people, are bits of news about the people whom we know and the incidents that occur in familiar situations. Only the patient's family and friends can bring him these. The nurse should remember that normal people are more interested in people than they are in things. If she can provide for satisfaction of this normal human interest, she has done much toward keeping her patient emotionally healthy and happy. If she can make him

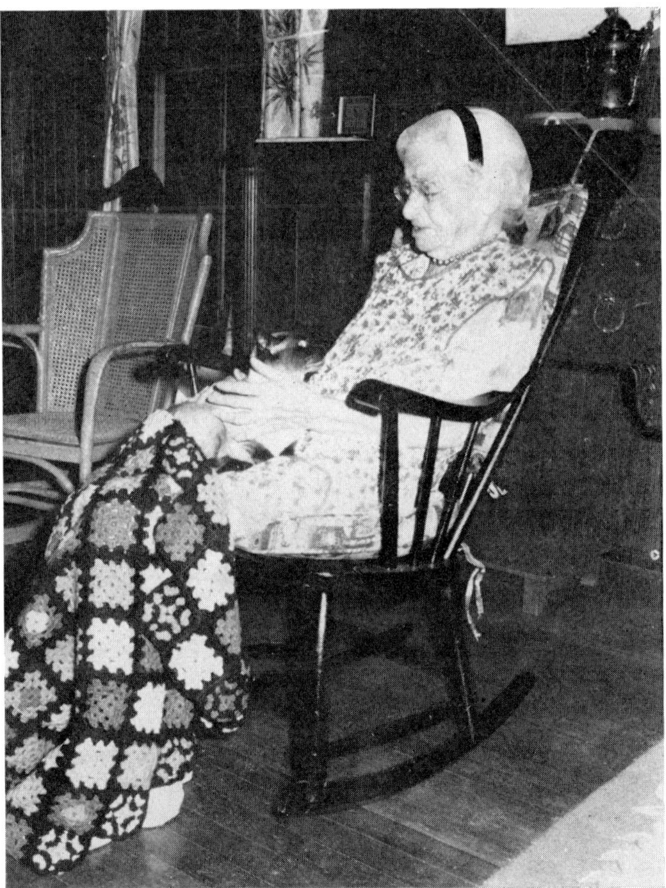

Figure 14. Pets can provide companionship for the elderly person who is alone.

feel that she is genuinely interested in the people he knows, talks about, and cares about, she will inspire his confidence and become his friend.

Satisfying use of free time is important in the mental hygiene of the aged. Every man, woman, and child should have a variety of hobbies, interests, and skills that will fit him to spend his leisure fruitfully if confined to bed for a period of time and in preparation for the time when he will have more leisure. Some hobbies that require group activity should be cultivated since association with others is essential to a normal personality. On the other hand, some hobbies should be those that can be carried on alone in case the individual is thrown upon his own resources entirely. Everyone should learn to enjoy something that does not require the use of the eyes; everyone should develop some interest, such as reading, that can be gratified without hearing.

Pets of any kind are helpful because their care feeds the ego of the caretaker and makes him feel essential. The affection and selfless devotion with which the pet responds brings comfort to the lonely older person. The antics and behavior of animals is also a source of entertainment.

It is distressing to see an older person who is partially blind, who cannot even hear the radio, and who has never learned any simple mechanical skill such as knitting, weaving, or carving that could be performed with the hands. One such old lady posed a real problem. She was completely blind, very deaf, and as the result of a cerebrovascular accident could scarcely move one arm and was unable to walk. Fortunately her mind remained active. She lived with a daughter who went to work every day, leaving the old lady completely alone except for the visits from the public health nurse twice daily. It seemed almost impossible to think of something to hold her interest. At the nurse's suggestion, a kitten was bought. Holding the kitten in her lap at intervals during the day gave the elderly lady a measure of happiness and companionship in her loneliness. This was, of course, very limited activity; yet even limited activity is better than none at all. Whether the old people are at home or in an institution, having useful tasks to perform especially for others or for the welfare of the family adds motivation and satisfaction to living.

REFERENCES AND RELATED BIBLIOGRAPHY

1. Accident facts, Chicago, 1964, The National Safety Council.
2. Allen, Edward F.: Dental aspects. In Cowdry, E. V. (editor): The care of the geriatric patient, ed. 2, St. Louis, 1963, The C. V. Mosby Co.
3. Austin, Catherine L.: The basic six needs of the aging, Nurs. Outlook **7**:138-141, 1959.
4. Carney, Robert G.: The aging skin, Amer. J. Nurs. **63**:110-112, 1963.
5. Cayer, David: Nutrition of the geriatric patient. In Johnson, Wingate M. (editor): The older patient, New York, 1960, Paul B. Hoeber, Inc., Medical Book Department of Harper & Row, Publishers.
6. Goodrich, Martha, and Schwartz, Doris: Some changes in the sleeping and eating patterns of fifty patients with long-term illness, J. Chron. Dis. **9**:63-73, 1959.
7. Krug, Elsie E.: Pharmacology in nursing, ed. 9, St. Louis, 1963, The C. V. Mosby Co.
8. Peszcznski, Mieczyslaw: Why old people fall, Amer. J. Nurs. **65**:86-88, 1965.
9. Peterson, Vera J., and Jerome, S.: The health of the aging. In Burgess, Ernest W. (editor): Aging in western societies, Chicago, 1960, University of Chicago Press.
10. Riese, Jacob A., and Damrau, Frederic: Use of activated charcoal in gastroenterology; value for flatulence and nervous diarrhea, J. Am. Geriatrics Soc. **12**:500-501, 1964.

11. Shafer, Kathleen Newton, and others: Medical-surgical nursing, ed. 3, St. Louis, 1964, The C. V. Mosby Co.
12. Soller, Genevieve R.: The aging patient, Amer. J. Nurs. **62**:114-117, 1962.
13. Stafford, Nova Harris: Bowel hygiene of older patients, Amer. J. Nurs. **63**:102-103, 1963.
14. Stieglitz, Edward J.: Principles of geriatric medicine. In Stieglitz, Edward J. (editor): Geriatric medicine, ed. 3, Philadelphia, 1954, J. B. Lippincott Co.
15. Thewlis, Malford W.: The care of the aged (geriatrics), ed. 6, St. Louis, 1954, The C. V. Mosby Co.
16. White, P. D.: The role of exercise in the aged, J.A.M.A. **165**:70-71, 1957.
17. Zeman, Frederic D.: Medical care of the normal aged. In Stieglitz, Edward J. (editor): Geriatric medicine, ed. 3, Philadelphia, 1954, J. B. Lippincott Co.

Chapter 7

Nutrition

Luigi Cornaro, who lived in Italy during the fifteenth and sixteenth centuries, believed that longevity might be fostered by a diet rich in eggs, meat, fish, and wine. He lived to be 98 years old and was one of the first to write at length on the subject of diet and length of life. Since that time an almost endless number of special diets that guarantee long life and health in later years have been advocated.

Nutritional needs of older people are only a little different from those of young adults. As activity decreases, fewer calories and therefore less carbohydrate and fat are needed. Protein and mineral requirements remain about the same, except that larger amounts of calcium are needed because of decreased absorption. Older people need a generous intake of vitamins, but total caloric needs are determined by the individual's weight and the amount of his activity. Caloric demands of the aged are roughly estimated at between 30 and 40 calories per kilogram of body weight per day. General nutritional requirements at various age levels are indicated in Table 2. Metabolic rate lowers with age. The Food and Nutrition Board recommends a reduction of approximately 3 percent of caloric needs at 25 years of age for each decade to 45 years of age, a reduction of 7.5 percent for each decade from 45 to 65 years of age, and of 10 percent for each decade thereafter.

There is abundant evidence that those who are below average in weight have a longer life expectancy than those who are overweight. Some authorities[4, 7] in the field of geriatric nutrition feel that the recommendations of the Food and Nutrition Board may be too high and too specific regarding the inclusion of certain items of nutrition. It is known that the general health improved and length of life was increased among some who lived during World War II on diets usually considered to be starvation diets and low in many items considered essential. Man's ability to conserve and to adapt to shortages in essential foods is probably much greater than is recognized generally.

CAUSES OF FAULTY NUTRITION

Physical changes of age may contribute to faulty nutrition, and both acute and chronic illness are responsible for poor nutrition in many instances. Other

	Age in years§ From	Age in years§ Up to	Weight in pounds	Height in inches	Food energy	Protein	Calcium	Iron	Vitamin A	Thiamine	Riboflavin	Niacin equivalent‡	Ascorbic acid	Vitamin D
					Calories	*Grams*	*Grams*	*Milligrams*	*International units*	*Milligrams*	*Milligrams*	*Milligrams*	*Milligrams*	*International units*
Men	18	35	154	69	2,900	70	0.8	10	5,000	1.2	1.7	19	70	
	35	55	154	69	2,600	70	.8	10	5,000	1.0	1.6	17	70	
	55	75	154	69	2,200	70	.8	10	5,000	.9	1.3	15	70	
Women	18	35	128	64	2,100	58	.8	15	5,000	.8	1.3	14	70	
	35	55	128	64	1,900	58	.8	15	5,000	.8	1.2	13	70	
	55	75	128	64	1,600	58	.8	10	5,000	.8	1.2	13	70	
Pregnant (second and third trimester)					+200	+20	+.5	+5	+1,000	+.2	+.3	+3	+30	400
Lactating					+1,000	+40	+.5	+5	+3,000	+.4	+.6	+7	+30	400
Infants‖	0	1	18		lb. × 52 ±7	lb. × 1.1 ± 0.2	.7	lb. × 0.45	1,500	.4	.6	6	30	400
Children	1	3	29	34	1,300	32	.8	8	2,000	.5	.8	9	40	400
	3	6	40	42	1,600	40	.8	10	2,500	.6	1.0	11	50	400
	6	9	53	49	2,100	52	.8	12	3,500	.8	1.3	14	60	400
Boys	9	12	72	55	2,400	60	1.1	15	4,500	1.0	1.4	16	70	400
	12	15	98	61	3,000	75	1.4	15	5,000	1.2	1.8	20	80	400
	15	18	134	68	3,400	85	1.4	15	5,000	1.4	2.0	22	80	400
Girls	9	12	72	55	2,200	55	1.1	15	4,500	.9	1.3	15	80	400
	12	15	103	62	2,500	62	1.3	15	5,000	1.0	1.5	17	80	400
	15	18	117	64	2,300	58	1.3	15	5,000	.9	1.3	15	70	400

*Adapted from Recommended Dietary Allowances, Publication 1146, 59 pp., 1964, National Academy of Sciences—National Research Council, Washington, D. C., 20418. Price $1.00. Also available in libraries.

†The Recommended Daily Dietary Allowances should not be confused with Minimum Daily Requirements. The Recommended Dietary Allowances are amounts of nutrients recommended by the Food and Nutrition Board of National Research Council, and are considered adequate for maintenance of good nutrition in healthy persons in the United States. The Minimum Daily Requirements are the amounts of various nutrients that have been established by the Food and Drug Administration as standards for labeling purposes of foods and pharmaceutical preparations for special dietary uses. These are the amounts regarded as necessary in the diet for the prevention of deficiency diseases, and generally are less than the Recommended Dietary Allowances. The allowance levels are intended to cover individual variations among most normal persons as they live in the United States under usual environmental stresses.

‡Niacin equivalents include dietary sources of the preformed vitamin and the precursor, tryptophan. 60 milligrams tryptophan represents 1 milligram niacin.

§Entries on lines for age range 18 to 35 years represent the 25-year age; all other entries represent allowances for the midpoint of the specified age periods.

‖The calorie and protein allowances per pound for infants are considered to decrease progressively from birth. Allowances for calcium, thiamine, riboflavin, and niacin increase proportionately with calories to the maximum values shown.

possible causes for malnutrition in the elderly are limited financial resources, psychologic factors such as boredom, edentia and its accompanying physical changes, lifelong faulty eating patterns, fads and notions regarding certain foods, and lack of sufficient knowledge of the essentials in a well-balanced diet.

Anatomic and physiologic changes. Anatomic and physiologic changes of age have not been found to be primarily responsible for malnutrition in older people. It is true that certain factors may affect appetite and digestion. The buccal mucosa may become less resistant to trauma, which will make coarse food less acceptable. Atrophy of lingual mucosa may make taste perception less acute. The quantity of saliva may be decreased and the quality changed; this may alter enjoyment of dry food that is eaten hurriedly.

Achlorhydria is quite common in older persons. Some studies show that free hydrochloric acid is absent in from 23.9 percent to 65 percent of all persons over 65 years of age. Since acid inhibits the growth of certain bacteria, antibacterial action in the stomach may be retarded.

The entire muscular tube of the gastrointestinal tract undergoes loss of muscle tone, although it is believed that it functions adequately into advanced age. A lack of tone in supportive voluntary muscles may interfere with adequate function. Poor posture may result in lack of muscle tone in abdominal muscles, with ptosis of the viscera and resultant impaired function. Attention to body alignment in bed and to sitting posture may bring remarkable results in improved appetite and digestion.

It is true that physical changes in the mouth lessen the desire to eat, that digestive motility is lessened, that atrophy of intestinal structures may seem to decrease absorption of food, and that arteriosclerosis may retard its utilization. However, the natural reserves of physiologic function seem to be such that, given adequate food in usable form, the aged body in good health can utilize sufficient amounts to maintain satisfactory nutrition. One study revealed that a group of older persons were able to utilize 86 percent of their intake of protein and 92 percent of their total intake of calories.

Blood protein levels in elderly people have been found to be consistently slightly lower than those in younger adults. Vigorous efforts to raise these levels have not appeared to contribute to improvement in the general health of the aged, however. This fact makes surgeons believe that it is necessary to check protein levels of aged patients very carefully before surgery is done and to raise the level if possible, because low levels may lessen the margin of safety for surgery and may delay surgical recovery.

The elderly person appears to be somewhat less flexible in his ability to utilize or dispose of carbohydrate that has reached the bloodstream; the glucose tolerance curve may be slower in rising in response to intake of glucose and slower to return to normal than in a young adult. Fairly frequently, elderly people develop hypoglycemia, which causes tremor, dizziness, fatigue, and headache and predisposes to accidents. It is generally believed that the blood sugar can be kept more stable in such instances by the patient's eating more protein, eating oftener, and choosing carbohydrates from those that take longer to absorb, such as those in fruits, vegetables, and cereals instead of syrup or sugar. This condition is described more fully in Chapter 22, Nursing in Diseases of Metabolism.

Edentia. The loss of natural teeth can interfere with the ability of a person to meet nutritional needs. By the time they are 70 years of age, approximately three fourths of all people have lost their natural teeth. Many people adjust poorly to the use of dentures and, finding them unsatisfactory, often refuse to use them. Scrupulous hygiene is needed in their care because unclean dentures and an unclean mouth may cause odors that destroy appetite and interfere with the flavor of food. Meals might be preceded by use of an alkaline or aromatic mouthwash, and dentures should be cleaned after each meal. Many times an older person will assume that this is not necessary since for years he may have cleaned his teeth only once a day. Provision for him to give frequent care to his dentures will often bring results in improved appetite. The nurse should report any dental difficulties so that necessary modifications in diet can be made, and the patient can be referred to his dentist, the dental department of the hospital, or the dental clinic.

Economic, social, and psychologic factors. Much attention is now being focused on the economic status of aging persons, and each year brings improvement in their incomes. The nurse, however, should know what financial resources are available to each individual patient and have a realistic approach to his actual situation. It is, for example, useless to plan a diet that is obviously outside economic possibility. The older person may benefit little from extra food if he is profoundly upset by either having to spend his cherished savings or having to accept charity.

Many elderly people suffer economic hardships. Some do not have enough money to buy sufficient amounts of necessary food. Some cannot afford the kind of food that they can masticate properly, and many cannot afford to buy enough protein, which is an expensive item in the diet. Some have no refrigerator where food can be protected from spoilage, and a large number live alone, which makes economic planning of meals difficult. Many aged persons do not have the money or energy to shop at the larger markets where foods are cheaper, and few can afford to have food delivered to their homes. Because of hesitation in spending limited funds, older people may put off necessary purchases until a considerable interval of time passes, during which food intake is not enough for health.

Emotional factors such as feelings of uselessness often dull interest in preparing and partaking of food. Many aging persons who live alone have little incentive to prepare complete or satisfying meals. The social aspects of eating, which are so important in normal daily living, are denied them. It takes great effort plus more than the average amount of ego-interest for the person living alone to prepare regular, attractive meals. Malnutrition produces lethargy, and lethargy, in turn, results in insufficient interest in food; thus a vicious cycle is formed.

Lack of employment or other satisfactory activity, lack of home and family all add to the older person's realization of his insecure place in the social scheme and rob him of the equanimity so necessary to good digestion. Until the aged are assured some emotional security and some satisfying experiences during all the years of life, the psychologic obstacles in the way of good nutrition must be recognized. Small, comfortable boarding homes with congenial surroundings and companionship are helpful for certain persons who suffer acutely from aloneness. Appetite and general health of many elderly persons improve when these are provided.

Age is not looked upon with favor in our culture, and older people suffer accordingly. In their desperate effort to stay young and to keep going, they attempt to find an acceptable reason for their increasing limitations and become ready victims for food cultists who offer miracles through diet. They may spend money they can ill afford on mineral water and obscure "vegetable and tissue juices" while not purchasing essential items of food. Insecurity increases introspection, and thus many older persons decide upon foods that cause gas, create an acid condition, cause constipation, give them headaches, and in many other ways do not agree with them. The remedy for these circumstances probably lies in economic and social rehabilitation since the person who is busy and happy has little time to worry about his indigestion, regardless of his age.

Quality of foods. Another factor that appears to complicate the meeting of nutritional needs is the inconstant quality of foods. Nutritional values depend not only upon when and how foods are prepared, but also upon where and how foods are grown. More attention must be paid by the government and other agencies to the prevention of soil erosion and to fertilization and replenishment of the soil if future generations are to be adequately fed. This is a serious national problem that needs to be better understood by individuals. The nurse as an active citizen in her community must be aware of these developing needs. From a practical standpoint she must in her everyday work remember that food values in vegetables, for instance, may vary with the quality of the soil in which the vegetables grew; that meat from cattle grazed on good land yielding a good quality of grass may be superior to that of cattle fed on grass grown in poor soil. The nurse cannot, of course, analyze each food item, but she can remember that safety lies in a wide variety of foods.

Sometimes a chronic multiple vitamin deficiency exists. Subclinical symptoms may or may not be present, and sometimes an increase in vitamin intake fails to give much improvement because permanent damage has already been done. Sufficient vitamins are helpful in preventing further damage from vitamin deficiency and will often produce some improvement. An adequate diet with careful attention to the essential foods will supply the needed vitamins, provided that physiologic functions are normal. Man is an omnivorous animal and should partake of a wide variety of foods in as near their natural state as possible. When loss of teeth and other factors make a wide selection less possible, special provisions must be made for modifications in the diet. When illness occurs, and intake and utilization of foods may be inadequate or restricted, extra vitamins must be supplied to supplement those obtained in food.

EATING HABITS

Food habits are usually established in youth and vary greatly with regional and national customs. When a person has reached 65 years of age, it is almost impossible to alter his basic eating habits by appeals to his intellect or reasoning powers. The nurse should recognize this in dealing with the aged—either in the home, the clinic, or the hospital. If she makes use of her understanding of the patient's need for companionship and inherent desire for approval and shows genuine interest in him, she may achieve success in getting him to eat adequate meals since he may, by her thoughtfulness, develop confidence in her suggestions. The nurse must be a good listener since food idiosyncrasies lose their importance in the mind of the patient merely by his telling them to a sympathetic audience.

It has been said that eating is a very personal matter. Before the nurse makes suggestions about diet, she should study the patient's eating habits carefully. She must remember that it is not important in what form or at what hour the patient gets certain foods, but it is important that at some time during each day he get some of all the basic foods. Some people may follow the same monotonous diet day after day; yet the analysis of the food intake, as dull and uninteresting as it is, may prove to be near to meeting their nutritional needs.

Uncle Dan is an example. Uncle Dan was a New England bachelor and was considered queer by many kindly relatives. He did heavy farm work and was in good health until the age of 72 years, when he died of a heart attack. His diet from young manhood until his death varied little from day to day. For breakfast he had a large number of muffins, "sass" (usually applesauce), and chocolate; dinner at noon consisted of a huge plate of potatoes, baked and served with butter (he ate the skins), a serving of meat, and bread. Two or three times a week he had either peas or squash. His supper was bread and butter, a huge dish of "sass" or else raw apples or berries, and more chocolate. For in-between snacks he had a barrel of crude maple sugar from which he took scoops at intervals.

Uncle Dan's diet appears to be low in citrus fruits, but he obtained essential vitamins in berries and other fresh fruit, as well as in applesauce. He never ate eggs as such, but received them in the muffins he consumed, and he got milk daily in the chocolate. This diet, though a little irregular on first inspection, was not deficient in essentials nor necessarily too high in carbohydrate for a vigorous working man. If Uncle Dan for some reason had had to restrict his activity in later years, his carbohydrate intake would have been excessive. If left to his own devices, Uncle Dan, like many older persons living alone, would probably have depended too much upon bread and sweets, which require less preparation and less chewing. He ate, however, one staple meal each day at the home of relatives, where a sister cooked and served him the meat and vegetables.

APPETITE AND FOOD REQUIREMENTS

Every effort must be made to stimulate the appetite of the older person who suffers from malnutrition. Appropriate exercise in the fresh air often stimulates appetite. Well-seasoned broths and various highly seasoned appetizers such as strong cheeses may improve the appetite. The aging person should have his meals in a quiet, pleasant, unhurried atmosphere. Tea and coffee should be permitted unless specifically contraindicated since they often stimulate appetite. Wines, beer, and other alcoholic beverages should be permitted in moderate amounts in the home or the hospital if they are desired. In the home the older

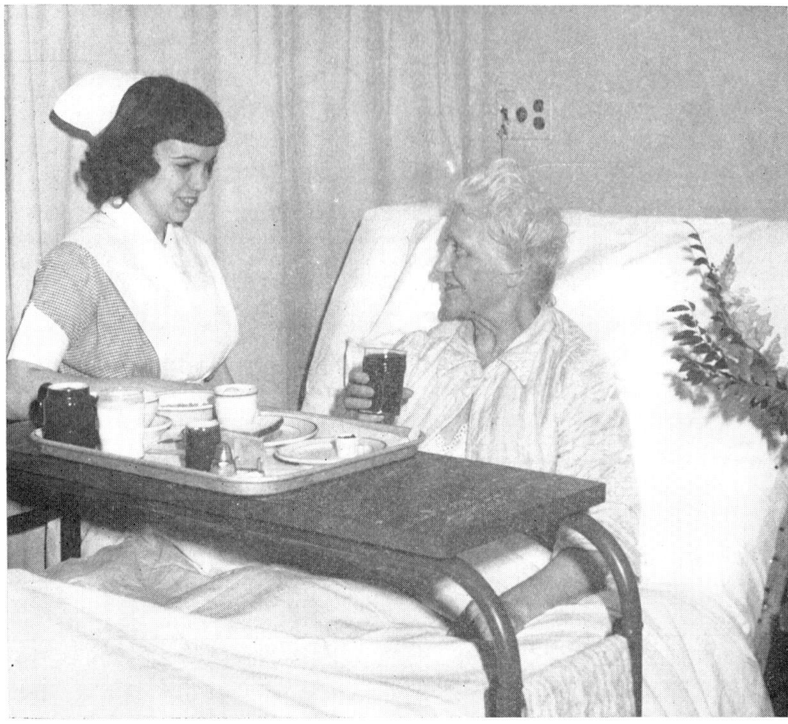

Figure 15. Appetite improves with pleasant, unhurried surroundings and companionship.

person should eat with the rest of the family. Special provision may be necessary for his needs, but these should be as inconspicuous as possible. The older person should never be made to feel helpless by having unnecessary attention drawn to circumstances like his need for ground or chopped meat, to the use of an extra napkin, or to his shaky hand.

In illness the greatest single stimulant to the patient's appetite is perhaps the serving of attractive meals with special consideration for individual taste and preference. The patient will relish a dish that caters to personal food customs or a special sauce seasoned at his own direction. Aged people are inordinately grateful for any small favor done them. An older lady will cherish a single flower on her tray or a special dainty salad. An older man may remember for years the nurse who made potato soup for him, using his mother's or his wife's recipe as he recalled it. A pleasant, unhurried environment is most important in ensuring a good appetite during illness. Cheerful conversation is also important. The thoughtful nurse will not tell the patient that he should eat certain foods because they are good for him. The patient may be struggling to preserve his identity as an individual and subconsciously will resent the implication that he no longer knows what is good for him. Best results will follow if he has small servings of attractive food that he likes, with no mention of the specific constituents of his meal.

Older people often need small meals with supplementary snacks to ensure generous amounts of protein, fluids, and vitamins. Large, bulky meals are not well tolerated, particularly if any limitation of heart action is present. Increasing protein in the meal may decrease appetite and tend to give the feeling of satiation, even when insufficient food has been taken.

Basic foods. The older person should have a minimum of one gram of protein per kilogram of normal body weight per day, and some physicians believe that larger amounts are advisable in order to ensure optimum repair of body tissues. Milk fortified with high protein concentrate or other protein hydrolysates may be ordered between meals when an increase in protein is desired. Skimmed milk, either fresh or dried, is an excellent and relatively inexpensive source of protein.

Fat is essential to supply the necessary vitamins A and D but should be used sparingly by overweight persons. Excessive intake of fat contributes to obesity and may cause damage to the liver and other vital structures. There appears to be growing evidence that diets high in polysaturated fats, such as the hard animal fats and the fat contained in milk and butter, result in higher cholesterol levels in the blood than when more of the polyunsaturated fats contained in vegetable oils such as corn oil and fish oils are used. A high cholesterol level in the blood is found often in those who suffer coronary artery disease and other vascular disease associated with deposits of abnormal substances in the blood vessels and with impairment of the clotting mechanism in the blood. The aged person who asks the nurse about the use of fat in his diet should be advised to consult his doctor on his next visit and to avoid diet fads. He should be advised to substitute oils for hard fats whenever this can be done without hardship. For example, corn oil can be used for frying and baking in place of butter or lard. Treatment of oils to cause hardening for the preparation of margarine increases the amount of saturated fat in the product. Peanut butter is often so treated to prevent the oil from rising to the top of the jar.

It is believed that the total fat intake of the average person in the United States may be too high for optimum health, and that it should be reduced. The national dietary intake of fat is at an all-time high. Approximately 40 percent of our dietary calories are derived from fat. Much of this comes from animal sources such as milk, butter, cheese, and meats. Our rate of coronary artery disease and other vascular disease is proportionately higher than in some other countries where less fat is consumed. Practically speaking, however, fat adds flavor to foods and is a necessary ingredient of most palatable food. For example, small servings of crisp bacon often add to an old person's appetite and enjoyment of breakfast.

The elderly person's diet should contain proportionately as much carbohydrate as that of a younger adult. Energy output may be reduced greatly, however, and the total calories should be reduced accordingly by decreasing proportionately both fat and carbohydrate. Calcium, iron, and other minerals are essential constituents of the diet, but usually they are provided for adequately if the older person eats a normal balanced diet consistently. In brief, the aging person needs all of the basic protective foods each day.

Foods containing essential constituents. The nurse must know what foods are considered essential and what substitutions for commonly eaten foods can be made in meeting basic food needs. Although people live to a healthful old age in other societies where milk is seldom used by adults and where the dietary intake of calcium is approximately one half what is considered optimum in this country, milk is considered an essential of an adequate adult diet in the United States. Without milk it is difficult to obtain sufficient calcium in other foods. Buttermilk is well tolerated by many elderly people who may not care for whole milk and who do not tolerate much fat. Hard or cheddar cheese is helpful, but must be eaten in fairly large quantities in order to provide the same amount of calcium as milk. One quarter pound of cheese equals a pint of milk in this respect. Dried milk is a good source of calcium and protein and has a lower fat content than fresh milk. It is often cheaper for the older person living alone since it keeps indefinitely. Small cans of milk are convenient for the person living alone, and canned milk keeps longer than fresh milk. Canned and dried milk can be put into muffins, cakes, puddings, and sauces if the patient insists on consuming large amounts of sweet foods and refuses to drink milk.

Protein foods are absolutely essential to retain body tissue. Meat is a desirable source of protein, but is not essential, provided that extra milk, eggs, cheese, fish, and legumes are eaten. Meat, though expensive, should be made available to older persons, even when mastication is difficult. Meat can be ground and liver can be minced before cooking. Pig liver is a good source of protein, minerals, and vitamins and is much less expensive than beef liver. Meats such as kidney and heart are often moderate in cost; either of these can be ground and seasoned to make excellent sandwich spreads. Fish is an unusually satisfactory protein food for the aged since it presents no difficulty in mastication. Sea foods such as scallops and oysters are good foods for the elderly and can be managed by persons with no teeth. Unless they are finely ground, clams are a poor choice when there is chewing difficulty, and lobster, crab, and shrimps are inclined to cause indigestion in some older persons.

Although no one of the plant protein foods alone contains all of the essential amino acids, often a combination of several of them will provide all the essentials.[4] For example, corn and beans taken together and in sufficient quantities provide nearly adequate protein. This accounts for the fact that some people who live largely on these two foods maintain adequate nutrition with a normal protein level in the blood. Legumes, in our country, are seldom taken in sufficient quantities to contribute substantially to protein needs. Soybeans are an excellent source of protein, and, when they are disguised in cakes, muffins, and wafers, they are acceptable to most people. Legumes, such as beans and peas, are sometimes indigestible for the elderly when they are cooked with large amounts of fat. Pea, bean, or lentil soup, however, flavored with lean meat and cooked with a minimum of fat is a good food for the old person.

Both leafy green vegetables and those grown underground are essential for health. The dental status of the older person often makes it hard for him to eat enough leafy and fresh raw vegetables in salads. Unless he has dentures that enable him to masticate properly, it may be necessary to grind or grate fresh vegetables. The need for fresh foods can be partially met by giving additional fresh fruits such as bananas, pears, oranges, melons, and tomatoes. If fresh vegetables are not eaten, the amount of cooked vegetables should be increased. There is considerable difference in the vitamin content of various vegetables. For example, broccoli, green peppers, and cabbage are higher in vitamin C than spinach and lettuce. It is not too important, however, just what vegetables the patient eats, provided he is able to take a variety in sufficient quantities. Turnip greens, collards, chard, dandelion greens, and beet tops are all excellent sources of daily vitamin requirements. It is important that the vegetables be lightly cooked in very little water and, if possible, that they be eaten either chopped or ground. Sieved or strained vegetables deprive the body of needed bulk in food and are generally lacking in appeal. When it is necessary to use strained foods, the canned baby foods may be used, but the fact that they are primarily produced as baby foods may be psychologically objectionable. Potatoes are an inexpensive item of diet that is easily prepared and easily eaten. Potatoes should be eaten in addition to green vegetables.

Some kind of whole-grained or enriched cereal food should be taken daily, but it does not matter whether this is in the form of cooked cereal, bread, hot muffins, buckwheat cakes, or oatmeal cookies, to name a few. Although whole-wheat bread is slightly higher in minerals and vitamins, many older people born in the United States like white bread and refuse to change. Many of our older generation have lived through an era when white bread was associated with a high standard of living. It may be impossible to change the kind of bread selected, but it may be possible to substitute a whole-grained cereal at least for some breakfasts.

Fruit requirements are not hard to meet since orange juice, tomato juice or cooked tomatoes, other fruit juices, and many fruits such as pears, peaches, and melons are easily eaten without the use of teeth. Bananas are an excellent fruit food for the older person, as also are applesauce and stewed dried fruits. Many older people do not eat enough fruit. This may be because fresh fruits are expensive or because many older people have notions about fruits not agreeing with them.

Fluids and electrolytes. Fluid needs of the elderly person do not differ substantially from those of the younger person. Most geriatricians believe that the elderly person should have a generous intake of fluid but that it should not be excessive. Some elderly people have taken limited fluids for a long time, and changes in this pattern should be altered only gradually.

The average adult normally takes between 2,500 and 3,000 ml. of fluid daily in moderate weather. Of this approximately 1,200 ml. is taken as liquid and the rest in food (1,100 ml.) and from oxidation of foodstuffs within the body (300 ml.). Approximately 1,000 ml. is lost through the skin and lungs, 1,500 ml. in urine, and 100 ml. in the stools. The elderly person who eats less food than the younger one receives less fluid from this source, and he loses less through the skin in perspiration.

Many elderly persons do not take enough fluid, and marked improvement in general health follows an increase in fluid intake. It has been noted in some in-

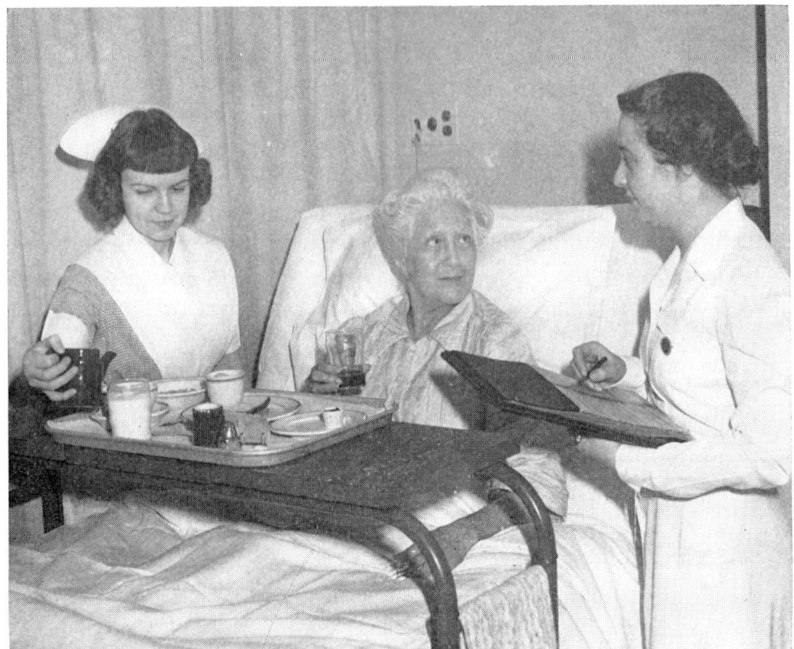

Figure 16. The meal tray provides a visual aid for teaching about nutrition and fluids.

stances that when fluids were increased, there was less constipation, skin texture was better, the patient's mouth felt less dry, so appetite improved, and urine no longer caused local burning and skin irritations.

Fluids must be spaced throughout the day and evening; consumption of large amounts at one time should be avoided. Giving large amounts of fluid either by mouth or parenterally or allowing intravenous fluids to run at a rate that replaces fluid faster than it can be excreted by the kidneys can cause pulmonary edema even in a healthy person. This can be a real danger in the aged, many of whom have marginal kidney function.

Before urging the elderly person to take more fluids, the nurse must be certain of what he is already taking. One elderly lady, for example, announced proudly that she hated water and never drank it at all. But a careful history revealed that she consumed two quarts of orange juice each day. Usually fluid intake for the healthy aged person and for the ambulatory patient can be increased satisfactorily if he can develop the habit of taking a glass of fluid of his choice in the midmorning and again in the midafternoon. He may need repeated reminders before this practice becomes an established routine.

The average person who eats a well-balanced diet gets the minerals and other essentials for normal electrolyte balance. When illness occurs and food cannot be taken normally, checking to observe signs of imbalance and assistance in administration of essential substances such as sodium and potassium becomes an important nursing responsibility. Problems encountered in the elderly do not differ substantially from those of the younger patient, except that the elderly patient withstands disturbances in electrolyte balance less well. This aspect of nursing is equally important for the patient ill with a medical ailment such as emphysema, in which acidosis may be developing from the retention of carbon dioxide and the patient undergoing surgery with loss of essential fluids. Since the subject is discussed fully in current nursing texts on medical and surgical nursing, it will not be covered here.[23]

Obesity. Obesity at any age should be avoided. It is comparatively rare in the extremely old since it is often not conducive to long life. Obesity may be the result of ignorance concerning the caloric value of foods and does not necessarily indicate overnutrition or even adequate nutrition, since extra weight may be the result of a diet high in fat and carbohydrate, yet lacking in other essential constituents. There is often an emotional factor present when overeating has become firmly established. The older person may wander about nibbling on a sweet roll mainly because he has nowhere to go and nothing to do. A rather large number of elderly people seek an outlet for their frustrations in the excessive consumption of poorly selected foods.

Obesity can have many consequences. Extra weight in the form of fat constitutes a burden to the circulatory system in that a blood supply must be provided for the excess tissue. The heart then has increased demands made upon it, and the kidneys are also taxed in excreting the waste products of additional metabolism. Even muscles, bones, and joints suffer from the tax of extra weight, which may be poorly distributed. Foot troubles, knee ache, backache, difficulty in breathing, and impaired circulation to extremities are a few of the conditions that may be caused in part by excessive weight. However, when marked obesity is found in persons 65 years of age or older, many geriatricians feel that it is not wise to deal with it too vigorously. The older person has physiologically adjusted to the condition and sudden change may be poorly tolerated.

PREPARATION OF MEALS

Older person in a family. For the happiness of all, it is important that the needs of an aging member disturb family meal planning and preparation as little as possible. The same menu can often be used for the entire family, with only a few minor modifications. Foods cooked separately are likely to be poorly seasoned, and their preparation takes extra time.

When meals are to be prepared for a family that consists of grandparent, parents, and children, it is well to plan roughly for the week. This tends to prevent omission of important constituents and contributes to economy. Several factors may have to be considered in planning menus. Foods might have to be prepared for an aging person who is not eating enough and who may have difficulty in chewing; calories may have to be limited for an adult member who is beginning to show obesity; and nutritional needs of growing children will have to be met. Menus for a family of five consisting of grandfather, father and mother, a 13-year-old boy, and a 15-month-old baby are given as illustrations. In these menus and in others that follow, it is assumed that whole wheat is used for bread, crackers, and breakfast cereals.

First day

	Mr. and Mrs.	*Junior*	*Grandfather*	*Baby*
Breakfast	Orange juice	Same	Same	Same
		Cereal with milk		Cereal with milk
	Toast with butter	Same with jam	Same	Same
	Milk and coffee	Milk	Milk and coffee	Milk
10:00			Vegetable juice	Cracker with milk
Lunch	Pea soup	Same	Same	Same
	Soybean cracker	Same	Same	Same
	Cottage cheese and pineapple salad	Same	Same (crushed pineapple)	Same (crushed pine-apple)
	Milk	Same	Same	Same
4:00		Peanut butter and jelly sandwich		Bread and butter
		Milk		Milk
Dinner	Baked halibut	Same	Same	Same
	Parsley butter	Same	Same	
	Baked potato	Same	Same	Same
	Broccoli with butter	Same	Same (chopped)	Same (chopped)
	Carrot and celery	Same	Same (grated)	Same (grated)
	Cherry cobbler	Same	Same	Banana
	Tea	Milk	Tea	Milk
8:00	Fresh pear	Same	Same	Same

Second day

	Mr. and Mrs.	*Junior*	*Grandfather*	*Baby*
Breakfast	Prunes	Same	Same (chopped)	Same (chopped)
	Toast with butter	Same	Same	Same
	Boiled egg	Same	Same	Same
		Cereal with milk		Cereal with milk
	Coffee and milk	Milk	Coffee and milk	Milk
10:00			Café au lait	Cracker, milk
Lunch	Cream of celery soup	Same	Same	Same
	Tuna fish sandwich with lettuce	Same	Same (no lettuce)	Bread and butter
	Fruit Jell-O	Same	Jell-O	Jell-O
	Milk	Same	Same	Same
4:00		Jam sandwich		Jam sandwich
		Milk		Milk
Dinner	Pot roast au jus	Same	Same (chopped)	Same (chopped)
	Mashed potatoes	Same	Same	Same
	Summer squash	Same	Same (chopped)	Same (chopped)
	Tomato salad	Same	Tomatoes	Tomatoes
	Custard pie	Same	Custard	Custard
	Tea	Milk	Tea	Milk
8:00	Whole orange	Same	Same	Same

Older person living in a hotel. Many elderly people live alone either in a furnished room or in a hotel and must have their meals in restaurants. Money may be limited, and it is often difficult to get adequate meals within the budget allowed. It is sometimes satisfactory for an older person to eat one good meal in a restaurant and have snacks in his own room for the remaining two meals of the day. If the weather is cool, evaporated milk in small cans, crackers, cheese, fruit, and even fresh vegetables such as celery can be kept for short intervals. Coffee and tea can be prepared in a single room, provided that the electric fixtures permit the heating of water and that it is allowed. Instant coffee and bouillon cubes are simple to prepare when a warm drink is needed. It is most important that foods be bought in small amounts and used within a short time, particularly in warm weather. Dried fruit is satisfactory in warm weather when fresh fruit spoils rapidly. It can be kept in glass jars with screw tops, which will not invite insects. Processed cheeses mold quickly in warm weather, and canned milk should not be kept over twenty-four hours without refrigeration.

The elderly person who eats in restaurants should guard against habitually going to hamburger shops, hot-dog stands, and coffee shops where vegetables are seldom served and where money can easily be spent for foods that are not essential. Certain items such as coffee, tea, and fresh fruit cost proportionately more in a restaurant than in a grocery store. The second cup of coffee, which is such a temptation to the confirmed coffee drinker, runs up the dinner check and may replace an essential food such as milk. The milk can be drunk in the restaurant, and a cup of instant coffee can be prepared when the person returns home, if this is practicable in the particular situation.

Care should be taken to obtain fresh vegetables, cooked green vegetables, and root vegetables in the restaurant meal each day. If money is short, the dessert may be omitted, and the person can eat fruit or a cookie upon returning home.

It is well to avoid certain foods in restaurants unless one can patronize restaurants with the very highest standards. Ordinarily, orange juice is not freshly squeezed. Prunes, other stewed fruit, and tomato juice are often good choices, and a whole orange can be eaten at home during the day or in the evening. Fricassees, stews, meat pies, meat "cutlets," and even meat loaf often have very little actual meat in the average serving and consequently do not go far toward meeting protein requirements. Suitable choices for a two-day period of restaurant dining might include the following.

First day

Breakfast	Tomato juice Boiled egg Toast and butter Milk and coffee or tea
Lunch	Clam chowder, other fish chowder, pea or bean soup Crackers or bread and butter Fruit dessert Milk
Dinner	Liver, pot roast, Swiss steak, chopped steak, or baked veal Potatoes, sweet or Irish

	Green cooked vegetable, e.g., string beans or spinach
	Lettuce or mixed vegetable salad
	Pudding or ice cream
	Milk, tea, or coffee

Second day

Breakfast	Grapefruit
	Scrambled eggs or cereal with milk
	Toast and butter
	Milk and coffee or tea
Lunch	Meat, egg, fish, or cheese sandwich with lettuce
	Fruit dessert
	Milk
Dinner	Baked fish, veal roast, lamb roast, or hamburger
	Potatoes, sweet or Irish
	Two green vegetables or one vegetable and tomatoes
	Pudding or ice cream
	Milk, tea, or coffee

Person living and cooking alone. Cooking for a single person presents difficulties, especially if funds are short. Some older people who live alone have relatives or friends fairly near and are able to share meals with them occasionally. This is helpful, particularly in breaking the monotony of rather limited menus.

The person living alone should avoid accumulating many foods that cannot be kept in sealed jars or tins. Cereals such as flour, cornstarch, oatmeal, and corn meal frequently become infested with insects if left uncovered, especially in warm weather. Prepared puddings that need only the addition of milk and an egg are often most palatable and are simple to prepare. Small cans of vegetables can be obtained and are helpful to older persons in planning meals. There is now a large variety of dried soups in small packages that make one or two servings, and soups are particularly acceptable if chewing is difficult. Quickly prepared soups should not be used regularly as the main item in the dinner, however, as they are likely to contain little or no meat, and protein inadequacy may result. Many products now available, such as TV dinners, are convenient although expensive and tiresome if used too often. They may be most useful for the elderly person whose energy is limited, but the older person who can develop an interest in preparing meals for himself will usually have better fare at a lower cost.

If money is limited, the same food may have to be eaten for two meals in succession or for two days in succession to prevent waste. It is important that meat and fish be cooked soon after purchase and that small amounts be bought at one time. The person who has facilities to do his own cooking is able to buy the cheaper cuts of meat and make stews, meat loaf, and those dishes that are not nutritionally satisfactory in restaurants. By lengthy cooking, the cheaper and tougher cuts of meat can be eaten, even by the elderly person with poor dentures. Cheaper cuts of meat yield the same amount of protein as the more expensive ones.

The older person cooking and eating alone would do well to make a hobby of learning about herbs and food seasonings. Most herbs and spices are quite inexpensive, and the possibilities they offer for variety and improvement in flavor of foods are endless. Care must be taken if any dietary restrictions are present. Occasionally someone who is on a restricted salt diet may think he has solved his seasoning problem by the use of celery salt or some other mixture containing salt.

Fresh vegetables should be bought in small amounts, washed, drained, and placed in waxed paper or a refrigerator bag in the icebox. An elderly person with poor vision who may be unable to prepare raw vegetables for cooking may use frozen vegetables quite satisfactorily. Liquids in which vegetables have been cooked can be used in preparing tasty soups.

Bread can be kept two weeks without spoilage if it is wrapped securely in a refrigerator bag and kept in the icebox. Hard cheeses keep longer than soft ones. Cottage cheese should be bought in small amounts since it does not keep well even when in the refrigerator. Prepared puddings that require only the addition of milk are now available; canned milk is usually satisfactory for these. Some elderly persons living alone have found that puddings prepared for infants and sealed in jars make wholesome and appetizing desserts that require no preparation and little or no dishwashing.

The older person living alone and cooking for himself should avoid the temptation to make a complete meal of coffee or tea and sweet rolls, toast, muffins, or hot dogs. He should plan meals systematically. Habit is an important factor, and the elderly person, like a person of any age, may find upon close scrutiny of his diet that he has fairly consistently omitted certain essentials of good nutrition. Shopping in a busy store may tire and confuse an older person, so a written list will help him to remember what he needs. Items forgotten on one shopping excursion may be done without in preference to making another tiring trip.

Suitable menus for a two-day period might include the following.

First day

Breakfast	Applesauce Toast and butter Soft-cooked egg Milk and coffee
Dinner	Tomato juice Hamburger Beet greens Baked potato Cabbage, raw or cooked Cookie and milk
Supper	Noodle soup Carrot sticks or cooked carrots Bread and butter Custard Tea

Second day

Breakfast	Grapefruit (one half) Soft-cooked egg Toast and butter Milk and coffee
Dinner	Beef stew with vegetables Lettuce and tomato salad Bread and butter Applesauce Milk
Supper	Cream of spinach soup Cheese and crackers Fruit Jell-O Tea

PORTABLE MEALS

Portable meals are of great help to feeble, aged persons. This service alone sometimes enables aged couples to remain at home together or makes it possible for an aged person living alone to remain in his own home and community. In addition to improvement in nutrition, many elderly people benefit emotionally from this service, since the delivery service provides a break in the monotony of their day and some individuals who may not speak to anyone else have at least one brief opportunity for a social encounter each day.

The plan for portable meals, first used in England about 20 years ago and called "Meals on Wheels" has been adopted slowly in the United States. In 1960 there were 22 cities in 13 states providing the service. Most portable meal programs provide one hot meal daily and unheated food for at least one other meal. Meals are planned and prepared in a central location under the supervision of a qualified dietition. Meals are then delivered daily by a messenger service; this may consist of volunteer groups in the community or be under the sponsorship of some voluntary or Red Feather agency. The local public health nursing service usually participates actively in the program by selecting suitable patients and by being a resource for the delivery workers who may encounter health problems when they enter an elderly person's home. The cost differs widely, ranging from a few cents to two dollars per day depending upon the sponsorship of the program and the extent of the service offered; some prepare special diet menus.

REFERENCES AND RELATED BIBLIOGRAPHY

1. Ackerman, P. G., and Toro, G.: Calcium balance in elderly women, J. Gerontol. **9**:446-449, 1954.
2. Allen, Edward F.: Dental aspects. In Cowdry, E. V. (editor): The care of the geriatric patient, ed. 2, St. Louis, 1963, The C. V. Mosby Co.
3. Batchelder, E. L.: Nutritional status and dietary habits of older people, J. Am. Dietet. A. **33**:471-476, 1957.
4. Bavetta, Lucien A., and Nimni, Marcel E.: Nutritional aspects. In Cowdry, E. V. (editor): The care of the geriatric patient, ed. 2, St. Louis, 1963, The C. V. Mosby Co.
5. Beeuwkes, Adelia M.: Studying the food habits of the elderly, J. Am. Dietet. A. **37**:215-218, 1960.

6. Buckley, Bonita Rice: Feeding the aged person, Amer. J. Nurs. **59**:1591-1593, 1959.
7. Cayer, David: Nutrition of the geriatric patient. In Johnson, Wingate M. (editor): The older patient, New York, 1960, Paul B. Hoeber, Inc., Medical Book Department of Harper & Row, Publishers.
8. Chinn, Austin B.: Some problems of nutrition in the aged, J.A.M.A. **162**:1511-1513, 1956.
9. Cooper, Lenna F., and others: Nutrition in health and disease, ed. 14, Philadelphia, 1963, J. B. Lippincott Co.
10. Fathauer, George H.: Food habits; an anthropologist's view, J. Am. Dietet. A. **7**:335-338, 1960.
11. Food guide for older folks, Home and Garden Bulletin No. 17, U. S. Department of Agriculture, Washington, D. C., 1959, U. S. Government Printing Office.
12. Fry, Peggy Crooke, Fox, Hazel Metz, and Linkswiler, Helen: Nutrient intakes of healthy older women, J. Am. Dietet. A. **42**:218-222, 1963.
13. Home-delivered meals for the ill, handicapped and elderly, Report of National Council on the Aging Committee on Guidelines for Home-Delivered Meals, New York, 1965, National Committee on the Aging.
14. Jones, Paul: Meals on wheels, Nurs. Outlook **3**:130-131, 1955.
15. Keyes, Ancel: Nutrition for later years of life, Pub. Health Rep. **67**:484-491, 1952.
16. Kountz, William B.: Therapeutic aspects of geriatric medicine, J.A.M.A. **153**:777-782, 1953.
17. Nutrition Service of Community Service Society: Foods for health as we grow older, New York, 1949, Community Service Society.
18. Nutritive value of foods: Home and Garden Bulletin No. 72, U. S. Department of Agriculture, Washington, D. C., 1964, U. S. Government Printing Office.
19. Phillips, Elisabeth Cogswell: Meals a la car, Nurs. Outlook **8**:76-78, 1960.
20. Piper, Geraldine M.: Nutrition in coordinated home care programs, J. Am. Dietet. A. **39**:198-200, 1961.
21. Piper, Geraldine M., and Smith, Emily M.: Geriatric nutrition, Nurs. Outlook **12**:51-53, 1964.
22. Pollack, Herbert: Nutritional problems in the aging and aged, J.A.M.A. **165**:257-258, 1957.
23. Shafer, Kathleen Newton, and others: Medical-surgical nursing, ed. 3, St. Louis, 1964, The C. V. Mosby Co.
24. Stare, Frederick J.: Overnutrition, Am. J. Pub. Health **53**:1795-1802, 1963.
25. Stare, Frederick J.: Good nutrition from food not pills, Amer. J. Nurs. **65**:86-89, 1965.
26. Swanson, Pearl: Nutrition needs after 25. In Food, the Yearbook of Agriculture, U. S. Department of Agriculture, Washington, D. C., 1959, U. S. Government Printing Office.
27. Zelman, Samuel: Relation of serum cholesterol to food and vitamin habits, J. Am. Geriatrics Soc. **11**:17-19, 1963.

Chapter 8

Prevention of illness

Prevention of illness in the elderly by early diagnosis and control of progression of chronic illness has become one of the most urgent problems facing both the health professions and our entire society. Illness in the elderly person is more protracted and more costly in economic and emotional resources than in the younger patient. In 1962, The National Health Survey showed that those persons 65 years of age and older had more than twice as many days of hospital care than those under 65 years of age. It showed also that the elderly had two and one half times as many days of inactivity restriction because of illness. Yet each year the proportion of elderly in the total population increases, the greatest increase being of those over 75 years of age; duration of illness and of hospitalization is the longest for this age group. At the same time the proportionate numbers of our population five years of age and under is increasing. They also make high demands on health services. While new technical procedures and a more knowledgeable public, most of whom have means of paying for health care, increase the demand for health services, many new fields of endeavor in our technologic age attract workers who might otherwise become members of the health professions. Although the number of nurses increases each year, it is not likely that professional nurses alone can give adequate care to all of the elderly who become ill. Therefore, the profession of nursing must give high priority to team participation with other professional workers to find and promote better means of preventing illness, dependency, and disability in our older population.

CONTRIBUTION OF PREVENTIVE PRACTICE

There is evidence that periodic health appraisal can and will contribute to better health for the elderly. Many public health medical officers recognize the important contribution that nursing can make in case finding and in appropriate referral of patients. Because of the relatively large number of nurses in proportion to other members of the health team, the variety of her functions, and her unique relationship to patients, she is in a strategic position to inform people of available services, explain the need, arouse interest, do initial screening, and ensure follow-up.

The public health nurse who is providing a generalized service and the nurse in the hospital, clinic, or related facility should ask herself three questions as she cares for any elderly person: What signs does the patient have that suggest need for further medical care by his attending physician or through him by a specialist? What education in general health maintenance does this patient need? What is the health status of other members of the family? She should then proceed according to her informed observations and her trained judgment to provide needed care or refer the patient to appropriate services.

The rules of health by which we live are important at any age, for they may well contribute to length of life and enjoyment of living. The nurse makes an important contribution to the teaching and carrying out of good principles of hygiene, not only in the critical period after 65 years of age but also in childhood, when the foundations are laid for a healthful and useful interval of life after 65. Interest in the study and correction of postural deviations in school children, guidance in the development of sound dietary patterns to avoid obesity, and encouraging the formation of habits of wise expenditure of physical energy are some of the aspects of nursing that will contribute to the prevention of illness and disability in old age. Emphasis must be placed on fostering sound practices in the formative years, since it is almost impossible to inculcate good patterns of daily hygiene in the aged who have not previously practiced them. With advancing age, fatigue and many other factors make it more difficult for the elderly to carry out good hygienic measures, even those who have had good habits in youth and maturity.

For many years an annual physical examination has been recommended for everyone, and it is agreed that periodic health appraisals should be part of preparation for health in later years. Regular health appraisals of infants and children, brought about by the need to give them immunization treatment, have led to the detection of signs of chronic illness and to early treatment in many instances. No such program, however, brings the elderly person to his doctor regularly. And indeed it is unlikely at this writing that there would be enough medical time available if every person 65 and over were to seek such care. It has been suggested by some members of the medical profession that all persons be supplied with a card or booklet that would include pertinent medical information from childhood as recorded by each physician who treated the patient. This practice, which is slow in being adopted, would be of substantial help to busy physicians caring for a mobile population.

MOTIVATION AND TEACHING

A real problem in a program of health education for the elderly is to motivate persons who consider themselves well to take an interest in positive health practices and to seek medical attention when that seems indicated. This may be a much greater challenge than was met by public health nurses in programs for antenatal, infant, and child care. The nurse's success will depend upon: (1) her genuine interest and feeling for the older person and how well she is able to show it; (2) her ability to transmit to him the real assurance that usually something can be done for symptoms he has; (3) her knowledge of the physical, pathologic, social, cultural, and emotional aspects of aging; and (4) her knowledge and understanding of each person with whom she works.

Before health education of the elderly can be successful, it is necessary for those involved in teaching to understand some attitudes and motivating forces affecting the elderly. Studies indicate that inconsistency—a human failing most of us succumb to occasionally—may reach a high peak in this age group's response to the need for preventive health care. In many instances elderly people who are limited seriously by several ailments state that they feel their health is good. Perception of the presence of illness or acceptance of the need for health care appears to be related more closely to concept of self than to actual signs and symptoms. The elderly gentleman, well dressed and setting out for a round of gratifying activities, may say he considers his health excellent while at the same time he may pop a tablet into his mouth to relieve anginal pain. The elderly person may say that he believes in health care, that it is a good idea for others but not for himself, and he may give as his reason the belief that he is well.

When faced with the need for some change of behavior that is not entirely pleasant, the elderly person will relate the value of the change to himself. What are the chances, for example, of his getting diabetes or heart disease if he continues to overindulge in food? What is the chance of having serious trouble if he continues to neglect safe practices of conduct as he moves about with less agility? And if he does encounter difficulties, what changes will they make in his life? Because the penalty for poor health practice is not certain, it may seem remote and not too important. A favorite reaction is the rationalization that probably he will be one of the fortunate ones who does not suffer any penalty for violating health practices. For some individuals the suggestion of consequences is so threatening that the possibility of their developing is rejected and nothing is done.

Yet many elderly people are concerned about their health and about keeping well. One Gallup poll taken in 1954 showed that 57 percent of a group of people 65 years of age and older listed good health as the first reason to be thankful.[22] Some will follow every suggestion given them of ways to stay well and thus be independent of others and able to participate and contribute socially. In this way some become prey to quacks or advertised tonics and the like or are misled by well-meaning but poorly informed friends.

Since the attitudes and thinking of their peers seems to influence the thinking of individuals, group discussions of health problems may be used much more in the future to teach health maintenance. Discussions could be held in day centers, housing projects for the aged, hospital outpatient clinics, or in a variety of other circumstances; there are groups specifically convened for this purpose, such as the Fitness for the Future classes under the sponsorship of the American National Red Cross. Subjects such as general nutrition, prevention or control of obesity, reasons for having a periodic health inventory, foot exercises and foot care, and prevention of accidents lend themselves well to group teaching. In one day-care center suggestions for group discussion are turned in by those attending and topics are selected from them.[17] Enrolling elderly persons and holding their interest is difficult, however, and will challenge the best efforts of the most imaginative and mature nurse. Day centers seem to have been singularly successful in bringing elderly people together for discussions of health care and in eliciting interest in individual health counseling. Perhaps the reason is that health teaching is made available in a pleasant environment that the participants associate with helpful experiences; studies would indicate that the teaching is more successful in such a setting than in a medical clinic like the outpatient department of a hospital because of its specific association with illness and its impersonal atmosphere.

A permissive, relaxed atmosphere is necessary in group teaching of the aged, and the informal discussion method is often used. Exhortation, or emphatically telling the person or the group what they should do will yield nothing. It is necessary to keep the content specific to the needs of those attending, to relate material to the actual life situation of the participants, and to stay within the context of the known and the familiar. The nurse must present material in the style and language that can be understood. She should remember that for the aged, learning takes time. Repetition is often necessary, and any appearance of hurry should be avoided. She should be keenly sensitive to group reactions and individual responses, since any frustration or failure to learn will produce apprehension and will delay learning still further. Movies, posters, and other visual aids are useful; a wealth of this kind of material is available. These should always be accompanied by commentary and discussion. It has been found that literature is far less effective in this context than person-to-person relay of information.

Individual health counseling by nurses also helps to prevent illness among the elderly. Group settings where this may be done include special disease-detection clinics, such as those for diabetes and glaucoma, multiphasic screening programs, and well oldster health clinics. In recent years there has been an enormous increase in day centers for the elderly, and health counseling has been found to meet a real need of many attending the centers. In the city of New York, for example, the number of health counseling interviews conducted by public health nurses assigned to day centers for the aged rose from 1,500 to 2,400 in the single year from 1962 to 1963.[17] The New York City Health Department has assigned public health nurses to day-care centers throughout the city.

Housing projects for the elderly designed and built with federal assistance have sprung up in all parts of the country, and health services are being established in many of them. These services vary a great deal. Some, such as the Destor Manor in Rhode Island, have a contractual arrangement with a local visiting nurse agency to provide the full services of a public health nurse. Screening programs are conducted in cooperation with the local health department.[17] Other housing projects have developed clinics in cooperation with a local hospital. These, although convenient and useful for the elderly residents, may not be in any sense focused on the prevention of illness. Health counseling often is not one of the functions of the nurse who is employed primarily to do laboratory work and give treatments in such clinics.

The nurse who participates in health counseling of the aged needs to have a thorough knowledge of the health resources of her community and the services that are available to the elderly. She must know, for example, whether or not homemaker service is available, whether portable meals can be provided, what rehabilitation facilities there are, and which social agencies provide help to the elderly person in such matters as housing. She must know the medical resources available and, if she works in a facility that does not include a physician on the health team, she should have written policies to guide her in referral of elderly persons to physicians.

In addition to maturity and a sound understanding of the psychosocial, economic, and cultural aspects of aging, the nurse must have a thorough knowledge of illness in this age group. Because the elderly patient may not have the typical signs of illness that occur in the younger patient, it is exceedingly difficult to detect early signs of disease. Another problem is that the elderly person usually has several chronic ailments, the symptoms of which complicate the detection of specific illness. The nurse needs to be a keen observer of small but important clues. She must conduct the counseling interview in a quiet and unhurried environment, with time to get to know the elderly person. Contrary to the belief of many, there often are early signs of such diseases as myocardial infarction and cardiac failure. Many patients who are questioned carefully reveal that they had a persistent cough more pronounced at night, or abnormal fatigue, or sudden awakening with dyspnea during the night, or occasional feeling of pressure over the sternum long before ankle edema or more pronounced symptoms appeared. The nurse is not a diagnostician, of course, but she can be most discerning and helpful in doing initial screening and referring potential patients to their physicians. A recent study revealed that in only 6 percent of the instances were nurses incorrect in appraising 112 abnormalities in 140 patients who were not under medical care at the time the patients became known to the nurses.[11] Fatigue, poor appetite, headache, and halitosis along with increased frequency of urination during the night may be present for months before the patient thinks he needs to visit his doctor. When he does he may learn that he has signs of renal failure.

Far too often, elderly persons and members of their families interpret nonspecific symptoms as the inevitable concomitants of advancing age. All who work with the elderly need to realize that changes of usual behavior or physiologic habits at any age are signs of maladjustment or homeostatic disequilibrium. Age may complicate the search for the cause, but age itself is rarely the primary cause. If treated early, most diseases are controllable; many are curable. If treated late, the chances of reversing the process or controlling disease in older persons is markedly decreased.

REFERENCES AND RELATED BIBLIOGRAPHY

1. Bozian, Marguerite W.: Nursing in a geriatric day center, Amer. J. Nurs. **64**:93-95, 1964.
2. Dolce, James A., Krauss, Theodore C., and Mosher, William E.: Preliminary report on a well aging conference in Erie County, J. Am. Geriatrics Soc. **11**:73-89, 1963.
3. Graber, Joe B.: Public Health Service programs on aging, Pub. Health Rep. **79**:577-581, 1964.

4. Grant, Murray, and Paupe, William E.: Countywide screening programs for chronic disease, Pub. Health Rep. **79**:767-771, 1963.
5. Haldeman, Jack C.: What the American public wants in health care, Pub. Health Rep. **77**:301-306, 1962.
6. Hess, Patricia: Home is where the nurse is, Amer. J. Nurs. **65**:116-117, 1965.
7. Kountz, William B.: Therapeutic aspects of geriatric medicine, J.A.M.A. **153**:777-782, 1953.
8. Kutner, Bernard: Health education in senior citizens' programs, Am. J. Pub. Health **48**: 622-626, 1958.
9. Kutner, Bernard, and others: Five hundred over sixty, New York, 1956, Russell Sage Foundation.
10. Morris, Robert: Chronic illness. In Lurie, Harry L. (editor): Encyclopedia of social work, ed. 15, New York, 1965, National Association of Social Workers.
11. Roberts, Doris E.: How effective is public health nursing, Am. J. Pub. Health **52**:1077-1083, 1962.
12. Ryan, Philip E.: Role of voluntary health agencies in planning to meet the health needs of older persons, Am. J. Pub. Health **51**:878-882, 1961.
13. Sargeant, Emilie G., and Carley, Catherine: Health and welfare of the aged, Amer. J. Nurs. **60**:1616-1619, 1960.
14. Shanas, Ethel: Medical care among those aged 65 and over; reported illness and utilization of health services by the "sick" and the "well," Research Series No. 16, 1960, New York Health Information Foundation.
15. Sheahan, Marion W.: Needed: reorganization for health services, Am. J. Pub. Health **52**: 393-400, 1962.
16. Skiff, Anna W.: Programmed instruction and patient teaching, Am. J. Pub. Health **55**: 409-415, 1965.
17. Smith, Emily M.: Health services in selected housing projects and day centers for the aging, Paper presented at the Annual Convention of the American Public Health Association, 1964.
18. Soller, Genevieve, R.: The aging patient, Amer. J. Nurs. **62**:114-117, 1962.
19. Stewart, William H.: Community medicine; An American concept of comprehensive care, Pub. Health Reports **78**:93-100, 1963.
20. Stieglitz, Edward J. (editor): Geriatric medicine, ed. 2, Philadelphia, 1954, J. B. Lippincott Co.
21. Thompson, Prescott W.: Let's take a good look at the aging, Amer. J. Nurs. **61**:76-79, 1961.
22. Wilbar, Charles L., Jr.: Keeping the aged healthy, J. Am. Geriatrics Soc. **92**:25-31, 1961.

Unit 3

General factors in care of the ill

Chapter 9

Housing during illness

During illness the elderly patient is housed in the general hospital, in the nursing home or related facility for chronic illness, or in his own home. It is agreed that the best place for the elderly patient is often in his own home, except in event of acute illness and for short periods during study and intensive treatment of chronic illness. Emphasis should be on creating a financial, environmental, and health situation that will help to keep acute exacerbations of disease at a minimum and avoid hospitalization.

Earlier and more frequent visits of public health nurses might help to prevent some of the situations that create need for hospitalization. Better clinic or ambulatory care that assesses and attempts to meet the total health needs of both well and ailing older persons would prevent much needless hospitalization. Sometimes financial assistance to ensure a better diet or homemaker service for a few hours a day is all that is needed to prevent episodes of illness.

Well oldster health conferences and multiphasic screening programs in health departments, housing projects and other housing or day care centers for the aging, and hospitals are now being tried. By this means, chronic illness may be prevented or be diagnosed in its very early stages, so that hospitalization will perhaps be avoided. Nurses can play a vital part in the success of these programs by referring patients, conducting health education conferences, and assisting with follow-up.

ACUTE ILLNESS

When the older person is acutely ill, he should be in a general hospital where specialists are readily available. The field of geriatrics embraces almost every disease known to man, and a single geriatric patient often requires the skill of several specialists. The atmosphere that pervades the general hospital is usually one of hope and optimism, which is psychologically beneficial to older patients. This is instinctively reflected in his own response to his illness. In the general hospital the aged patient is less likely to feel resigned to his condition than if he remains for a long period in an institution housing only the chronically ill. The atmosphere is progressive there; it is a situation in which the nurses and

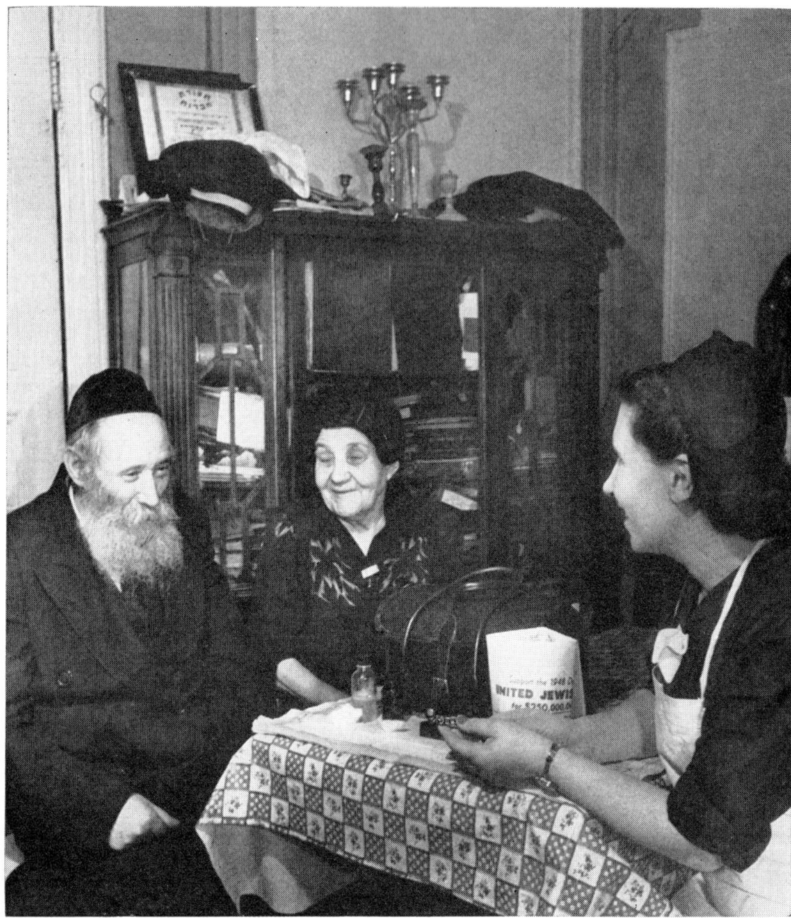

Figure 17. Health supervision by the nurse may help prevent illness that could lead to separation of the older couple. (Courtesy Visiting Nurse Service of New York; photograph by Hazel Kingsbury.)

doctors are gaining experience, and the patient benefits from the stimulation of new faces and new enthusiasms. Change, however, must not reach the point where the patient feels that no one really knows his story or is interested in his particular nursing needs. It should be remembered that many of the very old resist hospitalization. They often believe that if they are sick enough to go to a hospital, they will surely die.

Older patients are typical of a cross section of human life, and in the hospital they should be considered as such. Many are stimulating and delightful; many are morose and difficult, demanding much tact and sense of humor on the part of persons caring for them. The patient who is extremely ill and who is incontinent may have to be segregated, but under usual circumstances it is well to mix the aged patients with others of lesser age. This tends to keep the patient as well as the personnel alert and interested. Many workers become casual and bored when caring only for aged or chronically ill patients for long periods of time. Every effort should be made to change the attitudes that lead to this behavior.

The general hospital should be equipped to give older patients adequate care. Its community sponsorship and community responsibility require that a general hospital recognize its obligation to care for the aged and chronically ill as well as for patients who have an acute medical condition or require immediate surgery. For example, the aged patient is likely to forget that he is in a high bed and may fall in attempting to get up. Yet, when he is acutely ill and requires much nursing care, it is necessary that the higher regular hospital bed be used for the convenience of persons giving care. Side rails should be used routinely on the beds. Side rails that are of lightweight metal and are easy to manipulate can be left on the bed while it is being made up and thus will save nursing effort. There should be more footstools in the general hospital for the use of patients when they are being assisted into bed and for use in elevating the patient's feet when he is sitting by his bed. Even greater safety is provided by the use of high-low beds that can be kept at normal bed height except when bed care is being given. There is need in many general hospitals for more comfortable chairs to replace straight-backed, armless chairs. Floors should have a surface that is not slippery or dangerous to the patient, rather than a high polish. There should be rails around the walls in the bathroom so that a feeble older person can get about more independently, and there should be a chair in the bathroom so that he can rest for a moment before returning to his bed. As the number of older patients increases, there is need in many of our general hospitals for more bathroom facilities. Schedules should be altered to permit more leisurely morning care and more time to eat breakfast. These patients often require more care than younger ones. That they have special needs should be understood, and they should not be made to feel that they are merely being tolerated. Under the pressures and demands of a general hospital's busy acute service, the care given is often less personalized than in a nursing home or chronic care hospital. All too often a patient admitted from a chronic care facility for a short stay in a general hospital returns with decubitus ulcers. Back rubs have been virtually discontinued as routine care, which may in part account for the problem. Or as one woman who had arthritis and who returned to the nursing home said, "They are just too rushed; they take the pan out before you can lift yourself off."

REFERRALS TO PUBLIC HEALTH NURSE

Since it disrupts their lives so completely, hospitalization for older persons should be as short as is consistent with sound medical care. If the hospital makes the referral to the public health agency before the patient leaves the hospital, he may be able to return home sooner than would otherwise be feasible. Nursing service in the home is a most valuable part of the complete care of many patients. This service is not too well known to the elderly and sometimes not even to professional workers. The nurse in the hospital should recognize the need for public health nursing care or supervision of the patient after he leaves the hospital and should not hesitate to suggest this service to the physician. Plans should be made before the day or hour of his departure from the hospital since it is necessary to discuss the plan for care with the patient. The careful use of referrals by persons in hospitals would reduce the period of hospitalization and thus the cost, would release beds needed for other patients, and would decrease the period of separation of the older person from his family. The success of this plan depends upon the use of referral forms that supply pertinent information to the nurse in the home as well as suitable forms on which the public health nurse can record observations and details of the patient's progress to be sent to the physician in charge and to the nurse in the hospital.

HOME CARE PROGRAMS

Home care programs vary widely in their plan of operation. For example, some are operated under the sponsorship of a local health department, although generally they are under the aegis of a hospital.

Characteristic features of home care programs include a centralized administration to coordinate the functions of medicine, nursing, social work, physical and occupational therapy, and, as needed, other special services. In a large number of home care programs, the general hospital continues responsibility for patients who leave the hospital. Occasionally a patient is admitted to the program from the hospital clinic. Nursing is provided by a contractual arrangement with a local public health nursing agency, and a nursing coordinator on the hospital staff provides the liaison with other personnel within the hospital. Usually the patient remains on the census rolls of the hospital, and a chart is kept as for any patient. Laboratory, x-ray, and other hospital resources are immediately available to the patient if they are needed, and provision is made for his transportation to the hospital.

Home care programs are not new. The first was established by the Boston Dispensary in 1796, and the University of Vermont has conducted such a program since 1925. A reawakening to the knowledge that many patients are happier and do better in their own homes has been a factor in their development. The increasing incidence of chronic illness and the high cost of hospitalization have contributed to the study of this method of care for all who are ill, but particularly for those who suffer from long-term illness. Despite the evidence that these programs are effectively meeting the needs of many patients and families, their potential for reducing costs of care, and federal assistance to encourage their development, a recent Public Health Service survey reported only 33 such programs in all of the United States. The trend toward more rapid organization for home care will be given impetus by provisions for assistance under the 1965 Medicare legislation. Medical and other professional education is seldom the reason for initiating a home care program, but many teaching institutions report these programs as an excellent teaching resource.

The needs and problems of home care for the elderly ill are given perspective by a number of studies. It is reported that hospitalization of 30 days or longer is more often because of social rather than medical reasons. In a study of 7,136 medically indigent patients who were judged suitable candidates for home care, only 47.3 percent had families or homes that were willing or able to accept them;

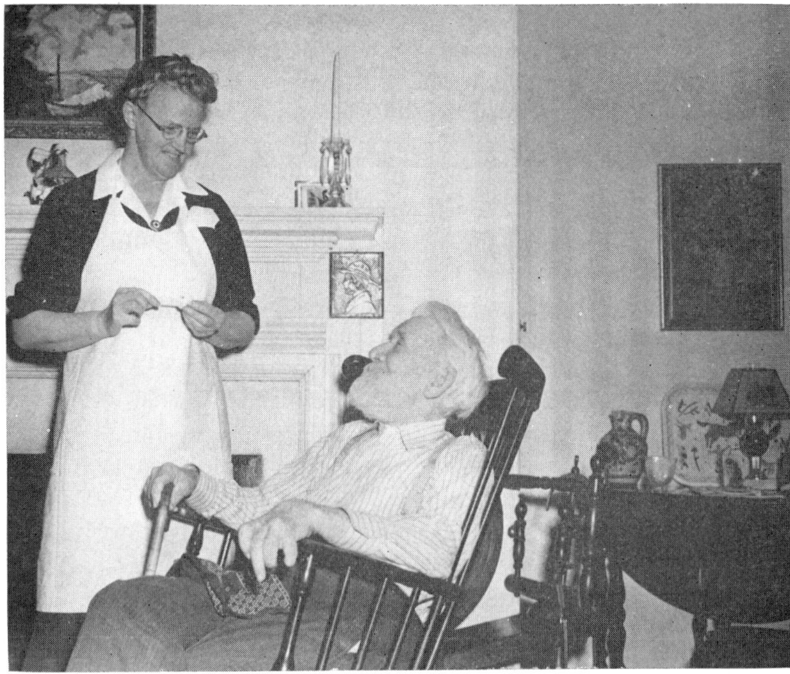

Figure 18. The visit of the nurse not only contributes to health but also affords a welcome break in the patient's day. (Photograph by Anne M. Goodrich.)

27.7 percent of the families were unwilling to care for patients at home, and 15 percent of the patients had no families. The remainder had families who were willing but not able to provide the needed care at home.[9] In New York City, a study of 2,000 home care patients revealed that 36 percent were over 65 years of age, while only 18 percent were below the age of 45.[25]

One widely reported home care program that has stimulated interest in these programs is the one conducted by the Montefiore Hospital in New York City. Others differ somewhat, but its practices are fairly typical of most hospital-based programs. In this program a department of the hospital takes responsibility for certain hospital patients who are permitted to return to their homes, but who are still kept on the patient census of the hospital. The patients chosen for release to their homes are carefully selected. The home is visited by a social worker before the decision is made to let the patient return home. An agreement with the visiting nurse agency ensures nursing care in the home. Housekeeping services are obtained and financed through the hospital budget. Records on all patients are kept by the hospital, and patients are visited regularly by members of the medical staff of the hospital. Medical staff members are on call for emergencies, just as they are for hospital patients. Hospital facilities (for example, x-ray and laboratory facilities) are available for the patients at home, as for those in the hospital.

There has been much discussion about the cost of home care, but reported costs are hard to compare and evaluate. It must be remembered that in home care, food, linen, and many other items normally provided by the hospital are provided by the family. Home care programs are fairly costly. It is agreed, however, that there is a substantial saving over general hospital care. In the effort to keep costs down for long-term care, Stiefel points out that standards of care must be maintained—that home care must not become the bargain basement of the hospital.[25] Cost is, or should be, a less important consideration than the comfort and peace of mind that home care programs so often provide. This is recognized and reflected in the provisions of the Medicare health plans that provide benefits for home care after hospitalization and, under the supplementary insurance benefits section, for home care without prior hospitalization.

CLINICS

Changes in our clinics to suit the needs of the older patient should be made. To him a clinic visit is often a frightening experience. Many elderly persons were brought up in the era of the family doctor. They feel shy and insecure about going to a large hospital clinic. Some do not know that clinics exist for persons other than those who are completely indigent. The idea of a public clinic suggests charity and to them is distressing since many have always been independent. It is disturbing to sit on a long bench for hours among strangers. They often see a different doctor each time they visit the clinic and have to explain their problems repeatedly. Sometimes they receive conflicting and confusing information and advice. The energy required to attend the clinic often exhausts an aged

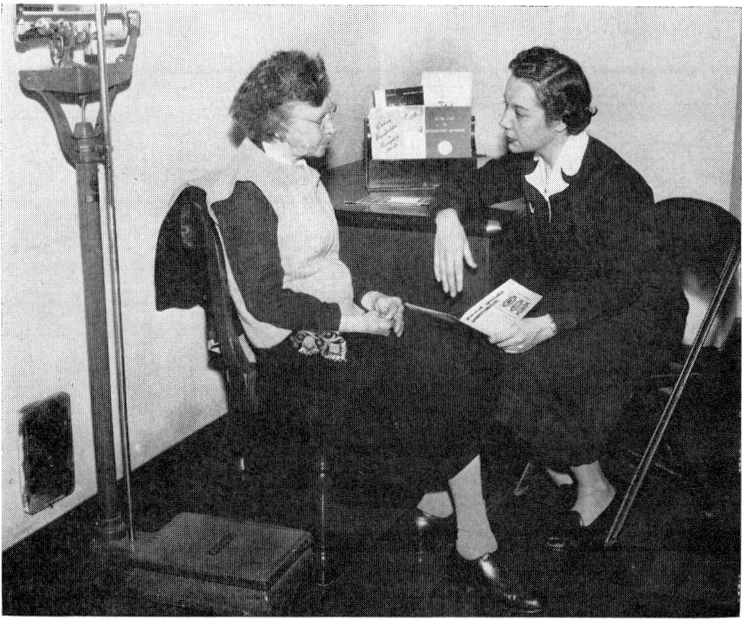

Figure 19. The nurse can be surprisingly successful in teaching health maintenance to the ambulatory patient. This patient, who has osteoarthritis, receives assistance in planning good meals that are within her financial means.

person, particularly if he is kept waiting for hours without food. Some physicians feel that a few days in a hospital where diagnostic procedures can be done more quickly and thoroughly is less strenuous for elderly persons than numerous clinic visits. Ambulatory services for the elderly are, however, receiving much attention. Comprehensive care clinics or general clinics, in which a patient is assigned to a single doctor but has access to the services of many specialists, are being encouraged.[30]

The number of visits to the clinic for treatment may often be decreased by having the nurse visit the patient in his home. For example, the nurse can check the weight record of a cardiac patient (bathroom scales may have to be arranged for through social or welfare agencies), supervise the diet, take the blood pressure, and administer drugs such as mercurial diuretics. A complete report can be sent regularly to the clinic physician so that he can follow the progress of his patient closely. This also helps the clinic nurse to give consistent information to the patient.

On the other hand, in some instances changes in clinic nursing can decrease the number of visits to the home that public health nurses must make. The potential for clinic nursing in the care of the elderly is enormous. An example of this is the Medical Nursing Clinic for the Chronically Ill opened recently at the Massachusetts General Hospital in Boston.[26] As the proportion of chronically ill aged persons in the general population increases, the emphasis will be more and more upon ambulatory management of disease. The elderly patient and his relatives may in the future receive much of the instruction necessary for self-care and home care during visits to the clinic. The nurse who has had experience in public health nursing as part of her preparation may be surprisingly successful in teaching the patient with severe diabetes, during repeated visits to the clinic, to give his own insulin and otherwise care for himself at home. Usually hospitalization is no longer necessary, and often a single follow-up visit to the home by the public health nurse is sufficient. The patient with osteoarthritis may learn much from the clinic nurse about accident prevention, weight reduction, and prevention of painful deformity. An elderly woman whose husband has had a cerebrovascular accident may get excellent suggestions on how to give him better care when she accompanies him to the hospital clinic.

INSTITUTIONAL HOUSING IN CHRONIC ILLNESS

The chronically ill person has been defined as one who is suffering from an incurable ailment that may or may not have remissions. Classification into three groups has been made and depends upon whether these patients require constant medical supervision and treatment, chiefly skilled nursing care, or simply custodial care. About 61 percent of the chronically ill persons in this country are over 45 years of age, and as the number of aged increases proportionately, the number of those chronically ill will increase. According to the National Health Survey more than 12,000,000 persons 65 years of age and over have one or more chronic conditions. Of these, nearly 2,500,000 are unable to carry on major activity, and approximately 4,500,000 have some activity limitation. The proportion of the population with activity limitation because of chronic disabling conditions increases with age. Only 2 of each 100 persons under 17 years of age are limited, whereas about 42 out of each 100 persons over the age of 65 have some degree of activity limitation.

When acute illness is over, the aged patient does not need the expensive facilities of the general hospital. Many chronically ill persons are kept longer than is necessary in wards for acute illness in general hospitals because there are so few suitable facilities to which they can be sent for the necessary medical and nursing care.

The selection of a suitable place for the aged chronically ill or convalescent patient is difficult in our society. Such institutions, though increasing in number, fall short of meeting the need in both quality and quantity. Some are located out of the city or town and have no affiliation with a medical center. From the patient's standpoint, this type of hospital is unsatisfactory because it removes him from his friends to a location where visitors can come only with difficulty. If it is a nursing home or elderly care facility, he is denied association with persons of various ages, and his life tends to become routine and monotonous. What is more, the confirmed city dweller does not desire or appreciate the satisfactions of living in the country. The city dweller who has gone to sleep with the roar of the subway for years does not want to live in the country any more than the country dweller wants to live in the city.

It is presently believed that the chronically ill aged patient, as well as all other persons who are chronically ill, should be housed (if not at home) in facilities closely associated with general hospitals, but designed, equipped, and operated with their special needs in mind. The Commission on Chronic Illness made this recommendation, and it has been repeated by leaders in the field. The Commission rejected the concept of chronic disease hospitals and also of *acute* general hospitals. The Commission felt that the general hospital should strengthen its position as the health center of the community and should concern itself with chronic disease—the number one health problem in the nation—as fully as with the acute emergency and the new operation. The Hospital Survey and Construction Act was passed in 1954 and provides some funds for construction of such facilities as part of general hospitals.

The Community Health Services and Facilities Act of 1961 greatly increased appropriations for all types of nursing home and chronic care facilities. Additional federal grants and loans are available for both new construction and remodeling of existing buildings. Although local community pressure and interest are needed to hasten these trends, real progress has been made in the past ten years. There are now 488 hospitals with nursing home units, 19 of which are Veterans' Administration Hospitals. The federal legislation for medical care of the aged will, when it begins functioning fully, hasten closer affiliation of nursing homes and hospitals and encourage hospitals to provide for the care of the chronically ill aged person.

The chronically ill person needs more complicated services than a person who has a short-term illness. When even a few of these services are listed, it is immediately apparent that they cannot be adequately provided in the small, isolated hospital for chronic illness or the nursing home.

The chronically ill patient often needs intensive evaluation and definitive treatment. He may have short-term exacerbations that require care in a general hospital. Housing the chronically ill person in a facility close by and related to a general hospital would permit him to move easily from one unit to another as the need arose and should provide the continuity of care presently in short supply. The patient needs long-term medical and nursing supervision by well-prepared staff members. Many times, he needs immediate rehabilitative services including physical therapy, social service, and vocational counseling; he needs a host of supportive services such as a recreational program, dental care, occupational therapy, and chiropodist services.

Care in a hospital rather than in a nursing home has been to the economic advantage of many persons because insurance plans have only covered that part of the care in a hospital or a hospital-related facility. More recently, however, insurance plans have begun to include some of the cost of care in nursing homes or other locations outside the hospital. In the future the economic advantages may influence the further development of hospital affiliated facilities for the chronically ill and elderly, because sharing of operating costs allows better use of buildings, equipment, and services.

NURSING HOMES

Because nursing homes have assumed such a vital role in providing care for the chronically ill, they are discussed at some length here. In the United States, there are more than half as many nursing home beds as total general hospital beds. Eighty-six percent of all the homes are proprietary or privately owned, and 71.6 percent of the beds are in privately owned homes. The average size of the proprietary home is 24 beds; of the voluntary home, 44 beds; and of the publicly owned home, 69 beds. This information was obtained from the Division of Hospital Services of the United States Public Health Service.[27]

Nursing homes belong to a group of facilities often referred to as *sheltered-care facilities.* Sheltered care for the aged usually means any kind of protective environment outside a hospital and outside a private home (their own or that of a relative or close friend). It includes homes for the aged, nursing homes, homes or hospitals for chronic illness, personal care homes, foster homes, and many other related facilities of varied names but similar function, regardless of sponsorship. Many of these resources elude accurate definition and classification. Overlapping of the services provided and confusion in terminology make it difficult for the professional worker and often impossible for the layman to distinguish the exact kind of services offered by a particular institution. The United States Public Health Service is currently attempting to define nursing homes more clearly. This would help enormously in their identification and subsequent inspection and control.

Many homes for the aged have an area set aside for residents who need close medical supervision and some skilled nursing. This is often referred to as the *infirmary.* In some homes this is a unit for the care of short-term acute illnesses only. If illness becomes chronic, persons are transferred to a hospital or nursing home. In others the infirmary is really a nursing home unit within the home for aged who are well. Two types of facilities are operated simultaneously; yet they vary a good deal in their medical, nursing, and other personnel needs and in their physical requirements. Homes of this kind are conducted mainly by religious and fraternal groups.

Nursing homes are also financed by public funds and operated as state, county, or municipal homes. These homes, which give care to the chronically ill, indigent, and homeless of any age, are partly hospitals for chronic illness and partly homes.

The really spectacular change in the past few years has been the extremely rapid growth in the number of *proprietary nursing homes* (operated for profit). Reasons for this increase are easily understood. Hospital construction did not keep pace with the population growth during and immediately after World War II, whereas prepaid hospital insurance and better knowledge of health and disease led to earlier and fuller medical treatment. Use of antibiotics and early ambulation reduced the length of hospitalization, but new methods of treatment (heart surgery, for example) continued to fill the hospital beds that were available. In 1937 there were 9,250,000 admissions to general hospitals, and by 1961 there were 25,500,000.[27] Pressure on general hospitals for available beds is so great that they are often reluctant to admit aged and chronically ill patients. Hospital costs have almost prohibited long-term care in general hospitals since the majority of retired elderly people do not have hospitalization insurance.

As these changes were taking place, communities did not generally provide care for long-term chronically ill persons, whose numbers were increasing tremendously and many of whom were aged. Hospitals, doctors, and individuals themselves looked desperately for places for patients to go. The result was that private individuals, many of whom at first took one or two persons into their homes for care, saw a good business opportunity and opened nursing homes that were run for profit. There is, therefore, a fundamental difference between proprietary nursing homes and a community facility such as the local voluntary hospital that operates without profit and serves all in the community, regardless of ability to pay and race, color, or other criteria.

In spite of the obvious need for chronic care facilities, both public and voluntary hospitals were slow to recognize either the economic or social advantages of opening units for the care of the chronically ill, who were filling beds in the general hospital designed for the acutely ill. Therefore, hospitals, private physicians, and welfare agencies were forced to turn to proprietary nursing homes because no other resources were available. Recently many voluntary hospitals, particularly those under Catholic auspices, have added nursing home annexes or units.

Sponsorship of nursing homes

Nursing homes under public auspices. Public funds may support nursing homes. The term *home* or infirmary is often used to identify what was once called a poor farm, old folks' county home, and the like. Old buildings discarded for other purposes and outworn wings of general hospitals have been used, and when new buildings are erected, they are often large, cold and impersonal, far removed from ongoing activities. Unfortunately, privacy for patients and respect for human dignity are hard to achieve in these homes, most of which are quite large. Although many fall far short of standards of good medical and nursing practices, most are improving. State health and welfare departments are providing medical, nursing, nutrition, and special therapy consultants. In most states today these homes must meet the same standards as required for the licensure of proprietary nursing homes or those units affiliated with voluntary hospitals, whichever is their equivalent. Policy has changed in recent years, and many public homes may now admit patients who have some income from Old Age and Survivors Insurance and other sources.

Nursing homes under voluntary auspices. Voluntary agencies such as fraternal, religious, and other philanthropic groups may administer nursing homes, although these comprise relatively few of the total nursing home beds. Those that are part of a home for the normal aged are overcrowded, and the higher cost of operation has not been adequately planned for. Residents in most voluntary nursing homes now pay a monthly fee based upon Old Age and Survivors Insurance and other income sources. Until fairly recently voluntary homes often took residents on a life-term contract basis. Thus, many homes were caught short when the lives of the residents were extended, and they now face serious financial difficulties.

Homes under voluntary auspices need the help and interest of specialized workers in this field. Some have shown remarkable foresight and leadership in setting a pattern of excellent care for the elderly. Others have developed slowly in practice of modern concepts of management and care of elderly persons. These homes are often superior to proprietary homes in home atmosphere and personal freedom for patients, but are often limited in health care facilities.

Nursing homes under private ownership. Proprietary nursing homes bear special mention because there are so many of them and because their kind of sponsorship is unusual in the health field. An estimated three fifths of the elderly persons who need nonhospital nursing care outside their own homes are cared for in these institutions. In 1961 there were approximately 8,297 proprietary nursing homes with a total bed capacity of 236,845. Relatively few proprietary nursing homes are operated by members of the health professions. A large number are operated by persons who have had no previous experience in a related undertaking, and even those who are from the health professions may have had no previous experiences that would necessarily qualify them for such an undertaking.

Fifteen years ago only a few states licensed nursing homes. Today all 50 states, Washington, D. C., and Puerto Rico require licensure. Under the present improved licensing programs and more stringent enforcement of standards for facilities, operation, and staffing, many poor proprietary homes have closed, although in some parts of the country—in urban as well as rural areas—old, rundown, outsized family dwellings or other converted structures that are unsuited and unsafe for their function are still to be found. They are gradually being replaced by new or reconstructed buildings. This has been made possible by a variety of federal grants and loans. There are still many substandard homes, but there are also many that provide high quality personalized, rehabilitative care.[3] The geographical location, per capita wealth in an area, the presence or absence of other facilities and consultant services, the level of community and professional interest, and the rate of payment by states for the care of public assistance patients all affect the quality of nursing home care.

The economic status of the patient is significant, for more than half of the patients in proprietary nursing homes are receiving public assistance. The costs of providing nursing care and limited rehabilitative services is quoted as being $8 to $10 a day or $240 to $300 per month. Payments for public assistance patients range from lows of $75 to $80 per month to maximums of $225 to $275 per month in a very few instances.[3] In one state in which proprietary care is very progressive, operators of proprietary homes have stated that a limit of 25 percent occupancy must be placed on welfare recipients if they are to operate without loss. This was stated as true, also, for the hospital-based nursing home. Since agencies of state governments both set the standards and determine the payments in many cases, it appears that they should work together for a solution of this problem. Until this social dilemma is solved, substandard nursing homes will continue to exist or gradually will be replaced by tax-supported facilities for the care of public assistance recipients. In the meantime broad generalizations about homes operated for profit can no longer be made. Some provide outstanding care, some are poor, and many are meeting at least minimum standards in their own states.

Classification of nursing homes. All nursing homes regardless of ownership are classified according to the type of care provided. These are skilled care nursing homes, personal care homes, and residential care homes. The skilled care nursing home provides the skilled nursing care as its primary and predominant function. Personal care homes are of two types: one provides some skilled nursing care but only as an adjunct to its primary personal care function; the other provides no skilled nursing. The residential care homes are similarly subdivided but have as their primary function residential or sheltered care.[28]

Present needs and recent developments

There are many heartening facts regarding nursing homes about which nurses should be informed, for they may greatly influence geriatric nursing. The Division of Hospital and Medical Facilities of the Public Health Service reported for 1961 a total of 23,000 nursing homes and related facilities. This is 2,000 less than estimated in 1954 in a Public Health Service inventory. In spite of this, there is an increase in the resident capacity of 32 percent. Over 338,000 of the beds are in 9,700 skilled care nursing homes; 207,000 are in personal care homes; the remainder are in 2,200 residential homes.

Figures that reflect the improving quality of care in those homes whose dominant service is nursing are the numbers of full-time nursing staff employed. More than 9 out of 10 skilled care nursing homes employ full-time registered professional nurses or licensed practical nurses or both. In 39 percent there are professional nurses only; in approximately 18 percent there are both professional and practical nurses; and in 39 percent there are licensed practical nurses only. A distressing figure still exists—13 percent of homes classified for skilled nursing care have no full-time registered professional or licensed practical nurses. Since no figures for use of nurses part time is available, it is not known whether this figure means total absence of persons with nursing preparation or if unlicensed but graduate nurses are employed.[28] The overall picture is improved, however, for in 1954 only 4 out of 10 skilled care nursing homes employed nurses.

The need for improved nursing is obvious when one looks at the patient population. The average age of patients in nursing homes is 80 years. Two out of every 3 patients have cardiovascular disease; 1 in 10 has a fracture; and about 1 in 20 has a mental disorder. Less than half of the patients can walk alone. Approximately half have periods of disorientation, one third are incontinent, and two thirds are receiving medications regularly. Many recent accounts of the effectiveness of nursing care and good teamwork among professional workers have amply documented what can be, and in many places is being, accomplished in nursing homes.[22]

There is great need for increased interest by both the nursing and medical professions in long-term care of the ill. In 1962, a geriatric nursing section was organized in the American Nurses' Association. The American Medical Association now has a Committee on Aging and is urging all state associations to do likewise. In 1958, a council, The Joint Council to Improve the Health Care of the Aged, was set up and included membership from the American Medical Association, the American Hospital Association, the American Association of Nursing Homes, and the American Dental Association. The American Medical Association has advised its state associations to set up similar councils within each state. Stated objectives of the Council are to identify and analyze the health needs of aging persons, to appraise available health resources for the aged, and to develop programs to foster the best health care of aging persons, regardless of their economic status. Unlike the Commission on Chronic Illness, this Council does not have representation from the American Public Health Association.

The increasing number of educational programs for all levels of nursing home personnel now being conducted throughout the country is evidence of the sincerity and interest of the proprietors of nursing homes. These programs are carried on cooperatively by nursing home associations, public health agencies, professional organizations, voluntary health agencies, universities, and hospitals. Emphasis is placed on improvement of administration and of patient care.

Probably the greatest impetus for the improvement of services to the elderly ill and of the facilities that provide care for them is the passage of the 1965 Health Insurance for the Aged (Medicare) legislation. The specific provisions as to requirements that institutions must fulfill in order to qualify for Medicare funds have motivated many homes to move more rapidly toward accreditation by making liaison and transfer agreements with hospitals, agreements with medical staffs, and by employing registered nurses and participating in community and interagency planning for implementation of this legislation.

The effects of this legislation; the leadership and assistance programs of the Nursing Homes and Related Facilities Section, Division of Chronic Diseases,

United States Public Health Service; and the accreditation and state licensure programs will undoubtedly be to upgrade standards of care.

Nursing responsibilities

Nurses should be informed about the kinds, distribution, quality, and control of nursing homes in their communities. The patient, his family, and his friends may look to the nurse for assistance in deciding to use a nursing home and for choice of the specific type of facility. They may ask her for sources of additional information and guidance. The nurse may help by giving needed reassurance that the selection of a facility recommended by the doctor or the social worker is the right one.

In the future, many nurses will contribute professional service to nursing homes. They may work as staff members in the homes; as public health nurses giving help on such matters as nutrition, accident prevention, rehabilitation, and general hygiene; or as nurses in larger hospitals and teaching centers or public health nursing agencies that offer staff education programs for persons who work in nursing homes. A publication titled *How To Be a Nursing Aid in a Nursing Home,* prepared by the United States Public Health Service, should be read by all nurses involved in teaching persons who work in nursing homes.[20]

The nurse who works in a community nursing agency may be—and many now are—called upon to give informal guidance to persons planning to operate nursing homes. She may work with other persons, such as a social worker, fire inspector, or sanitary engineer, in the inspection, licensure, and control of these institutions. If she is going to meet the challenge of this area of nursing responsibility, she must know a good deal about the needs of the elderly persons, both individually and collectively, as well as about nursing homes and other related facilities in her local area and throughout the nation.

At present all states and territories except for Guam and the Virgin Islands license nursing homes. In 46 states and territories the licensing agency is the state health department; in 3 it is the state welfare department; and in 2 an agency other than health or welfare has this responsibility. Regardless of where within each state the responsibility rests, there is usually a separate unit or division responsible for licensing nursing homes and homes for the aged.

Most licensing authorities consider education an essential element in the enforcement of standards. They provide a wide range of consultation services to established nursing homes as well as help and guidance to individuals who are contemplating opening new nursing homes.

The state authority usually sets up standards that are acceptable to the federal government (Department of Health, Education and Welfare), but which are essentially minimal. Licensure does not mean that a home is ideal, by any means.

Licensed homes are required to renew their licenses periodically, although the interval between renewal varies with the states. Additional inspection visits may or may not be made, depending upon the staff available. Occasionally, because of staffing shortages, a serious complaint prompts additional inspections. If the facility is part of a home for the aged, it must still meet the state specifications for a nursing home and is licensed as such. Local agencies concerned with community planning, such as community councils, sometimes have a list of approved homes, and occasionally, the homes in the community are classified alphabetically as to quality.

Licensure and accreditation programs

In January, 1966, the Joint Commission on the Accreditation of Hospitals assumed the function of accreditation of nursing homes and facilities other than hospitals that give extended care. Prior to this time the American Hospital Association conducted one approval program, and the National Council for Accreditation of Nursing Homes, sponsored by the American Nursing Home Association and the American Medical Association, carried out an accreditation program for proprietary nursing homes. The Joint Commission will continue the practice established by the National Council for the Accreditation of Nursing Homes of having qualified professional nurses make the appraisal visits to homes that apply for accreditation.

Selecting a nursing home

In 1953 and 1954 the National Social Welfare Assembly published two pamphlets on standards of care for older people in institutions,[24] that may be useful to nurses in helping patients and in solving problems in their own lives that are related to care of elderly family members and friends.

If the patient is hospitalized and has a private physician, placement is usually arranged by the physician, the patient, and the patient's family. If he is on ward service, arrangements are usually made by the social worker who works with the doctor, the nurse, the patient, and the patient's family. The nurse can help by reporting the patient's reaction to plans as they progress to the social worker and the doctor. Because she is with the patient more than anyone else, she may learn from him or his family some of the misinterpretations and fears that he may not express to others. The nurse should avoid making adverse comments to the patient or his family about the facility under consideration. To do so might increase immeasurably the work of the social worker who may already have an exceedingly difficult assignment because of eligibility restrictions as to race or color, or financial status, waiting lists, and many other factors.

If the patient is entering a nursing home from his own home, placement may be made by the physician, the social worker, or welfare worker, all working closely with the patient and his family. In small communities and in rural areas particularly, the public health nurse may assist in this. In some instances the patient's family determines the placement, with little or no assistance from others.

If he is physically and intellectually able to do so, the patient should participate in the selection of a suitable nursing home. In most instances family members should be encouraged to discuss plans with the individual concerned and to avoid assuming that, because he is old and chronically ill, he should have little to say about his disposition. If placement is being arranged with little consultation from the patient or his family, it is important that persons making the arrangements know the patient fairly well. Careful placement based on the individual patient's needs contributes greatly to his adjustment and to his family's peace of mind.

Sponsorship of the facility under consideration should be known, and it should be borne in mind that there are good homes and poor homes under all kinds of sponsorship—public, voluntary, and proprietary. Sponsorship should not cause one to limit careful observation if he visits the home or to refrain from seeking pertinent information. One must learn whether the home in question is licensed by the state and whether the license is current. If it is not, it is reasonable to assume that it does not meet even minimum standards.

If the nursing home is a proprietary one, it is particularly important to meet and learn something about the person who operates the home. What is his standing in the community? What is his previous experience? How long has he been in this field? What appear to be his attitudes toward his responsibilities and toward his staff? Fairly often operators of small private homes show attitudes and behavior patterns that do not contribute to the acquisition or retention of capable professional staffs. Because of unfavorable location, low salaries, poor personnel policies, and other causes many homes fail to attract and to hold competent nurses.

Medical care. Medical care is often a scarce commodity in nursing homes. One should know whether the home has a board with licensed medical representation that helps to set policies regarding admittance of suitable patients, pre-entrance medical examination, frequency of medical checkups, and the like. Many larger voluntary homes have such a board and have an attending physician designated by the board who gives overall medical supervision, gives medical care to persons who have no personal physician, and serves in emergencies if the private physician cannot be located. Some states require that proprietary nursing homes, however, admit only patients who are under the direct medical supervision of their own private doctors.

The United States Public Health Service study of nursing homes showed that the largest number of patients had a diagnosis of cardiovascular disease; yet one fifth had not been seen by a doctor in six months and one tenth had not been seen by a doctor for a year or more. The operators and "nursing staffs" of some proprietary homes did not know the diagnosis of some patients. Pertinent questions include the following: What are the lines of communication between the nurse and the patient's doctor? Where does the charge nurse take any medical care problem in the absence of medical supervision? Are medical and nursing records kept? What standing orders are used and who prepares them?

Nursing staff. The nursing home should provide skilled nursing care around the clock. Unfortunately, the written regulations in many states are not explicit and leave room for loopholes in conforming to regulations. These are taken advantage of by some persons who operate homes, since graduate nurses must be paid more than other less highly skilled workers. For example, the statement that there must be a graduate nurse for a specified number of patients may not clearly state that there must be a relief nurse when she is ill, on vacation, or having regular days off. To get a real idea of the amount of nursing care given, one must learn whether the nurse is really caring for patients and supervising patient care or whether she is relieving the administrator when he is away and is perhaps cooking meals when the cook is off. Salaries and personnel policies give good clues to nursing care. The administrator of the home may complain that nurses are not available, when an appraisal of policies may show clearly why the home cannot possibly compete favorably with other institutions employing nurses.

It is well to know whether the home has any planned, ongoing training program for aides and attendants, whether it seeks help in nursing from outside agencies such as the local public health nurse, and what contact the nurses employed have with neighboring hospitals and with their professional organizations. The kind and quality of medical care are also good indications of the quality of nursing, since qualified nurses will seldom remain in institutions in which they do not have orders and direction from licensed physicians for the medical aspects of their work.

Other staff and related services. Food is important to almost everyone, sick or well. Small homes may provide better food than large ones, since it is almost impossible to prepare good appetizing food when it must be cooked in very large quantities. Reading menus, talking to patients, and eating a meal in the home help one to judge the food. The imagination and interest of the staff are shown in other ways. Some homes collect the favorite recipes of residents and feature them with appropriate publicity on suitable occasions. One might observe how meals are served, that is, whether patients eat at a common table when they are physically able to do so, and one should learn the time interval between breakfast and supper. Usually supper is served far too early; there should be at least ten hours between breakfast and supper, and bedtime nourishment should be served.

Housekeeping is an essential service in the home, but it should not be carried to extremes and thereby detract from a homelike atmosphere. There should be provision for individual untidiness if that is the way a particular patient has always lived. It is well to find out whether the aides and attendants who clean inpatient units are included in the figures for personnel giving nursing care.

Specialists such as nutritionists, social workers, physiatrists, occupational therapists, and nursing specialists are usually available to nursing homes that really seek their services. They may be available on a part-time fee basis or as consultants from community agencies, in which case their services may be free. Whether they are called upon depends primarily upon the interest of the home and its attitude toward the patients and toward rehabilitation. If the attitude is one of maintaining the status quo for each patient rather than fostering his improvement, then their services will not be used. Actually some proprietary homes find it good business to keep the patient in bed, because in some states the allowance for his care is lowered if he becomes ambulatory. Most progressive homes today are finding it more important and lucrative to provide activity programs that stress the maintenance and restoration of self-help and independence.[3]

It is important to learn what recreational facilities are available to persons living in the home. If the home is a proprietary one, is it willing to pay something for entertainment? Does it have an organized activity or rehabilitation program? Is it receptive to visits from individuals who serve without pay, such as friendly visitors, American Red Cross volunteers, or other voluntary groups?[4]

Physical structure. Despite the fact that state regulations usually contain details as to space per patient and other building requirements, the state of housing in many established homes is a sorry one; these regulations seem to apply primarily to new homes as they are established. Many homes throughout the country are operated in structures that were not intended for their present purpose or have facilities that are totally inadequate by present-day standards: narrow steep stairways, lack of elevators, shortage of plumbing and heating facilities, and lack of fireproof construction or emergency exits. A myriad of questions about the physical structure could be asked: adequacy of lighting, the number and location of bathrooms, provision for privacy, recreational space, dining area, and presence or absence of conspicuous accident hazards such as slippery floors are only a few. In 1956, the Committee on Aging of the National Social Welfare Assembly sponsored an Architectural Competition on nursing homes. The results were published in the magazines *Modern Hospital* and *Architectural Record* in 1956 and thus gave help to persons building new homes. Model plans and construction and safety standards are presently available from all health departments.

Rates. A patient should understand the rates thoroughly before he enters any kind of nursing home. If the facility is under public sponsorship, a regular daily rate usually covers whatever the patient needs. The voluntary home may have a contract that states what is provided and what must be paid for additionally. Physicians' fees, personal laundry, and medications are examples of what may be charged for separately. Sometimes a down payment is required, which is held in reserve to pay for sudden needed hospitalization.

The proprietary nursing home seldom has a contract prepared, and it is necessary to determine specifically what is provided. Details such as the amount of space, single or multiple room, kind and amount of nursing, laundry, medications, use of equipment such as special beds, special diets, and barber service should be considered when rates are being arranged. If the patient's family is making the arrangements, they should be urged to obtain from the doctor specific information as to what the patient needs.

The patient's relatives may need help in selecting a suitable home in terms of cost. They should be cautioned against assuming that the most expensive home is necessarily the best one. Expensive appointments within the home are much less important than kindly, patient staff members and a homey atmosphere. Family members sometimes place the patient in an expensive home and find later that they cannot continue the payments. Changes to less attractive surroundings and to new people may be upsetting and demoralizing to the patient. Occasionally one family member acts impulsively without consulting the group, each of whom may be expected to assume a share of the financial responsibility.

Atmosphere. The right atmosphere is one of the most important things to look for in a nursing home. Atmosphere may be easy to sense yet difficult to evaluate objectively. It depends largely upon the understanding that the persons who are responsible for management and service have for the patient's basic human needs and upon their ability to translate this understanding into actual practice. Some regulations are necessary in any kind of communal living, but people who really understand and care about the patients in nursing homes realize that the frustrations they face are already enormous and try not to add to these. Respect for the dignity of the individual is essential in the creation of a good atmosphere. This may be demonstrated in the respect that is shown for the patient's privacy—the patient's right to send and receive mail unopened, to have a drawer and a cupboard that is his and that is not subject to casual inspection, to go or to stay away from religious observances. Consideration of staff members that shows attention to the individual regardless of age, infirmity, or attractiveness contributes to atmosphere. As one 84-year-old lady said, "I don't mind the dust—I can't see that, but I do mind when they don't come and talk to me."

The home that has a good atmosphere will take pride in what the patients are doing, such as the entertainment programs they plan or the committee they themselves select to determine the rules by which they all shall live. Such activities as these will have much more interest to them than a set of shiny new chairs in the hall or the waiting room.

The policy of the nursing home on visiting and its attitude toward visitors provide a clue to the basic attitudes of the staff and to the care given. Homes that really understand the patient and his needs welcome visitors and are glad that they find the time to visit. When a home discourages visitors, restricts them, and prepares patients especially to receive them, one may suspect that the real spirit of a true home is missing.

REFERENCES AND RELATED BIBLIOGRAPHY

1. Alt, Edith (project director): Standards of care for older people in institutions, sections i and ii, New York, 1953, The National Committee on the Aging, National Social Welfare Assembly.
2. ANA statement of standards for nursing care in nursing homes, New York, 1960, American Nurses Association.
3. Beaumont, William E., Jr.: ANHA, its role in improving nursing home conditions, Nurs. Homes **13**:11-12A, 21-22, 1964.
4. Bengson, Evelyn M.: A guide to planning and equipping a handicraft facility for a nursing home activity program, Washington State Health Department, Olympia, Washington, 1964.
5. Cherkasky, M.: The Montefiore home care program, Am. J. Pub. Health **39**:163-166, 1949.
6. Crawford, Eugene B., Jr.: Ambulatory services, Hospitals **39**:41-44, 1965.
7. Dolce, James A.: Raising nursing home standards; a community approach, J. Am. Geriatrics Soc. **10**:360-366, 1962.
8. Drake, Ronald A.: Accident prevention in the nursing home, Nurs. Homes **13**:11-12, 1964.
9. Elconin, A. F., and others: An organized hospital-based home care program, Am. J. Pub. Health **54**:1106-1109, 1964.
10. Graber, Joe B.: Public Health Service programs on aging, Pub. Health Rep. **79**:577-581, 1964.
11. Kovell, Joyce: A home care program for King County, Am. J. Occup. Therapy **18**:255-259, 1964.
12. Littauer, David: Home care programs. In Cowdry, E. V. (editor): The care of the geriatric patient, ed. 2, St. Louis, 1963, The C. V. Mosby Co.

13. Lovelace, Bryan, Jr.: Areawide planning for health facilities, Hospitals **39**:45-49, 1965.
14. Madden, Barbara W., and Affeldt, John E.: To prevent helplessness and deformity, Amer. J. Nurs. **62**:59-61, 1962.
15. Morris, Robert: Chronic illness and disability. In Lurie, Harry L. (editor): The encyclopedia of social work, ed. 15, New York, 1965, National Association of Social Workers.
16. Morris, Stephen M.: Long-term care, Hospitals **39**:115-119, 1965.
17. O'Connor, Paul G.: The logistics of physical therapy rehabilitation in nursing homes, Nurs. Homes **13**:5-6, 1964.
18. Ranck, Margaret: From consultant to owner, Nurs. Outlook **7**:152-153, 1959.
19. Randall, Ollie A.: Selecting a nursing home. In Cowdry, E. V. (editor): The care of the geriatric patient, ed. 2, St. Louis, 1962, The C. V. Mosby Co.
20. Reese, Dorothy Erickson (Public Health Service, U. S. Department of Health, Education and Welfare): How to be a nursing aid in a nursing home, Washington, D. C., American Nursing Home Association, 1346 Connecticut Ave., N. W.
21. Rogers, Edward S.: Medical assistance for the aged. In Lurie, Harry L. (editor): The encyclopedia of social work, ed. 15, New York, 1965, National Association of Social Workers.
22. Savage, Peggy G.: It's no longer over the hill to the poor house, Nurs. Homes **13**:7-10, 20-21, 1964.
23. Sheps, Cecil G., and Bachar, Miriam E.: Nursing medicine, emerging patterns and practice, Amer. J. Nurs. **64**:107-109, 1964.
24. Standards of care for older people in institutions. Sec. i, Suggested standards for homes for the aged and nursing homes; sec. ii, Methods of esablishing and maintaining standards in homes for the aged and nursing homes, New York, National Social Welfare Assembly, 345 East 46th St.
25. Stiefel, Joseph B.: Home care, Hosp. Progr. **45**:82-84, 1964.
26. Stoeckle, John D., and others: Medical nursing clinic for the chronically ill, Amer. J. Nurs. **63**:87-89, 1963.
27. U. S. Department of Health, Education and Welfare, Public Health Service: Areawide planning of facilities for long-term treatment and care, Report of the Joint Committee of the American Hospital Association and Public Health Service, Washington, D. C., 1963, U. S. Government Printing Office.
28. U. S. Department of Health, Education and Welfare, Public Health Service: Nursing homes and related facilities fact book, Public Health Service Publication No. 930-F-4, 1963, U. S. Government Printing Office.
29. U. S. Department of Health, Education and Welfare, National Health Survey Vital and Health Statistics: Chronic conditions and activity limitation, United States, July 1961-1963, Washington, D. C., 1963, U. S. Government Printing Office.
30. Walker, James E. C.: General clinics can serve patients better than specialty units, Hosp. Topics **42**:47-48, 1964.

Chapter 10

Care in the patient's own home

The number of chronically ill and elderly persons who are living at home cared for largely by family members and friends is much greater than the number cared for in institutions of all kinds. Studies for the period of July, 1959, to June, 1961, showed that in the United States there were approximately 19,000,000 persons who were disabled partially or totally by chronic illness and who were not in institutions. Of these, 7,000,000 or approximately 37 percent were 65 years of age and older.[16] Of the 7,000,000, one third or 2,300,000 were totally disabled. Reports for the same time show that institutions of all kinds, including mental hospitals, nursing homes, nonprofit homes for the aged, Veterans' Administration hospitals, and related institutions housed and cared for only a little over 660,000 elderly persons.

Public health nursing is not available to all chronically ill and incapacitated elderly persons living in their own homes or in substitute noninstitutionalized facilities. In 1961 only 70 percent of our cities with a population of over 25,000 had public health nursing service available.[15] No figures are available as to the situation in smaller cities and towns and rural areas, but it is known that public health nursing in the home is not available in many communities. At the present time there are approximately 35,000 nurses employed in public health nursing and about one third of these are working in schools. Because of lack of personnel, lack of financial support, and other reasons, public health nursing has not kept pace with growing and widely recognized needs.

It is apparent that a tremendous burden for the care of the aged who are chronically incapacitated is carried by the patients themselves and by their relatives. As the proportion of elderly persons increases, it is likely that the number of chronically ill aged persons who remain in their own homes will increase further. Care in his own home is generally recognized as best for the patient and best for all concerned in the majority of cases.

Some aged persons who are chronically ill are seldom seen by doctors and are unknown to nurses. This situation may change somewhat in coming years. Health counseling services in day centers for the elderly may help to inform some friends or relatives about available resources. Recent improvements in hospitalization insurance for the elderly, especially the new federal Medicare legislation, will enable more of them to enter the hospital for periods of intensive treatment. Voluntary insurance programs have experimented with providing insurance benefits for care of patients in their own homes under certain circumstances, and there are signs that this may be general practice throughout the country within a few years. This practice would give great impetus to the development of home care programs in which the patient remains under the medical supervision of the general hospital, with nursing care provided—usually on a contractual basis with a public health nursing agency. Lack of any broad insurance policy to cover medical and nursing care for the patient who is ill at home has been a major obstacle in providing adequate care. This has become a serious problem in recent years because inflation has caused a tremendous increase in service costs, whereas the income of the retired person from pensions or annuities is often fixed.

Major causes of disability in the aged include cardiovascular and renal disease, nervous and mental disease including senility, arthritis, blindness, accidents, tuberculosis and other chronic diseases of the lungs, diabetes, and cancer. The patient who remains at home may receive medical care from his private physician, from a hospital outpatient department, or from an organized home care program (Chapter 9, Housing During Illness).

The nurse has a serious responsibility to help the chronically ill patient and his family. This means that she must sharpen her teaching skills, broaden her general knowledge of resources available, and be alert to make the best use of each opportunity that arises. Nurses who work in hospital inpatient units, in the hospital clinic, and in community public health nursing agencies should all give assistance. Some patients are referred to the public health nursing agency directly from the doctor's office and are not admitted to a hospital; others visit the general hospital clinic; and many spend various lengths of time in the general hospital.

It should be the practice for the nurse in the hospital to have a review and planning conference with every chronically ill and aged patient or with his family before he leaves the hospital. This should not be a casual, "Are you ready to go home?" kind of conference, but should be planned for carefully. It should be conducted in a private conference room if the patient is in a ward with other patients. Content of the conference would vary with the particular situation. For example, it might include the following: a review of the ability to change dressings or carry out treatments as ordered by the physician; an inventory of equipment that is needed and how it may be obtained; making sure there is understanding of the nature, purpose, and frequency of exercises if they have been ordered; plans for the purchase and preparation of food; suggesting changes in living arrangements in the home that may be necessary; making future appointments at the clinic or doctor's office and giving information about the availability of the public health nurse. If there appears to be need for special services such as homemaker service, the social worker should be consulted. The patient with a chronic illness should be referred to the social worker during his hospital stay. She is the person called upon when the patient has no home or for some reason must go to a nursing home or related institution. It is well to remember that she can often give real assistance to the patient returning to his own home.

In the hospital clinic a similar conference should be conducted with the chronically ill person on his first visit, and there should be follow-up conferences as they are necessary. Conference content must be recorded on the patient's chart in order to make the best use of conference time at future visits. The practice of a formalized conference with antenatal patients during a clinic visit has long been accepted as good clinic nursing. The realization that this is just as necessary for the chronically ill patient has been slow to find favor in medical and nursing care in hospital outpatient departments.

SPECIFIC ASSISTANCE TO FAMILIES

Specific assistance can be discussed here only in general terms and illustrated with a few examples. Each situation is different, and each patient is an individual. Much of the nurse's success will depend upon her interest, her imagination, and her resourcefulness. At the risk of appearing repetitious, it is emphasized again that *all* nurses share this responsibility. Too often the public health nurse is called when the patient and his family are in serious difficulty. She may arrive in the home to find that unsuitable although costly supplies have been bought, that errors in treatment have been made, and that the family's confidence in their ability to manage has been severely shaken. Many unhappy situations could be avoided if the nurse in the hospital would review the situation, consult with the doctor and the patient, and make the referral to the public health nurse *early*, before the patient is about to leave the hospital. The public health nurse may then either visit the patient in the hospital or visit the family and plan with them for his return home.

Assistance to the family in planning. Careful planning when the patient leaves the hospital or when he first becomes ill at home helps to prevent difficulties later on. Family members should be encouraged to discuss together their common problem and joint responsibilities and not to forget that the patient's wishes should be considered also. They should, at this time, face their own feelings realistically. Sometimes this requires the assistance of a psychiatrist or of a medical social worker. For example, if a son or daughter is obviously emotionally unstable and unable to face illness or impending death, it may be better for him to contribute financially instead of housing the patient and giving the necessary care. All legally responsible relatives should be encouraged to contribute in some way. This forestalls the tendency for one family member, who may have an unconscious desire to be a martyr, to assume all or too much of the burden. Vacations or periodic rest for the person tied down with the physical care of the patient, the cost of changed living arrangements or housing, the extra cost of food and drugs, and the cost of special equipment are examples of matters that should be considered.

Elderly couples often show a real reluctance to turn to their children when one member becomes chronically ill. There are probably many reasons for this. They may appreciate their children's need to maintain high standards of living in our culture, and they may feel that their own period of usefulness to their children is over, that they can only be a burden. A lack of close understanding and an estrangement may occur when in-laws are of different nationalities or come from distant geographic locations. The recent trend toward larger families is another cause. Old people often comment that their children have too many problems of their own. Brothers, sisters, and cousins can sometimes help; some of them have a need to be needed and welcome an opportunity to help relatives of their own age.

A carefully conducted conference by a professionally prepared person will usually reveal financial worries when chronic illness occurs. It is really amazing how poorly informed some elderly people are about their financial rights as citizens. Some live in a tiny world of their own, and, despite the numbers of newspapers published, they are quite uninformed on such matters as the social security laws. One elderly lady who fainted on the street and was admitted to the hospital with a diagnosis of malnutrition had been living meagerly on savings since the death of her husband ten years before. She had almost exhausted her savings but had no idea that she was eligible for old-age assistance or that such a thing even existed. She did not know about her husband's social security coverage, which entitled her to a small income monthly. Some elderly couples who are receiving old-age assistance do not know that there are special allowances for persons with disability to which one member may be entitled when he becomes chronically ill. One 79-year-old lady continued to care for her bedfast and incontinent 83-year-old sister, doing all laundry by hand in an old-fashioned bathtub until she collapsed. She firmly believed that her own home would be taken from her if she sought public assistance for her sister.

The patient and his relatives need to know what community resources are available to them. For example, homemaker service is badly needed by some aged couples if or when one of them becomes ill. This service is developing rapidly throughout the country and is described in a booklet published by the Children's Bureau[13] and in a bulletin published by the American Medical Association.[1] In many communities it has been used almost exclusively to keep families with small children together in the event of illness of the mother. Its value for the aged is becoming widely recognized. One community* has developed a homemaker service primarily because of the needs of the aged, although it serves all age groups.

The patient should know what public health nursing service is available and how he goes about obtaining this service. In most communities the patient or his family may initiate the request for the public health nurse, but he must be under a doctor's care. It is customary for the nurse to get in touch with the doctor before visiting his patient in order to verify orders and obtain general information that will be useful.

American National Red Cross Motor Corps service is available in many communities to take patients to and from hospital clinics, doctor's offices, and the like. In most instances the original request must come through a public health

*Summit, N. J.

nursing or local welfare agency. Local chapters of the American Cancer Society render an extremely valuable service in many communities by supplying clean, unsterile dressings for patients with cancer; usually the original request for dressings must come through a doctor's office or public health nursing or other public agency. Portable meals are being provided in more and more communities each year, and the nurse must know whether this service is available in her community and how it is secured. Some communities have established sheltered workshops, in which elderly persons can engage in full- or part-time productive activities, or have opened shops to sell the products made by chronically ill persons in their own homes. The community health council or similar coordinating agency in a large city and the county or local health department in smaller communities are good sources of information for nurses in their efforts to give clear, accurate information.

Relatives often need help and guidance so that they will not overdo and thereby lessen their usefulness to the patient. Sometimes their solicitude is too great in the beginning, but is not sustained during a long-term illness. At other times they continue to insist upon doing too much themselves and become so worn out that their emotional reactions are most unfortunate for all concerned. Several publications are available that may be useful to family members. They include the *Red Cross Home Nursing Textbook*, prepared by the Nursing Service of the American National Red Cross, *Home Nursing and Medical Care* by I. J. Rossman and Doris Schwartz, and *You and Your Aging Parents* by Mabel Stern. The state division of mental hygiene can often supply helpful pamphlets and booklets that have been prepared by insurance companies such as the John Hancock Mutual Life Insurance Co. and the Metropolitan Life Insurance Co. These pamphlets deal with the care of patients in the home and are available without charge. Many organizations such as the American Heart Association and the American Cancer Society have free pamphlets available to patients and to their families.

In addition to reading publications, many family members need very badly to have some person, such as a social worker or a nurse who is outside the family circle, with whom they can discuss their actual situation and what it means to them.

Understanding the patient's behavior. Family members are sometimes shocked and deeply hurt because a chronically ill family member seems not to appreciate but to resent their solicitous care. They must be helped to understand why the patient behaves as he does. By far the best treatment for the irritability and resentment that any chronically ill person feels at his limitations is to help him develop the ability to care for himself, particularly in meeting his most personal needs, such as eating, using the bathroom, and getting in and out of bed (Chapter 11, Rehabilitation). Family members who direct their efforts toward helping the patient to help himself are often amazed to discover how much happier the patient becomes and how much better the entire situation is for all the family.

Actually, one can never truly put himself in another's place and know exactly how the other person feels. There is ample evidence, however, that the limitations in meeting basic personality needs (Chapter 3, Basic Sociopsychologic

Needs) that chronic illness imposes are usually extremely difficult for the patient to face without experiencing serious traumatic effects on the personality. The chronically ill aged person may wish to participate in life around him as much as persons who are well; yet it is a fact that chronic illness imposes serious obstacles.

Thoughtfulness in planning family activities often helps. For instance, it is sometimes possible to have several chairs in the patient's room so that family members may form the habit of gathering there for a time each evening. Here conversation should not center around the patient but should deal with general family matters; this helps to keep the patient from feeling out of things. Bringing samples of food and a complete verbal report from outdoor excursions and other social gatherings also helps to allay the resentment that is felt when the chronically ill family member cannot attend. As one old lady said to the niece with whom she lived, "Yes, you're going to a picnic again, but I'm not going to a picnic, I'm just going to die here." Vacations and outings for persons who are tied down with care of the chronically ill patient are surely necessary, but provision must also be made for the care of the patient left at home. Plans should be made for someone who is completely familiar with the situation to be in attendance, and special food or other special treats may also be planned. The literature mentioned previously is useful to the nurse and to the family members in discussing individual reactions of patients.

Teaching physical care. Family members can learn to give physical care from several sources. They can learn from the hospital nurse at the bedside of the patient in the general hospital, provided that visiting rules are flexible and provision is made for this in the nursing program in hospitals. It appears to be an unfortunate reality that the larger the hospital and the higher its standards so far as some medical aspects are concerned, the more formal its organization becomes and the less communication there is between family members and the nursing staff. Visiting hours, for example, are looked upon often as a time when nurses can have hours off or "catch up on charting or other desk work." They are seldom viewed as an opportunity for the nurse to get to know those who may be responsible for the patient when he leaves the hospital.

There is real need for serious studies of priorities in nursing functions in hospitals, with emphasis upon what things must come first in meeting total patient needs both during hospitalization and in preparation for his continued care.

Family members can learn about care of the patient with chronic illness from the nurse in the hospital clinic, provided the clinic is set up with this as an accepted and planned-for part of the nurse's function and provided the nurse herself has orientation to this phase of her work. At the present time, the majority of outpatient clinics are so designed, operated, and staffed that the nurse seems to spend most of her time directing traffic and keeping mechanical details in order so that the clinic operates smoothly. She may be so concerned with keeping the physicians' equipment in order and maintaining a steady flow of patients that she scarcely sees the individual patient, much less knows about his nursing needs.

Family members are often taught by the public health nurse in the home.

This is the most widely used method at the present time, although it is known that there are not enough public health nurses to give all the instruction that is needed. More organized and effective early teaching by nurses in the hospital followed by additional instruction and supervision in the home would probably lead to better care for patients and more efficient use of the limited public health nursing time available.

The American National Red Cross has rendered a valuable service in preparing an instructor's guide for the Red Cross home nursing instructor in teaching care of the aging and chronically ill.[2] Courses such as those in home nursing offered by the American National Red Cross are extremely helpful to family members who will have to care for a chronically ill person.

If possible, the patient who is confined to bed for all or most of the time should be downstairs. This saves steps for the persons providing care and makes the patient feel more a part of the family. Patients confined to upstairs rooms often complain that they are put away and isolated. On the other hand, arrangements should not be such that normal social life for the rest of the family is restricted by making a bedroom out of the main living room. If possible, the patient's bed should face a window; shades can be drawn if there is too much light.

Body mechanics. It often becomes the nurse's responsibility to teach family members how to move and lift a helpless person. It is important that the younger person understand body mechanics so that she may avoid injury and have energy left to devote to the rest of the family. The principles of body mechanics are the same as those that apply in care of the patient in the hospital and should be so familiar to the nurse that she can protect herself from injury and demonstrate them to family members with ease.

It is important that moving and lifting the elderly person be done with as little effort as possible. Apparent difficulty in these procedures increases the patient's feeling of helplessness. Before turning, lifting, or moving the patient, the nurse should take time to explain to him what she proposes to do. This will prevent needless fear and tension that might interfere with the ease of moving the patient.

A few basic principles of body mechanics must be understood in order that one work effectively. The correct application of these principles will prevent back strain and general fatigue. An object should never be lifted when it can be drawn or moved. Lifting means that the entire weight is raised against gravity, whereas in moving only friction or resistance must be over overcome. This principle is applicable to such activities as raising the patient in bed and drawing him to the side of the bed. An example of poor application of the principle is the common habit of reaching across the patient and lifting his hips in an attempt to center his body in the bed. The nurse should reach completely under the patient, bend her knees, and draw the patient toward her.

In correct standing posture, a line passing through the ear, the shoulder, the hip, and outer malleolus of the ankle represents the line through which weight falls. The base of support can be increased and improved in stability by placing the feet well apart, as is commonly done by workmen in anticipation of heavy lifting. Any pull exerted to draw the body from its base of support alters the center of gravity and, to prevent complete loss of balance, is compensated for by muscular effort. The result may be muscle fatigue and muscle and joint strain if the pull has been excessive. Hence the need to hold heavy objects close to the body as, for example, when raising the foot of the bed on shock blocks or when lifting or assisting the patient to a wheelchair.

The nurse will save herself much fatigue if she remembers to use the heavy muscles of the thighs for lifting and moving, instead of the smaller muscles of the arms and shoulders. In order to lift, she must assume a squatting position, with the back straight and the knees and hips bent. She must lift by rising to a standing position, making use of the strong muscles of the legs, thighs, and pelvic girdle and not lift directly with her arms, which should be used mainly to steady the object lifted. To move an object, use the same principles. The nurse must bend the hips and knees and stabilize the pelvis by tightening the abdominal muscles. With her arms well under the object, she can draw it toward her, again using her arms chiefly to grasp the object. Work is mainly accomplished in this instance by a shift of position assisted by momentum as the nurse's weight is transmitted from the forward foot to the back foot. To raise the patient's head, replace a pillow, turn the patient on his side, or move him to the side of the bed, the nurse should remember to move rhythmically, make use of momentum, stand near the bed, and bend the knees slightly to take strain off the lower back.

Working with the trunk bent forward places an excessive strain on the back muscles and ligaments. To avoid this the nurse should do her work at a comfortable and efficient arm level, standing, sitting, or stooping with the trunk erect. Stooping rather than bending to adjust a footstool is an example of correct use of the body.

When continuous bedside care must be given to a patient in the home, it is more satisfactory to raise the bed to a suitable work level than to stoop each time it is necessary to care for the patient. Beds can be raised effectively by removing the castors and mounting the bed on blocks. The only disadvantage is that the older person, if forgetful, is likely to attempt to get out of bed during the night and may fall from the high bed and injure himself. Beds that can be mechanically raised and lowered can be purchased or rented for home use in many communities.

Medications. It is not unusual for the elderly person who is chronically ill to have half a dozen or more medications prescribed to be taken daily. Recently it has been found that a really alarming number of errors are made by patients administering their own medications.[11] The nurse in the hospital or in the patient's home should anticipate this problem and plan with the patient so that medications will be administered as prescribed. Carefully written instructions can be given to the patient if the medicine is obtained while he is still in the hospital. In the home the nurse should check all medicine bottles carefully to see that the dispensing instructions are understood by the patient and that he has an appropriate system for assuring that they are being carried out accurately. A chart or large calendar with room for writing is helpful for some patients, particularly when they are receiving drugs such as hormones or diuretics that may be prescribed to be taken for several days and then discontinued for several days. Many elderly persons find it useful to establish a particular time of day, such as when preparing for bed or at the breakfast hour, as the time to take medicine regularly; sometimes, though, this method is not effective, since, for example, the elderly person may not recall at the end of an evening's preparation for retiring whether or not he took the drug. Often more accuracy can be obtained if the patient places the drugs for one day in a glass and sets it in a conspicuous place, such as by the kitchen sink or at his place at table.

The elderly person caring for himself at home or the close family member, who may be elderly also, should be encouraged to write down any particular responses the patient has or believes he has to medications taken. General symptoms may also be recorded. Many persons forget to mention symptoms when they see the doctor or else are uncertain as to their time of occurrence and their duration. Such events as spells of dizziness, sudden nausea, falls, or bouts of diarrhea should be noted briefly with the date included.

Obtaining and selecting equipment. Nurses should know about community resources through which the patient at home may borrow or obtain equipment that is needed. Sometimes equipment must be rented from supply houses or other similar establishments. More often it is available on a loan basis from a variety of agencies such as the local public health nursing agency, the volunteer ambulance or "rescue squad" service, or one of several women's groups.

Hospital beds may be purchased or may be borrowed on a long-term basis if the patient's illness is likely to be a long one. High-low beds are very expensive but may now be borrowed. If a firmer foundation than the mattress provides is needed, bed boards should be used. Pieces of lumber three fourths to one inch thick are best for this. The bed should be examined and measured. Boards must rest on metal cross pieces at top or bottom or metal pieces on the sides; they must not rest on the springs since this will give poor support and will damage the springs. The boards sold by supply houses are often made of thin plywood or plasterboard material that sag under normal weight. If they are to be used, their length must be carefully checked since some are too short to be effective. Adjustable or high-low beds cost about three times as much as regular hospital beds, but they are extremely useful since they can be raised to accommodate the height of the person giving care and thus prevent much physical strain; they can be lowered to a normal bed height at other times.

Bed rails can be rented or bought; they cost from $25 to $50. They are difficult to improvise in the home. Boards on the sides of the bed are unsatisfactory in that they prevent the patient from seeing about.

The mattress should be firm and covered with heavy ticking. Sponge rubber mattresses are good, particularly for very old, debilitated patients, for patients who are paralyzed from a disease such as carcinoma involving the spine, and for patients sensitive to dust or hair. They do not give a patient as good support for leverage for moving about independently as a firmer mattress, and their odor is distasteful to some people. The mattress must be protected from soiling. Rubber sheeting or one of the thinner plastic materials may be used. Shower curtains or pieces of oilcloth can also be used. Care must be taken not to have seams in the center of the bed since they may be uncomfortable for the patient and may not protect adequately from enuresis or wash water spilled accidentally. Contour sheets give a firm fit to the lower sheet if they can be used properly, but they do not permit the top sheet to be changed to the bottom, which saves linen. Drawsheets can be made from sheeting bought by the yard. Usually, however, a standard bed sheet can be folded and used for a drawsheet as is done in many hospitals. Cotton flannel bath blankets used as sheets are often comfortable for the patient. These also may be used as rolls or pads to maintain the patient in good body alignment.

Enamel basins are more satisfactory than the plastic ones, which spill easily and tend to retain odors. The bath basin must be large enough to soak the patient's feet comfortably. Enamelware is perfectly satisfactory for urinals, emesis basins, and bedpans used in the home and is much cheaper than stainless steel utensils.

Commodes can be borrowed from a community resource such as the public health nursing agency, rented, or improvised in the home. Lightweight portable and collapsible commodes made of aluminum are available and are cheaper than the box-type ones made of wood. Any family member with a little carpentry skill can improvise a commode from an old chair. The chair should, if possible, have arms, and the height should permit the patient to rest his feet firmly on the floor. The simplest commode is made by removing the caning or any soft seat material, nailing a piece of board over the seat of the chair, and cutting a suitable opening in this. A bucket that can rest on the floor is then all that is needed. A more easily moved commode is made from a chair with a cross stretcher on which the bedpan or other receptacle may be placed; the receptacle may be secured with pieces of wood attached to the chair legs or the seat. Wooden grooves into which the pan can be slid can be attached to the underside of the chair seat. The appearance of the commode may be improved by adding a hinged seat, which can be lowered when the chair is not in use. Waterproof chintz, used for a ruffled drape around the lower part of the chair, makes this improvised commode a respectable piece of furniture in the patient's room.

Panties that have snap fasteners, zippers, or lacing at the sides are available from commercial companies for use by incontinent patients. Most of them have a pocket for an inner lining of disposable cotton. Commercial companies also supply bed liners or large disposable pads that can be used directly on the bed under the patient or inside panties if the patient is up and about. These devices are quite expensive for use by the long-term patient. Panties can be made at home by anyone who has even a moderate amount of sewing skill. In fact, panties made by family members usually fit the patient better than those purchased. They should fit rather snugly and have elastic around each leg and at the waist. If a waterproof lining is used, it should turn outward at the leg openings so that the edge does not become dampened, which would require frequent changing. These panties, laced and knotted at the waist, are sometimes quite effective for a senile person who is untidy in his personal habits and inclined to soil himself and his surroundings after defecation. This patient usually has poor hand coordination and does not untie knots easily. The cotton lining must be changed frequently. Large rolls can be obtained much more cheaply than when pads are bought already cut and ready for use.

Gauze is available in 10-yard, unsterile rolls from which small dressings can be made by the patient's family. They can be taught to wrap the dressings in paper and bake them in the oven at 350° F. to make them sterile for use. Thicker cotton dressings or abdominal pads are also available in rolls and can be cut and cared for in the same way.

Much equipment is available or can be improvised to help the patient maintain good body alignment, be fairly active, and take care of many of his personal needs. There should be a footboard on the bed if he spends many hours in bed. This should be adjusted to the patient's length so that he may push his feet firmly against it to obtain foot and leg exercise. A sandbag in a box or a board at the end of the mattress merely keeps covers off the feet. A wooden box such as an orange crate can be cut down and can sometimes be supported firmly with blocks to withstand pressure from the patient's feet. The best foot support for any patient is made individually for him and consists of a firm board from which supports extend to rest against the foot of the bed.

A bed table may enable the patient to wash his face, feed himself, shave, and enjoy recreational activities that may be impossible if he must hold equipment in his hands or twist sideways to use a table beside the head of the bed. Adjustable tables similar to those used in operating rooms are very helpful. A wooden box such as an orange crate can be made satisfactory by knocking out the two side panels. An ironing board, particularly if it is the adjustable kind, makes an excellent overbed table. The leaf of a dining room table or a piece of smooth lumber can rest on the backs of two chairs placed on either side of the bed.

Metal walkers without wheels can be purchased for less than $20 for use by

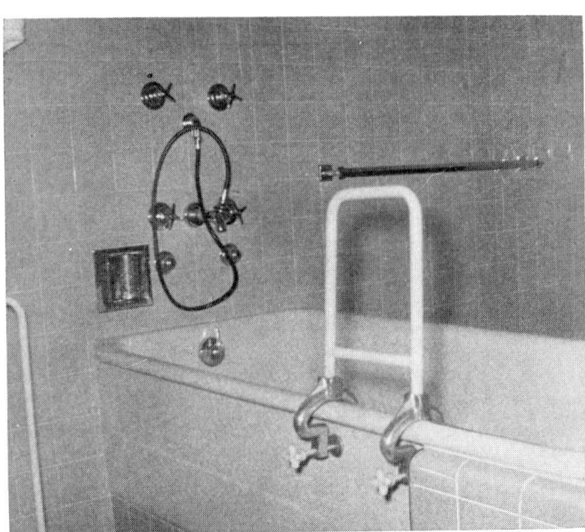

Figure 20. Lifeguard appliance attached to the side of a tub. (From Gubersky, Blanche D.: In Cowdry, E. V. [editor]: Care of the geriatric patient, St. Louis, 1958, The C. V. Mosby Co. Courtesy Miss Gubersky and the Home for Aged and Infirm Hebrews of New York.)

a person whose gait is unsteady. Lightweight folding wheelchairs can be purchased at a relatively reasonable cost and permit easy transportation of helpless persons in and out of cars, up steps, and the like. There are many kinds of wheelchairs—some are intended purely for use outdoors, and others are for indoor use. Family members should be advised to investigate thoroughly before making purchases. For example, a collapsible wheelchair may not be secure enough for a heavy patient, and it may not provide as good support as the more conventional wooden one.

Small alterations in and about the home may help the patient to be independent. Metal rails installed on the walls around the bathtub and bars such as the Lifeguard with two hand grips clamped to the side of the tub may enable the patient to handle himself safely. Armrests can be attached to toilets to provide safety and security. Ramps can sometimes be built either at the back or front door, and thus the chronically ill person is able to get outdoors. A firm wooden rail should be built along the ramp if the patient is ambulatory.

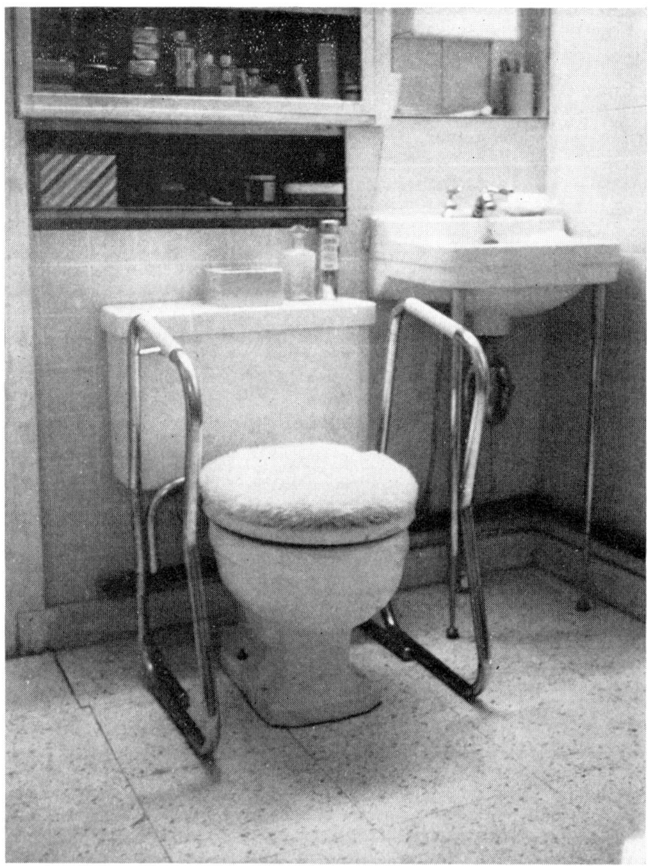

Figure 21. Improvised or available manufactured bars at the toilet contribute to the independence and safety of the infirm or disabled person at home.

The chronically ill person usually spends a good deal of time sitting. He should have at least one chair that is comfortable and that meets his particular needs. When he is at the dining room table, he should be so seated that he may safely lean on the table as he gets up. Many individual adjustments have to be made for each patient. For example, a patient who has joints that are ankylosed in a sitting position may be better able to get into a chair that does not have arms as he attempts to get out of bed. A patient who has stiff knees or who must wear a back brace is often helped by using a stick with a hook on the end of it or a tiny dustpan and broom to pick up small articles that have dropped to the floor.

Family members need help in planning and preparing meals, particularly when special diets must be prepared. Occasionally a patient enjoys being different and causing extra trouble in preparation of food, but usually foods can be prepared as for the rest of the family, with minor adjustment. Food planning and preparation are discussed in Chapter 7, Nutrition.

Family members who care for ill relatives at home must sometimes be cautioned about buying gadgets that are of little use and are often costly. For example, commercial devices are now available that are fixed to the bed yet enable the patient to sit up on the side of the bed. This may have advantages over getting the patient out of bed and into a comfortable chair beside the bed in certain circumstances, but these are rare. Special devices for lifting patients have limited usefulness in many homes when space is limited.

REFERENCES AND RELATED BIBLIOGRAPHY

1. American Medical Association Council on Medical Services in cooperation with the Executive Committee of the National Conference on Homemaker Services: Homemaker services bulletin, first issue, 1960.
2. American National Red Cross: American Red Cross home nursing care of the aging and chronically ill instructor's guide, Washington, D. C.
3. Austin, Catherine L.: The basic six needs of the aging, Nurs. Outlook **7**:138-141, 1959.
4. Delagi, E. F., and others: Rehabilitation of the homebound in a semi-rural area; a two-year experience with 120 patients, J. Chron. Dis. **12**:568-576, 1960.
5. Henley, Barbara M.: Helping the elderly find community services, Amer. J. Nurs. **63**:89-92, 1963.
6. Jaschick, Eva, and Olsen, Catherine: Nursing care of the arthritic patient at home, Amer. J. Nurs. **55**:429-432, 1955.
7. Kurtagh, Cathryn H.: Which bed to buy, Amer. J. Nurs. **58**:208-210, 1958.
8. Morgan, Elizabeth M.: A push, anyone? Amer. J. Nurs. **58**:821-833, 1958.
9. Randall, Ollie A., and others: The problem of extended illness and old age, Amer. J. Nurs. **54**:1220-1225, 1954.
10. Rossman, I. J., and Schwartz, Doris R.: The family handbook of home nursing and medical care, New York, 1958, Random House, Inc.
11. Schwartz, Doris: Medication errors made by aged patients, Amer. J. Nurs. **62**:51-53, 1962.
12. Shanas, Ethel: Family relationships of older people, Research Series No. 20, New York, 1961, Health Information Foundation.
13. U. S. Department of Health, Education and Welfare, Social Security Administration: Children's Bureau Folder No. 46-1958.
14. U. S. Department of Health, Education and Welfare: Health manpower source book, section 18, manpower in the 1960's, U. S. Public Health Service, Washington, D. C., 1964, U. S. Government Printing Office.
15. U. S. Department of Health, Education and Welfare: Report on nursing care of the sick

at home, Public Health Service Publication No. 901, 1962, U. S. Government Printing Office.

16. U. S. Department of Health, Education and Welfare, Public Health Service National Health Survey: Chronic conditions causing limitation of activities, United States, July, 1959–June, 1961, Health Statistics Series B-No. 36, 1962, U. S. Government Printing Office.
17. Wiles, Margaret: Financing nursing care of the sick at home, Nurs. Outlook **9**:687-691, 1961.

Chapter 11

Rehabilitation

The nurse must be concerned with rehabilitation of the older patient. Rehabilitation of an aging population has been named as one of the most important problems confronting our society today, and recent active interest in the subject is one of the most hopeful signs of our generation. Rehabilitation means the restoration of the individual to the greatest personal, social, and economic usefulness and independence of which he is capable. Lifelong maintenance of good physical, mental, and social habits is the best preventive measure, for it may help to avoid the need for more intensive rehabilitation later in life.

Gradual loss of functional ability is the hardest burden that aging persons must bear. Awareness of decreasing physical abilities usually begins in the early fifties when, for example, a person becomes aware of using stair railings, pausing before stepping off a curb, or stopping part way up a flight of stairs. Eyes begin to lose accommodation ability, and reading glasses or bifocals are needed. At about the same time it may be noticed that a whole day spent with small children, groups of friends, or relatives is wearing, and behavior that once was accepted becomes irritating. A woman may postpone inviting friends for dinner or invite them only for dessert and coffee to conserve her energy. Often these changes are only slowly progressive and are not particularly troublesome even at 65 or 70 years of age until or unless an acute illness or an emotional or social crisis occurs. Adaptation to many such situations becomes more difficult and may exhaust the old person's energy reserve temporarily.

Many chronic ailments exaggerate and add to the older person's declining functional abilities, but may not result in a complete loss of function. Maintenance of physical, mental, and social functional abilities and capacities requires their continuous use. How to conserve and budget energy is one of the most valuable lessons the aging can learn. If learned and applied, this practice can help a person live more fully and happily and also prevent or delay deterioration.

The need to maintain all possible function becomes increasingly important when an acute illness, accident, or chronic disease occurs. When a patient is confined to bed at home or in the hospital, as pointed out in other chapters, the effects of inactivity become apparent within a few days and may compound the disabilities that result from the injury or illness.

Restoration of the organic capacity for function may take time. But while caring for the elderly person the nurse should keep constantly in mind that the goal of therapy is rehabilitation—the achievement of functional ability. Within the limits imposed by the therapy essential for recovery, she should provide for and encourage maximum use of the affected and unaffected parts or organs. If the medical plan does not clearly indicate the extent to which physical, social, or other activities may be encouraged, the nurse should ask the physician to define the essential limitations imposed by the primary diagnosis and any other health problems. Many physicians today assume that preventive measures and activities will be provided in the nursing care of the patient as automatically as are cleanliness, comfort, and other basic care needs. Other physicians may not, but when approached with a request for guidance or a plan of nursing care that includes active therapy, may readily give permission or specific orders for such nursing care.

Depending upon the resources of the institution or community, special therapy in addition to rehabilitative nursing may be prescribed. Whether this specific care is physical, occupational, recreational, speech, psychiatric, or other therapy, the nurse should cooperatively plan her care to supplement or complement it. Coordination of care is essential in order to bring to the patient the maximum benefits of total therapy. Immediate salvation for many of our aged patients lies in control of their chronic ills and in rehabilitation services for their restoration as self-sufficient individuals and perhaps useful members to society.

Rehabilitation of the chronically ill older person may sometimes make employment possible and will often enable the person to live fairly happily and still contribute socially. Many times, if it cannot make him employable, it may make him more independent in meeting his personal needs and spare him the experience of being a burden to his family or to others. Many individuals are placed in institutions because the care they need at home is such that a family member would have to stop outside work if the patient remained at home, or because there is no one in the home who is physically able to give the necessary care. If the patient can learn to care for his personal needs, he can often remain in his own home and with his family.

The average cost of rehabilitation or restorative services is difficult to determine, but the cost of rehabilitation is thought to be considerably less than the cost of one year of custodial care. The nonmonetary values to the patient and potentially to society are so great that every patient should be considered a possible candidate for rehabilitation. If even the smallest amount of self-care can be learned, the patient should be given hope and encouragement as to his future. Teaching self-care or the activities of daily living is rehabilitation in its best sense, even when no more can be taught because of the patient's age and his disabilities.

The concept and practice of rehabilitation is not new. There are evidences that the ancient medical practitioners of Egypt and Greece showed remarkable ingenuity in improvising substitutes for absent body parts and knew the basic principles of rehabilitation. What is new about rehabilitation is that the fragmentary services of the past have been replaced by a unified team approach to the problems of each patient. Success in rehabilitation depends upon teamwork. Many people and many agencies are needed to get the patient back to maximum self-sufficiency. The nurse, to function effectively, must be an active part of the team. She must know the goal for each patient and share responsibility with persons in physical medicine, social service, occupational therapy, psychotherapy, vocational rehabilitation, and others for helping the patient achieve it.

Rehabilitation of the aged must often be carried out in the general hospital, the nursing home, or other sheltered-care facility, or in the patient's own home and without the personnel and equipment of the specialized rehabilitation center. This is because specialized centers are still not available to the majority of aged patients in spite of a large increase in their numbers during the last five years. The rehabilitation team may, therefore, be available for only a short time on a consultation or part-time basis, if at all. The nurse must often rely upon her own resources and must sometimes teach techniques that in large centers are taught by specialized workers such as physical therapists. In the large center, self-care activities carried on at the bedside are usually taught by nurses with the assistance of an occupational therapist, whereas the techniques needed to climb stairs and open doors when a patient uses crutches are taught by a physical therapist. In the patient's home or the small nursing home, the nurse may teach all these activities.

The past ten years have been ones of rapid increase in the number of rehabilitation centers and improved care facilities for the aged that provide such services. Impetus was given by the passage of the *Community Health Services and Facilities Act* of 1961, which increased the provisions and appropriations for construction of rehabilitation facilities, hospitals, and nursing homes. Programs to promote the improvement and increase of services and research and to raise the number of trained personnel for care of the aging have expanded in the United States Public Health Service, the Vocational Rehabilitation Administration, and the Welfare Administration. Greater emphasis is being placed on the needs of the older disabled worker, the recipients of Old Age and Survivors Disability Insurance, and the healthy aged. Many out-of-hospital services for the aged and chronically ill have been stimulated and assisted by federal grants. These include coordinated home care programs, half-way houses, and foster home care. The home care and nursing home programs that focus on rehabilitation supplement the still insufficient hospital and special facilities services. An increasing number of consultant services by qualified rehabilitative nursing specialists, physical and occupational therapists, and others are available to nurses through state and local health agencies. The nurse in a local health agency or community hospital or nursing home no longer needs to feel that she must depend entirely upon her own resources. The nurse still is and will probably continue to be the professional worker who provides the bulk of rehabilitative care to the elderly both in and out of specialized centers. Physical and emotional readiness are being given more attention as important prerequisites for intensive rehabilitation, as is the patient's motivation to participate in his own care. Helping him attain these is a nursing responsibility. More activities such as teaching or supervising the activities of daily living, ambulation, and recreation are being shared or interchangeably carried out by nurses and physical and occupational therapists. Particularly in geriatric rehabilitation, the concern of all professional persons is not so much who provides the special services but that they are provided on a continuing basis.

The nurse needs good basic knowledge and good judgment to seek appropriate assistance as necessary and to carry out her responsibilities. Geriatric rehabilitation offers wide opportunities to nurses for the fullest use of their professional talents.

REHABILITATION OF THE GERIATRIC PATIENT

Rehabilitation for aged patients differs in several ways from that for younger patients. Long-term objectives may be different. Although these should not alter the positive approach and the application of basic principles in the least, from a practical standpoint they do affect the time and money that can be expended.

The elderly patient may have several chronic ailments, and this places an added burden upon the doctor in charge and upon the nursing staff to observe the patient closely for sudden changes in general health. Unusual dyspnea, change in color, dizziness, change in quality of the pulse after normal exertion, and complaints of pain or discomfort are symptoms and signs that there may be an impending exacerbation of a chronic illness or that maximum physical capacity has been reached. This is especially true when active exercise or social programs are being undertaken. Studies of the physical energy output that can be expected in elderly patients are limited. One study[11] showed that none of the study group of patients had more than 70 percent of the predicted normal vital capacity, whereas the vital capacity of the majority of patients was below 50 percent of the anticipated normal. Despite individual potentials to make enormous adjustments to bodily changes, it is obvious that the margin of safety in supplying the oxygen so necessary for safe cardiac action was small in this group of patients. It is no wonder that some very old people find that dressing themselves and attending to a few other personal needs is an entire morning's work.

Perhaps the most important difference in geriatric rehabilitation is that older patients may need more encouragement and more stimulation than younger ones. Many elderly patients have withdrawn almost completely from association with others, and with this withdrawal has gone the normal desire to do for themselves and to be independent. Sometimes it is necessary to work intensively to develop the patient's sense of personal worth before any steps toward rehabilitation can be taken. This is now termed the *repersonalization* of the patient; he must learn again to think of himself as a personality and as an individual. It has been found that the will of the patient (based upon his own feelings about himself) is the most important element in rehabilitation; without it no amount of skill in teaching technical procedures and no amount of special equipment is effective.

Repersonalization can be accomplished only by the earnest efforts of every member of the rehabilitation team, including all auxiliary nursing personnel who help in patient care. Some large institutions have a part-time or resident psychiatrist to work with members of the staff and with patients in meeting

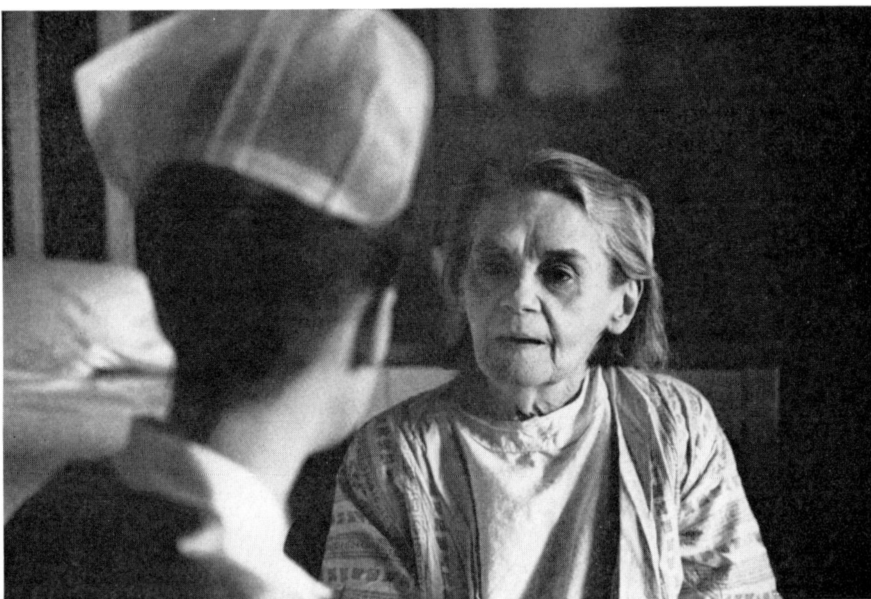

Figure 22. A nurse can help to restore the patient's sense of personal worth and strengthen the will, which are essential elements for achieving rehabilitation. (Courtesy American Journal of Nursing; photograph by Robert Goldstein.)

personality needs. This is extremely helpful. Much can also be accomplished if all nursing personnel will analyze their procedures, their routines, and their conduct toward patients. They should constantly ask such questions as: "How can this routine be changed to stress the individuality of each patient?" "Is this what I would like if I were in the patient's situation and circumstances?" "How can we change this procedure to foster the patient's feeling of importance?"

The older patient becomes discouraged, particularly when he is attempting to learn (or relearn) skills after a long period of dependence and inactivity. As one elderly lady said, "I don't know why I try really. It's not that I'm morbid, but so many who are younger and more useful have been taken." This comment is typical of the thinking of many aged patients and must be compensated for by real interest and encouragement from persons who work with them. Competitive activity is sometimes used, but must be used with care, as disappointment and frustration may sometimes follow when persons cannot succeed as fast as their colleagues. New abilities bring new desires that may be beyond achievement. Unless careful treatment is given, retreat and regression may occur.

NURSING RESPONSIBILITIES IN REHABILITATION

The nurse has several distinct functions in rehabilitation. These functions, in varying degrees, are components of good nursing care of any patient and should not be reserved for the patient identified especially as one who is being rehabilitated.

One of the most important and most often neglected functions of nursing in rehabilitation is that of assessment of the patient's condition, abilities, and disabilities. This should be done by the nurse despite the fact that assessments are also made by the physician and others of the rehabilitation team. Each views the patient in different perspective. The sum of their observations is a more reliable and more complete appraisal on which to base judgments and plans. If the patient has a family or companions with whom he lives, they too should be assessed for their abilities to participate in the total care plan. Often the social case worker participates actively in this, but the nurse should take every opportunity available to get to know the patient's relatives and friends and thus be able to add appropriately to the assessment.

It may take very little time to assess the patient's physical abilities and health practices. It will take a longer period of observation and interaction to appraise how he feels about his illness, how he views himself, his behavior, and his wants. The nurse is in an enviable position to learn to know the patient and his family well and thus can often interpret the patient's reactions, aspirations, and needs to other team members who know him less well.

Because nursing is a continuous service, nurses must consider all of the patient's needs. The nurse acts as a coordinator of services to assure not only that the patient's specific therapeutic needs are met, but also that they are equated with his other health needs. Unless the basic needs for food, elimination, rest, sleep, and comfort are met, the value of special treatments will be greatly decreased. Some people cannot be rushed and rarely can be held to a strict appointment schedule. Some must rest after a short period of activity. The nurse must be flexible and able to adjust and individualize care. However, she must keep the program for each patient directed toward the goals he has helped to set. The nurse fosters, maintains, and encourages emotional responses and attitudes that enable the patient to want to help himself. The patient and all persons who work with him must think of what he can do and what he will be able to do. It is useless and demoralizing to dwell even briefly on the activities that are permanently beyond the realm of possibility. Out of the myriad activities available to man, there are almost always some that are accessible to every individual, regardless of the extent of his physical inconveniences or his mental misfortune.

The nurse must help to establish and maintain the communications that are the lifeline of continuity of care. Such communications must be meaningful and during all hours of the day keep nurses, doctors, and others informed about the patient and his progress. They must be transmitted to the family. Although many aspects of geriatric care and even the development of warning signs of changes in condition may seem slow, startling changes can and often do occur rapidly. Many elderly persons are maintained in precarious balance for years of happy, useful living by alert persons who know how to make the needed adjustments at just the right time. This may be accomplished more easily if good records are kept. Although much informal and formal verbal communication may be encouraged, written records are invaluable. They are needed for legal purposes, and they also serve as sources of motivation. A daily record of progress helps a person view in perspective the road he has traveled. The nursing care plan is an important link in the communication chain from nurse to nurse and can be used or modified for the use of the patient and his family when he goes home or for the use of the public health nurse or nursing home nurse when the patient is discharged to their continuing care. Any device that will make transition from one situation to another smoother helps avoid the too often observed setbacks in the patient's progress.

The physical and social environment in the institution is the nurse's responsibility, although it, too, may be shared with others. When the objective of geriatric care is the maintenance or restoration of functional ability, the environment can be an important motivating force. The physical plant requirements that meet patient's needs for privacy, safety, freedom, and protection will not be described because they are discussed in Chapter 5, Housing in Health, and in Chapter 9, Housing During Illness. Publications that describe this subject and model plans are available through departments of health and hospitals, and nursing home and rehabilitation center associations. However, the social climate is so dependent upon the nurse that it merits consideration here. The attitudes of the nurse about aging and old people, her commitment to the goals of active therapy and rehabilitation will influence the total care program. They determine to a large degree how the physical facilities are used, what policies are made and how they are carried out. For example, will family members be welcome at any time or be permitted and helped to assist with the care of their relatives? Should learning self-care include teaching the patient how to take his own medications, permitting him to assume responsibility for his own actions and decisions about his care, making his own appointments, and deciding the extent of his social participation or recreational activities? It has frequently been demonstrated that the full effectiveness of special therapy and recreational activities can only be achieved in a dynamic goal-directed nursing program. The physical therapist, for example, can help the patient regain the physical strength and coordination to perform useful activities, but unless he is permitted and encouraged to perform them in his daily life, the objective of the treatment fails.

In a rehabilitation setting, the nursing role is to help, to teach, and to permit the patient to do all that he can and may do for himself. The most difficult orientation that most nurses and families have to achieve is to let the person do for himself. This is contrary to all human impulses and to much of the training nurses have had. When one sees a person having difficulty in performing a task the natural tendency is to give help. Sometimes help is needed and should be given. Geriatric rehabilitation requires the development of a fine degree of judgment—to know when and when not to intervene. Also, it becomes important to know how to intervene without destroying the person's motivation and sense of personal accomplishment, usefulness, and pride. When an old person resists treatment or refuses to engage in activity, the nurse must be able to judge whether his behavior is simply a need for attention—a desire to be coaxed, or is because of fatigue or incipient physical or emotional problems of greater significance. Skill in making such judgments is learned through experience in working with old people.

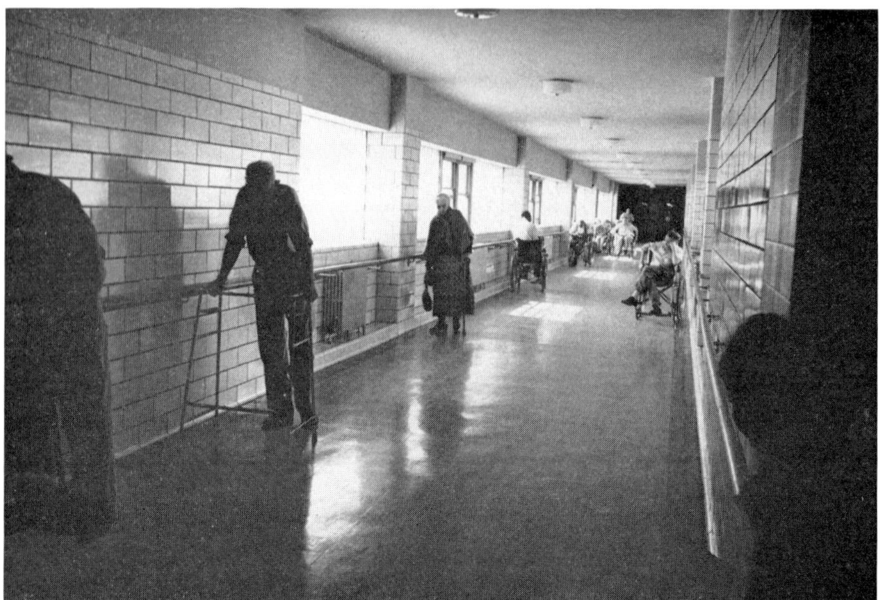

Figure 23. Independence can be encouraged and ambulation made safer by the use of aids: wheelchairs, canes, walkerettes, and corridor handrails. (Courtesy American Journal of Nursing; photograph by Robert Goldstein.)

In addition to the basic health and hygiene needs mentioned in earlier chapters, the nurse is responsible for teaching conditioning exercises and sometimes therapeutic exercises. These are discussed with relation to specific conditions in other chapters of this book and in other texts and manuals.[9, 15] It is important for the nurse to recognize that although many intelligent elderly people in reasonably good physical health can learn exercises quickly and assume responsibility for carrying them out independently, many others will need to be retaught at each exercise session and cannot, even though alert and intelligent, be expected either to remember how to perform them or to do them regularly. Many persons can perform movements automatically but cannot volitionally perform the same movement on command. For example, if a person is directed to bend his elbow he may do less well than if asked to touch his nose. Moving a part toward a perceived object elicits a better response than a simple directional command. Voluntary deep breathing and coughing are particularly difficult for many older persons. The use of some simple technique such as blowing through a straw placed in a glass of water may be much more successful. In spite of these difficulties, exercise programs can often improve the general condition of many older persons.

Similarly, the nurse should be prepared to repeat directions for getting out of a chair, or she can provide the stimulus of long-established habit patterns and sensations to encourage other functional activities. Older persons who will not voluntarily feed themselves will often do so if they are seated at a table and a spoon is placed in the hand; or a person who will not readily drink fluids may automatically drink if a glass in placed in his hand.

It takes considerable ingenuity and imagination to help old persons preserve or recover normal abilities. Many of the aids to rehabilitation of the geriatric patient are simple and easily available and need only nursing interest and initiative to sponsor their use. Many useful devices and home adaptations are described in nursing and rehabilitation publications and will not be repeated here.[7, 9] By using to the fullest their professional knowledge and skills, nurses can fulfil the major role of rehabilitation of the geriatric patient that is expected of them. Not the least of these skills is employing the aid of the many available professional consultants and the family and using the resources of equipment, materials, and information that can be found in most situations.

REFERENCES AND RELATED BIBLIOGRAPHY

1. Asher, Richard A. J.: The dangers of going to bed, Brit. M. J. **2**:967-968, 1947.
2. Dahlin, Bernice: Rehabilitation; fact or figure or speech, Nurs. Outlook **12**:34-37, 1964.
3. Dahlin, Bernice: The homebound adult, Nurs. Outlook **10**:592-593, 1962.
4. Goda, Sidney: Communicating with the aphasic or dysarthric patient, Amer. J. Nurs. **63**:80-81, 1963.
5. Graber, Joe B.: Public Health Service programs on aging, Pub. Health Rep. **79**:577-581, 1964.
6. Hartigan, Helen: Nursing responsibilities in rehabilitation, Nurs. Outlook **2**:649-651, 1954.
7. Lawton, Edith Buchwald: Activities of daily living for physical rehabilitation, New York, 1963, McGraw-Hill Book Company.
8. Mead, Sedgwick: Rehabilitation. In Cowdry, E. V. (editor): The care of the geriatric patient, St. Louis, 1963, The C. V. Mosby Co.
9. Rehabilitative nursing techniques: (1) Bed positioning and transfer procedures for the hemiplegic; (2) Selected equipment useful in the hospital, home or nursing home; (3) A procedure for passive range of motion and self assistive exercises, Minneapolis, 1962, Kenny Rehabilitation Institute.
10. Render, Helena W.: My old age, Nurs. Outlook **12**:31-33, 1964.
11. Rose, Donald L., Shires, Edward B., and Alyea, William S.: Physical measures in the aged, J.A.M.A. **162**:1524-1526, 1956.
12. Rusk, Howard A.: Rehabilitation belongs in the general hospital, Amer. J. Nurs. **62**:62-63, 1962.
13. Spencer, Marian G.: The aged patient in a chronic disease hospital, Nurs. Outlook **10**:594-595, 1962.
14. Steinberg, Franz U., and Frost, Thelma: Geriatric rehabilitation in a general hospital, Geriatrics **18**:158-164, 1963.
15. Terry, Florence Jones, and others: The principles of rehabilitation nursing, St. Louis, 1961, The C. V. Mosby Co.
16. Zimmerman, Muriel E.: Self help devices for rehabilitation, Dubuque, Iowa, 1958, William C. Brown Company, Publishers.

Chapter 12

Special treatments

MEDICATIONS

Most human beings treasure the hope of cure that medications offer them when they are ailing. Since the earliest times man has brewed herbs and sought innumerable panaceas to combat discomforts arising from illness and other causes. Especially is this so with the aged, who look for a magic power to mitigate their ills. During the last generation there has been promise that some of their dreams might be fulfilled. There has been an enormous increase in drugs available for treatment of a variety of ills. It now seems hard to believe, for example, that thirty years ago the ataractics (tranquilizers), antibiotics, and adrenocorticosteroids were not available. The bacteriostatic drugs were just coming into use, but drugs that might lower blood pressure were not known.

The tremendous increase in the kinds of medications being used has enlarged nursing responsibilities proportionately in this area of treatment. It is not unusual for elderly patients who are ambulatory and not ill enough to require hospitalization to be taking as many as a dozen kinds of medicine, all prescribed by a well-qualified physician. Help must be provided the ambulatory patient or his family members so that dosages of drugs will be accurate and so that failure of response or untoward reaction will be reported. In the hospital the patient must be observed carefully for signs of unusual reaction. Many elderly patients do not respond to drugs in the expected manner. Furthermore, many drugs now prescribed, though they had been tested experimentally, are found, sometimes after years of use, to have unexpected effects upon patients.

Unprescribed medications. The consumption of unprescribed medications by elderly persons is large. Diseases of old age are most often chronic (for example, osteoarthritis, bursitis, neuritis), and at the present time little real help for them in the form of medication therapy is available. Sufferers may turn to the newer trade preparations of iron, calcium, vitamins, and the like, which are especially named as being effective for the aged and which are relatively expensive. The aged are ready and willing victims for the promises of patent medicines in their efforts to find relief where no true relief is to be found. A conservative estimate reveals that in the United States the public spends about

$360,000,000 each year on patent remedies. Much of this money comes from the limited resources of the aged. Each year brings new preparations to drugstore windows, titled and advertised to bolster specifically the failing resources of the aged. Many of these, although harmless, are expensive and provide nothing that could not be attained more cheaply in another form.

The best approach to teaching the public about the menace of patent medicines should be found in the wide field of general health education. The services of the local pharmacist should be used in projects planned for local community education. The nurse in her community has an obligation to teach the dangers and uselessness of many patent remedies. She should be interested in the existing legislation and that which is pending to control the advertisement and distribution of patent remedies. The nurse in the hospital can also teach the patient, although by the time he reaches the hospital he is in the hands of a good physician and protected from the indiscriminate use of such medication. The delay in bringing his problems of failing health to proper medical attention, prompted by the false hope of cure from patent medicines, may have seriously impaired the chance for recovery. In any event, valuable time will be lost and funds will have been dissipated needlessly.

Attitudes toward medications. In contrast to those who eagerly seek use of large numbers of drugs, there are some older people who do not believe in medications at all. These patients will frequently not argue with the doctor, the nurse, or relative, but will not take the medication offered. It is good nursing practice to offer the patient a glass of water with the medication and remain at the bedside until he has taken the ordered dose. These patients may hold fluid medications in the mouth for a minute or so and then expel them surreptitiously. Tablets, capsules, and other forms of solid medication may remain unswallowed until the nurse's attention is diverted, and then the patient removes and hides them. Precious time may be lost in treatment of disease if medications are not taken as ordered. Furthermore, there is always the possibility of suicide if hoarded sedative drugs are in the possession of a patient. The danger of this is greatest on a convalescent ward, where patients may not be observed by the nurse frequently during the night.

Another reason why the older patient may not wish to take needed medications is his belief that medications are not good for him. It is surprising how many older people have the fixed idea, for example, that aspirin is injurious to the heart. Some patients of a particular religious faith are afraid to take medications because of the possibility of breaking a dietary law. The older person who has definite convictions about not taking medications needs explanation from the nurse. Many times a few words of explanation, simply expressed, about either the ability of the physician, the prestige of the hospital, or the important purpose of the medication will satisfy the patient and result in his taking medications willingly.

Administration of medications. The nurse needs to be familiar with the expected action of the medication she administers and certain that the correct dosage is given. Reactions of aged persons to drugs may be bizarre and entirely out of proportion to the nature of the drug and the dosage given. Generally speaking, older patients, like the very young, require smaller doses of many drugs, particularly sedatives, although larger doses of stimulating drugs are required for therapeutic effect as age advances.

Differences in rate of action and in rate of excretion or destruction of drugs may occur. When circulation is less active, the effect of medications given hypodermically or intramuscularly may be delayed. Kidney or liver function may be impaired, and the normal excretory rate may be decreased, with the result that cumulative effects of the drug may appear. For example, careful supervision of the patient receiving digitalis is necessary since any storing of the drug within the body may result in a fatal heart block. Bromides may accumulate in the tissues of the older person who has limited excretory function, and toxic signs of overdose of the drug may appear.

Drug groups prescribed widely

Sedatives and analgesics. Most geriatricians believe that sedatives should be used with the utmost caution in treatment of the aged. Reactions to sedative drugs are often bizarre and completely unexpected. Their overuse in the institutionalized care of the elderly may lead to restlessness, sleeplessness, and confusion. Sensibilities may be dulled so that incontinence occurs more often and predisposition to accidents is increased. The simple yet surprisingly effective nursing measures that may give peace of mind, relaxation, and sleep should all be tried before drugs prescribed to be given as needed are resorted to.

Attention to warmth, ventilation, lighting, and elimination of noise helps to allay apprehension and induce sleep. A warm drink such as tea or chocolate, which the patient enjoys, often helps. Conversation with an elderly patient, the nurse showing interest in his particular worries or problems, is often more effective than sedatives to induce sleep. Perhaps because he is often alone and has fewer close human contacts than younger patients, the elderly patient is more in need of actual tactile contact with nursing and related personnel. A backrub is often unusually effective in producing a feeling of well-being and relaxation that will lead to satisfactory sleep.

Chloral hydrate is considered one of the best sedatives for the elderly patient who must be given a drug for sleep. It produces normal sleep with a minimum of toxic effects and seldom causes a delayed reaction of headache, drowsiness, or confusion. Sometimes it is prescribed to be given in capsules to camouflage its disagreeable taste, and occasionally it is given rectally. Paraldehyde is also a relatively safe sedative that produces normal sleep. Its distasteful odor and irritating properties when taken by mouth limit its use. Occasionally it is given intramuscularly or rectally in oil. Because it is believed to be destroyed by the liver, it is seldom prescribed if the patient has liver disease. Some of the drug is excreted by the lungs, increasing bronchial secretions and causing the odor of the drug to persist about the patient. It is seldom prescribed if the patient has any respiratory ailment.

Bromides are relatively safe as far as toxic systemic reactions are concerned, but they are likely to cause other reactions such as skin eruptions. Excretion of this drug may be slow in the elderly patient, so that cumulative reactions may occur. Bromides supply one of the constituents of many sedative drugs that can be obtained without a prescription. The ambulatory patient who is taking a prescribed sedative should be questioned about his use of any other medication obtainable at the local drugstore, and its use should be made known to the doctor.

The barbiturates have been found to be much safer and more effective than many of the newer drugs in treatment of the elderly patient. They are also much cheaper. Barbiturates may be ordered to combat some of the minor annoyances of the aged such as sleeplessness, nervousness, itching of the skin, and general anxiety. Fine eruptions and generalized itching of the skin may characterize excessive barbiturate therapy. Persistent drowsiness and headache are other symptoms. Appearance of these symptoms in the aged may be due to entirely unrelated causes but should be noted and reported to the attending physician. When a barbiturate is prescribed for a patient living at home, the nurse must emphasize to the patient or to the persons responsible for his care the danger of increasing the dosage without consulting the physician. In the hospital the nurse must check carefully to see that the patient is not using sedatives he may have brought with him in addition to the ones being administered there. Barbiturates are likely to have a cumulative effect in older people and may in some instances produce the opposite reaction from that desired. Restlessness and even maniacal states may accompany a cumulative or secondary effect of the drug or be a personal idiosyncrasy to its use.

Alcohol is an excellent relaxant, and, contrary to the opinion of many patients, it is a sedative rather than a stimulant in that its action depresses the central nervous system. Its moderate use tends to relieve worry and nervous tension. Modern nursing of the aged demands that the nurse have a tolerant attitude toward the use of alcohol. Studies have failed to demonstrate any ill effect from prolonged use of small amounts of alcohol. Many of the serious effects attributed to its use, such as cirrhosis of the liver and neuritis, have been found to be the result of the nutritional deficiency that often accompanies excessive use of alcohol, rather than of the alcohol.

The geriatrician usually feels that a moderate use of alcohol should not be denied the aged patient if he is accustomed to it and believes it essential to his well-being. The older person, however, should not be encouraged to take alcoholic beverages. In some hospitals it is now permissible for a relative to bring the elderly patient his nightly bottle of beer. Furthermore, some doctors believe that a bottle of some form of alcoholic beverage should be kept handy in the home where old people live.

The ataractic drugs (tranquilizers) are sedative drugs, but in the strictest sense they are not somnifacients in that they do not induce sleep, although their relaxing effect often makes sleep possible. These drugs are used widely in the care of medical and surgical patients, although their greatest use is in the field of psychiatry. Chlorpromazine is a synthetic tranquilizer that is very frequently ordered, and the list of newer drugs is endless. Perphenazine (Trilafon), meprobamate (Miltown, Equanil), and chlordiazepoxide (Librium) are other examples of tranquilizing drugs prescribed widely. It must be remembered, however, that these drugs are relatively new and that dangers from their use may not yet be known. There is accumulating evidence that many toxic effects can occur. Some may be habit-forming or lead to dependence upon them, others are known to be contraindicated in alcoholism, and others cause confusion. Instability of gait may occur with their use, and this predisposes the elderly patient to accidents. The nurse must never be tempted to give tranquilizing drugs, which are often prescribed to be given as necessary, when nursing measures such as allaying fears and anxieties and paying close attention to physical comfort might make their administration unnecessary.

Reserpine, the alkaloid present in Rauwolfia serpentina, lowers the blood pressure and causes relaxation and a feeling of well-being when the crude drug is used. Toxic signs include nasal congestion, flushing of the skin, gain in weight, diarrhea, and neurologic and skin reactions. Fatigue, confusion, and nightmares can occur and appear more often in older patients than younger ones. The United States Public Health Service has recommended that elderly patients not be given more than 0.25 to 0.5 mg. ($\frac{1}{250}$ to $\frac{1}{125}$ gr.) daily.[12]

Morphine sulfate may be used when a painful disease such as carcinoma has developed beyond surgical aid. The dosage is usually 8 to 10 mg. ($\frac{1}{8}$ to $\frac{1}{6}$ gr.). Before and especially after the administration of morphine, the respiratory rate is noted carefully. It must be remembered that any prolonged slowing of respiration may result in an accumulation of secretions, with aspiration and pneumonia. If, for any reason, a rather large dose of morphine has been given and the patient is sleeping soundly, the nurse should change his position often. Patients under sedation neither aerate pulmonary tissue adequately nor alter their position freely. Under these circumstances pneumonia may develop, or a thrombus may form from the possible slowing of the circulating blood and from pressure of the body weight on blood vessels.

Demerol Hydrochloride (meperidine hydrochloride) is an important analgesic-hypnotic drug that may be preferred to morphine in some instances. The dosage is usually 50 mg. ($\frac{3}{4}$ gr.) given either hypodermically or by mouth. Although the tendency of Demerol to promote addiction may be less than it is with morphine, a patient may easily become addicted to the drug. Dependence upon these agents is to be avoided if possible. Both Demerol and morphine come under the federal narcotics regulations. Local interpretations of these regulations must be observed when the drugs are administered.

Antibacterial drugs. Emphasis in geriatrics should be upon the prevention of infection so that use of drugs for treatment of infections can be minimized. Nurses working in hospitals have a very real responsibility in carrying out effective medical and surgical aseptic techniques so that infections are not spread within the hospital. For persistent chronic infections of some duration, many clinicians believe treatment should first consist of drugs of known although somewhat limited value. The more specific, more potent agents should be reserved for times when other medications fail or when an acute infection that may be superimposed can be treated with an antibiotic specific for the organism involved. An example is the early treatment of a urinary tract infection with mandelic acid. This may be followed by a sulfonamide drug or even an antibiotic if it has been determined that the organism involved does respond to these drugs. It is now believed that antibiotics should never be given indiscriminately to patients suffering from viral disease alone, since viruses are not controlled by these drugs.

The sulfonamide drugs are being used more extensively as the reactions to antibiotic drugs increase and as organisms appear to become more resistant to them. Although they are often prescribed for the elderly patient, there is the danger of poor excretion and of additional damage to already poorly functioning kidneys. If these drugs are given, the nurse must be certain that adequate fluids are taken as ordered and that the urinary output is measured carefully and is consistent in amount with the high fluid intake. Decreased urinary output and any other abnormal signs such as apparent blood in the urine must be reported to the physician at once. Gantrisin is the sulfonamide most often ordered for elderly patients because it is more soluble and more easily excreted than other related preparations.

Many antibiotics are given intramuscularly, and the nurse should be certain that only the sharpest of needles is used. Because the older patient has lost much subcutaneous fat, the penetration of the needle through loose skin and resistant connective tissue is often difficult and painful. In older people who are thin, it is safest to give any intramuscular injection into the buttock rather than the thigh or the deltoid region. The site of injection should be inspected at intervals for signs of pain, induration, or inflammation.

Cathartics. Hippocrates (ca. 400 B.C.) advocated the use of oil to "lubricate the bowels" in old age. Constipation is fairly common, and older people are often vitally concerned with their elimination. The patent medicine trade finds its largest number of credulous customers in this field, and many people come to the physician suffering bowel damage from years of abuse from regular, drastic, catharsis. In 1939 Mulengracht reported a study showing that the cathartic habit may cause calcium deficiency as well as other difficulties.

Habitual use of cathartics over a period of years may have established physical and psychologic dependency that is hard to break. For discussion of the treatment of constipation, see Chapter 6, General Hygiene.

Cathartics, wisely controlled, do have a place in the treatment of the elderly. If the patient has had an attack of coronary artery disease, has an aortic aneurysm, has sustained a stroke, or has a symptomtic hiatus hernia, it may be important that he avoid straining at defecation, and a cathartic may be needed. Sudden illness that causes the patient to be inactive, as when a stroke or a hip fracture has been sustained, may upset the normal pattern of elimination and necessitate the use of a cathartic.

If the patient has not taken cathartics regularly and has not built up a tolerance to them, smaller doses than for the younger adult may suffice. Saline cathartics are seldom ordered since they cause dehydration and are often too drastic in their action. Mineral oil is often ordered when it is important to prevent straining. Because it absorbs vitamin A from the intestinal tract before it can be utilized, mineral oil usually is not given over a long period of time, and the doctor may order that it be given several hours after meals. The mild bulk-producing cathartics prepared from agar and psyllium seed given with extra fluids often produce satisfactory results and are often prescribed for elderly patients. Occasionally a small amount of mineral oil is combined with these preparations.

Bisacodyl (Dulcolax) is a relatively new laxative that is extremely popular at the present time. It acts by reflexly stimulating peristalsis when it comes in contact with the intestinal mucosa and can be taken by mouth or used as a suppository inserted high in the rectum. The drug is inactive in a neutral or alkaline solution, so that dosage should not follow too closely the administration of antacids. To date there appears to be little difficulty with a tolerance to the drug and the need for increase in dosage. Bisacodyl suppositories have been found to be very satisfactory to assure complete emptying of the lower bowel before examinations and before surgery. Although this drug should never be used routinely to take the place of serious attempts at bowel retraining of the elderly incontinent patient, the regular use of bisacodyl suppositories for severely deteriorated patients who are totally incontinent has reduced the amount of soiling and the resultant skin irritation.[10]

Adrenocorticosteroids. The adrenocorticosteroid drugs are fully described in current texts in pharmacology and pharmacology in nursing.[6] Because of the well-known inability of elderly patients to withstand stress as well as younger persons, they are often given these preparations for several days preoperatively and may be given large doses if emergency surgery must be done. The adrenocorticosteroids are also ordered for medical emergencies and for infections and other lesions of almost every part of the body. Since the outcome for the patient may be influenced profoundly by response to adrenocorticotrophic hormone and adrenocorticosteroids, it is an important nursing responsibility to see that the administration of these drugs is not overlooked. Serious difficulties have arisen, for example, when a patient who has been taking the drug sustains an accident and is operated upon without continuance of the medication. The nurse can help in such situations by asking the elderly patient what medications he is taking, since he may forget some of them in the confusion and excitement of a trip to the emergency department of a hospital.

PHYSICAL THERAPY

Physical therapy, an indispensable adjunct to the treatment of many acute and chronic diseases of the aged, may be defined as the treatment of disease by the use of physical measures such as heat, massage, and therapeutic exercise. Rapid and spontaneous cure of disease is less common in age than in youth. Such conditions as arthritis, bursitis, fibrositis, and residual hemiplegia yield in part to physical measures since slowing the process of disease, preventing further complications, and alleviating discomfort can often be achieved by physical means, even if complete recovery is not possible. Some diseases of older people such as hypertrophic arthritis are not too serious to life and are sometimes termed the "nuisance diseases" in that they are a burden to both the patient and the physician. These diseases, however, in terms of human comfort are far from trivial and make the contribution of physical therapy invaluable.

Physical therapy is ordered by the physician and carried out by the professionally prepared physical therapist. Every nurse should be familiar with the physical medicine department in her hospital or the physical therapy resources in her community. If she understands the physical therapy program and keeps informed about the available facilities, she can often give pertinent and helpful information to the patient and can help him carry out the principles taught by the physical therapist.

Some of the same precautions must be observed in physical therapy treatment for the aged as are noted in the administration of medications. Problems in use of physical therapy are presented by age changes such as decreases in sensory perception and circulatory efficiency. Because body systems in older persons are not geared to cope with sudden physical changes, smaller amounts of physical treatment are administered than in maturity, and untoward or unusual responses to treatment must be anticipated. Sudden changes in body temperature and circulation may produce collapse and exhaustion.

The nurse should assume responsibility for reading the physical therapy prescription on her patient's chart and knowing what treatment he is receiving in the department of physical medicine in order that she can better care for him on his return to the ward. After the patient has received physical therapy treatment, he should rest and be protected from drafts and chilling. It is the nurse's responsibility to watch the patient closely and to report pertinent observations such as marked fatigue, diaphoresis, cyanosis, pain, or other change following treatment. Aged patients are extremely sensitive; they feel that because they cannot get about as freely as formerly they are a burden. Thus they hesitate to report symptoms to the doctor that might warn of future untoward developments.

Heat. Physical therapy application of heat gives aid to the elderly, but extreme care to prevent burning and exhaustion is necessary. Burns occur easily, and recovery from burns in very old persons may be tedious or even impossible. If high-frequency current is used to produce heat, it is applied with caution to the aged. The best method of application of heat is by convection and radiation as, for instance, the use of the infrared lamp. Even with this method, the greatest care must be taken to have the lamp at the prescribed distance from the delicate skin to avoid burns. A very old or unconscious patient must be watched when a heat lamp is used for treatment of a pressure area since he may move nearer the lamp and be burned.

In most instances it is dangerous to supply heat by conduction, such as the direct application of a hot-water bottle to the body. One useful method of giving heat by conduction is the paraffin bath, which produces a penetrating form of heat with little danger of burning. Orthopedic specialists often order this treatment for conditions such as arthritis and bursitis in the elderly. The paraffin bath is heated, and the temperature is tested with a fat thermometer; it must not be over 54.6° C. (130° F.). The affected hand or foot may be immersed in the bath, but, when this is not possible, paraffin may be applied by means of a brush or padded tongue blade. After six to twelve coats of the wax have been applied, the part is usually wrapped in waxed paper, plastic, or a towel for about twenty minutes. The wax is then peeled off and can be washed and reused. After application of heat by means of paraffin, other physical therapy such as massage and stretching or exercise may be employed. Chilling after the use of paraffin must be avoided, and the part is usually wrapped in a light, warm covering for about thirty minutes. The paraffin bath is usually given in the department of physical medicine where special equipment for the melting of paraffin is available. If for any reason it is used on the ward or by the nurse in the home, the greatest care is needed, since paraffin is inflammable and has been known to cause severe damage by fire when it is overheated. In the home it is best to melt the paraffin slowly in a double boiler away from an open flame. Handles of pans must be turned away from the edge of the stove since severe burns can be caused by spilling overheated paraffin.

Massage. Massage is valuable in the treatment of many older patients. Massage should not be too vigorous in most instances since subcutaneous tissue is diminished and trauma and pain may be produced. It must occasionally be vigorous on special prescription when certain conditions such as fibrositis are being treated. Massage following a heat treatment helps to improve circulation, prevent or reduce contractures, and maintain a normal range of joint motion for the patient who is confined to bed. It has little value in the maintenance of muscle

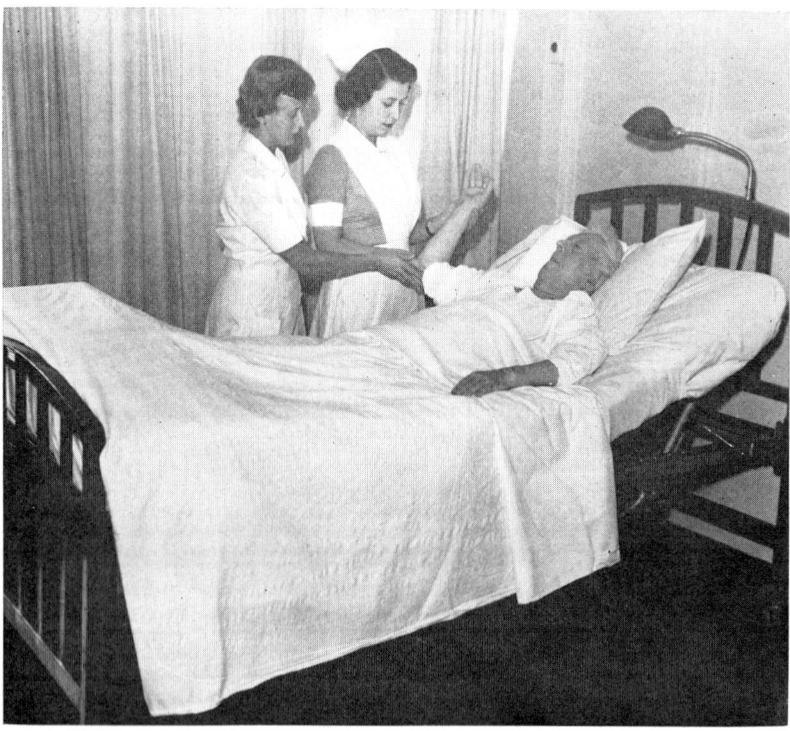

Figure 24. The physical therapist can be of help to the nurse in reviewing normal range of joint motion. (Photograph by Robert Waldeck.)

tone since this is almost wholly dependent upon active muscular exercise. Massage to the muscles of the extremities of any patient is never given by the nurse unless it is specifically ordered by the physician, though gentle massage to joints such as those of the toes, ankles, and knees may be safely carried out.

Hydrotherapy. Hydrotherapy such as alternate hot-and-cold immersion of an affected extremity may be ordered for the older patient, though complete immersion in tubs is seldom used because of the danger of exhaustion. In such a treatment the water should not be warmer than 40.5° C. (105° F.). After hydrotherapy, a mild lotion should be used on the skin, which may become excessively dry from the treatment. In many hospitals that have no department of physical medicine, procedures such as sitz baths or soaking an extremity in a tub of warm water are carried out by the nurse. The nurse must be aware of the specific precautions observed by the physical therapist. The elderly patient must not be left alone while a sitz bath is being taken, and signs of faintness, dizziness, profuse diaphoresis, or apprehension are indications for stopping the treatment. Assistance in getting out of the bath is needed in order to prevent accidents. When a limb such as the foot and leg is to be immersed in a tub of water, it is important to provide a comfortable stool for the patient so that he need not sit in a cramped, awkward, fatiguing position. Any water spilled on the floor should be removed at once since it may contribute to accidents.

Therapeutic exercise. Therapeutic exercises are used when there is bone, joint, muscle, or nerve damage to a part. These exercises are prescribed by the physician and are carried out by a qualified physical therapist. Certain specific therapeutic exercises may occasionally be given by the nurse when she is carefully instructed by the physician or when she is working under the supervision of the physical therapist. An even brief explanation of definite therapeutic exercises is beyond the scope of this chapter. Nonspecific exercises are described in Chapter 6, General Hygiene.

OCCUPATIONAL THERAPY

Occupational therapy, or treatment by occupation, is an essential adjunct to good geriatric care. The history of occupational therapy goes back many years. In 172 A.D. Galen said, "Employment is nature's best physician and is essential to human happiness." Since then many other leaders in the field of treating human ills have recognized the need for occupational therapy. Mr. Thomas Eddy, soon after the founding of the Society of the New York Hospital in 1771, read a paper in which he said, "Those kinds of employment are to be preferred, both on a moral and physical account, which are accompanied by considerable bodily action, most agreeable to the patient and most opposite to the illusion of his disease." In fact, it is surprising that, with the long-known value of suitable occupation to almost all who are ill, development of this form of treatment has been so slow. Many of our large general hospitals today do not have occupational therapy departments.

Occupational therapy has been defined as any activity, mental or physical, that is medically prescribed and professionally guided to aid a patient in recovery from disease or injury. The aims of occupational therapy are to improve

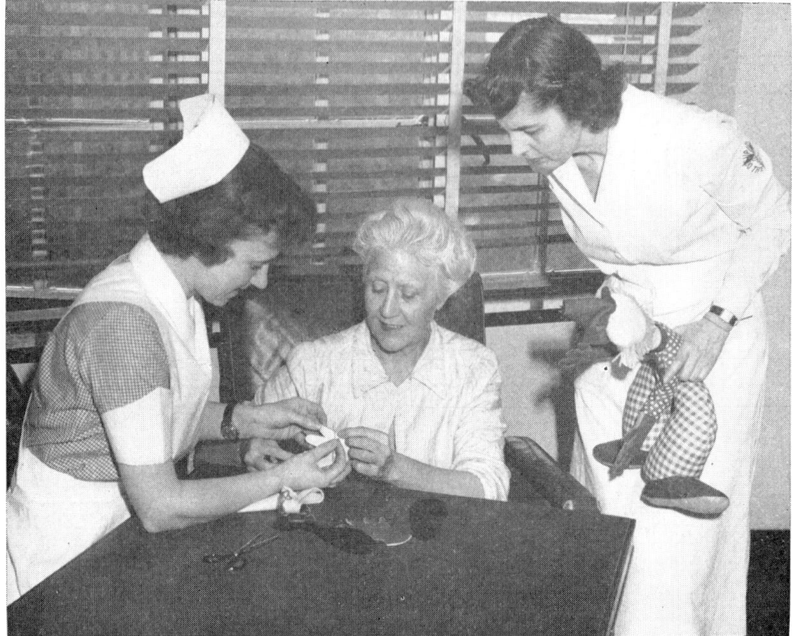

Figure 25. Occupational therapy adds to the patient's contentment and assists in rehabilitation.

or restore specific physical functions and give psychologic benefit. The patient's interest is stimulated to perform an activity that will require the correct use and development of an affected part. Some overlapping exists between occupational therapy and allied therapies. The nurse will avoid some confusion if she remembers that occupational therapy is not prevocational, though it may create interests that may in turn lead to vocational placement, and that it is not primarily recreational or diversional, though recreational activities may be used for a specific therapeutic purpose.

Specific remedial occupational therapy is a form of treatment prescribed by the physician for an individual patient and carried out under the supervision of a prepared occupational therapist, either at the bedside in the hospital or home or in the department of occupational therapy.

Nurse's role in the occupational therapy program. Some hospitals have only a few occupational therapists, and it is often impossible for one of them to be on the ward at the time the doctor sees his patients. The nurse can be of assistance in securing specific outlined and signed instructions from the physician. She can be of help to both the physician and the therapist by informing them of the particular interests of the patient so they can select suitable activities that are in line with these interests. When the patient is going regularly to the occupational therapy department, it is helpful if the nurse can see that the department is notified if the patient is unable to keep his appointment. The occupational therapist should also be informed when plans for the patient's release from the hospital are being made, since it not only enables her to collect equipment and avoids confusion and misunderstandings after the patient has left the hospital but also allows her to give instructions for activity at home.

The nurse has a responsibility to understand what the occupational therapist is trying to accomplish. She can be invaluable in reporting any special difficulties the patient may have in carrying on the prescribed activity. She should give encouragement to the patient in his activity and should help make any needed adjustments in his environment so that the activity can be undertaken and continued. Often a small detail such as changing the type of overbed table will enable the patient to carry on some activity satisfactorily. Newspapers may be needed to protect the bed and table if paints are to be used. A little rearrangement of equipment may allow two bed patients to carry on some activity of common interest and benefit. An extra wastebasket beside the patient's bed may be all that is needed to make his pastime less disrupting to the general ward.

There are many criteria by which the therapist judges the general suitability of various activities for the patient. The activity must be safe for the patient and to persons around him. For example, knives used for some crafts might not be safe in psychiatric wards. The activity must not produce eyestrain either from the position in bed or by poor lighting. It must not cause poor body alignment and strain. The patient may have to be instructed to stop at intervals to take deep breaths and to stretch. The activity must be one that suits the patient's mental and physical abilities sufficiently to challenge interest and creative ability. Yet it must not result in too much activity or cause frustration from the inability to complete a project undertaken. Occupational therapy for a patient with tuberculosis may be just the opposite of that for a patient with arthritis in that it may aim to lessen activity and thus facilitate rest, whereas in the patient with arthritis it may challenge him to use atrophied muscles and involved joints. The nurse should know some of the criteria by which the therapist judges the activities for each patient.

For almost every clinical entity that may be found in geriatrics, there is some form of occupational therapy that would be beneficial. The patient with cardiac illness may benefit from graded activity to increase strength and resistance; the patient with a fracture needs something active and interesting to do while his fracture is healing; the patient with skin disease needs activities to divert his mind from himself and his symptoms. Occupational therapy can often be of value to the patient struggling to adjust to a hearing loss or to the use of a hearing aid.

Occupational therapy gives to the hospital situation an atmosphere of normalcy. It helps the patient remain satisfied, to some extent at least, and therefore more receptive to treatment. Thus, it aids in recovery generally. The need for this type of therapy in the general medical and surgical wards of our hospitals and in the homes for the aged is now becoming well known.

Diversional activities. No sharp dividing line exists between occupational therapy of physical and psychologic therapeutic benefit and that which is largely diversional or recreational. Diversional activities might well be under the supervision of an occupational therapist and carried on largely by others. In many institutions this type of activity is left to the nursing service, but, if the services of an occupational therapist are available in the hospital or in the community, they are invaluable to nurses in planning ways to keep the patient gainfully occupied. From her store of knowledge and skills the occupational therapist can usually devise some activity that will be satisfying to each patient.

Generally speaking, diversional activities for the aged should be those that allow for moving about freely since long sitting and long standing are not good for older people. They should demand little in energy output and should not produce poor posture, stiffness, or deformity. Diversional activities could include movies, cardplaying, even dancing, and much of the so-called busy work such as knitting, crocheting, and making flowers and other knicknacks. Photography, gardening, light carpentry work, collecting recipes, and answering radio quiz programs are but a few of the many diversional activities in which the aged may participate. More and more attention is being given to the beneficial effects of good music. Recreational centers in large cities have literary and art contests for older people that are highly successful.

Diversional activity is of tremendous importance in the happy living of the aged who are confined to the hospital or any other type of institution. Many older people live at home, and they, too, are greatly benefited by appropriate diversional therapy. One of the reasons why the older woman adjusts better to living alone in her home is that she has innumerable small activities in which she may engage, whereas the older man, frequently less self-sufficient about the house, finds that time hangs heavy on his hands.

Persons who care for the patient should not pass judgment on his selection of how he occupies himself. They must not apply their own yardstick of value to the product of his efforts but must permit him to apply his own. Many of the articles produced by the elderly person may not be attractive or even useful by some standards, but if they please and occupy the individual, they have served a useful purpose. The nurse and the occupational therapist must make use of their knowledge of psychology, remembering that no activity is good if it is forced upon the patient, but that it is often possible to motivate him to want to do something suitable and constructive.

Many of the hobbies developed in youth and middle age assist immeasurably in helping older people to adjust to physical and emotional restrictions. Activities such as weeding the garden and doing carpentry or tool work provide both physical and mental diversion and contribute greatly to the prevention of maladjustment and unhealthy preoccupation with oneself. Some people like to cook at the end of a busy day for the change and relaxation this activity affords. Others like to come home from a busy day and trim hats to relieve mental fatigue. Still others may pore for hours over a record collection, cataloguing it perfectly.

CANCER

Cancer certainly is not strictly a disease of old age. Indeed it is the second cause of death (next to accidents) among those aged 4 to 24 years. The incidence of cancer, however, increases with age, and cancer in several locations—for example, the skin, the prostate gland, the stomach and esophagus, and the lower bowel—occurs most often in the later decades of life.

Nurse's attitude and general nursing care

The nurse who cares for the older patient with cancer must often analyze her own thinking and sometimes revamp her sense of values. Her attitude toward malignancy must be positive. She must remember that she is likely to see in the hospital and in the home the serious and recurrent cases of malignancy. Reliable figures show that there are many patients who have had freedom from recurrence extending beyond a five-year period. Carcinoma in the elderly usually develops more slowly than in the younger person. The prognosis is better, provided that detection can be made and treatment started early. The importance of noticing early symptoms and urging the patient to seek medical attention cannot be overemphasized.

Sometimes the nurse may be inclined to feel that it would be better for the patient to die rather than to face the mutilating operation that is necessary. Particularly is this thinking likely to occur when the patient is elderly. We must remind ourselves constantly that age alone does not alter individual basic feelings about living. One lady of 91, for example, was a real source of aggravation to her doctor and the nurse. She was eager to avoid atherosclerosis and sought precise answers as to the relative safety of various diets. On the surface this might appear ridiculous for someone of her age. Yet this lady was maintaining her own apartment herself and studying Spanish. Her interest in participating in life experiences was as keen as it had been in her youth and in this way she never thought of herself as at the end of her life. The nurse must remember to think of what the patient wishes and not of what she happens to think she would want if she were in the same circumstances. The will to live is exceedingly strong in most of us. Persons who have had a great deal of experience in dealing with patients who have cancer tell us that most patients want to live regardless of how disfiguring may be the operation that makes living possible.

The sense of enjoyment and appreciation of many of the things that life offers is greater in age than in youth. It is absolutely impossible ever to say whether the manner of life for another person, lived as another may have to live it, is worthwhile. The patient who has an entire jaw removed, who cannot talk, and who cannot eat normally can still enjoying hearing a full day of beautiful music, can spend an entire and happy evening looking at art masterpieces, or view a sunset with delight. There is no end to what can be seen and done and felt, no matter what feature may have been removed or what physical liberty may have been restricted by illness.

The nurse must give her patient hope. The patient with cancer does not want pity. Neither does he want immature thoughtlessness. He does want, above all, the unquenchable hope that whatever physical activity left to him by the necessary treatment may be continued. The question of whether to tell the patient that he has cancer is a matter of opinion among physicians, and the decision must come from the physician for each individual patient. Many times the patient will not mention the word *cancer* though he may know quite well the nature of his illness. Persons who have studied the matter carefully feel that some patients do not really want to know the complete truth, that some of them, though they may ask a question, hasten to answer it themselves in a manner that is acceptable to them. Some very definitely avoid conversation that may lead to their having to face acknowledging that they have cancer. Usually the patient's questions are such that a tactful, roundabout answer can be given without one's seeming to be unnecessarily evasive.

Some patients are utterly depressed either by the fear that they have cancer or by the confirmation of their fears and the physical limitations that the disease has imposed upon them. One principle which must guide the nurse in her care of such patients is fundamental in all rehabilitation. It is that the nurse cannot permit her patient to become preoccupied with things that are no longer possible. She must help the patient to give attention to that which can be accomplished in the present, without dwelling in the past or peering too far into the future.

The patient with cancer needs encouragement. He needs this early when he is perhaps struggling to accept the radical surgery the surgeon has told him may be imperative. He also needs it in the slow return to health and strength. He needs uplift to his morale, particularly when a series of radiation treatments is necessary and if malignant cells have escaped medical control and the disease is progressing unfavorably. Radioactive isotopes, hormones, and the alkenylating and antimetabolic drugs have extended life for some patients. Many times, however, side effects cause new discomforts that require the most thoughtful and understanding care.

When all measures available for treatment have failed and the patient is in the terminal phase of cancer where no participation in any life experience is possible, many physicians and also ethical leaders believe that continued attempts to prolong life in this condition benefit no one.[11]

Early discovery. The success of medical measures now available for the control of cancer are based on an early discovery of the disease. Cancer detection clinics are now being held in various parts of the country and serve a most useful purpose in educating the public, as well in discovering incipient cancerous lesions. The American Cancer Society has also done a great deal toward educating the public to be on the alert for the early signs of cancer. All patients, particularly elderly ones, have a tendency to postpone seeing a physician or going to a clinic in the hope that signs or symptoms may disappear and they will be spared the bother and the expense that medical attention involves. Metastasis may develop beyond medical control during this period of procrastination. The problems of diagnosis in the elderly are compounded by the fact that often they have a number of ailments so that their complaints are more difficult to relate to a single cause. Also, symptoms may not be those typically seen in younger patients, and while pain may bring them to the doctor, it is more likely to be a late sign, the disease far advanced by the time it occurs.

Treatment. The treatment of cancer for the aged is the same as for the patient of any age. The best hope for cure lies in early and complete removal of the tumor and the surrounding tissue. Difficulties encountered in the treatment and nursing care are those applying to elderly patients who undergo extensive surgery for any cause. They are described in Chapter 13. The nursing care needed when radiation therapy is used or hormones and other drugs are given is similar to that for younger patients and is described fully in current medical and surgical nursing texts.[9]

REFERENCES AND RELATED BIBLIOGRAPHY

1. Ayd, F. J., Jr.: Tranquilizers and the ambulatory geriatric patient, J. Am. Geriatrics Soc. **8**:909-914, 1960.
2. Bender, A. Douglas: Pharmacologic aspects of aging; a survey of the effect of increasing age on drug activity in adults, J. Am. Geriatrics Soc. **12**:1114-1134, 1964.
3. Goodman, L., and Gilman, A.: The pharmacological basis of therapeutics, ed. 2, New York, 1955, The Macmillan Company.
4. Johnson, Wingate M. (editor): The older patient, New York, 1960, Paul B. Hoeber, Inc., Medical Book Department of Harper & Row, Publishers.
5. Jones, Thomas H.: Chlordiazepoxide (Librium) and the geriatric patient, J. Am. Geriatrics Soc. **10**:259-263, 1962.
6. Krug, Elsie E.: Pharmacology in nursing, ed. 9, St. Louis, 1963, The C. V. Mosby Co.
7. Lehyr, D.: Problems of chemotherapy in the older age group, J. Am. Geriatrics Soc. **3**:355-366, 1955.
8. Litin, Edward M.: Mental reaction to trauma and hospitalization in the aged, J.A.M.A. **162**:1522-1524, 1956.
9. Shafer, Kathleen Newton, and others: Medical-surgical nursing, ed. 3, St. Louis, 1964, The C. V. Mosby Co.
10. Warman, Seymour: Standardized treatment of chronically constipated dependent geriatric patients, J. Am. Geriatrics Soc. **9**:285-287, 1961.
11. Warren, Richard, and others: Surgery, Philadelphia, 1963, W. B. Saunders Co.
12. Yow, E. M.: A reevaluation of sulfonamide therapy, Ann. Int. Med. **43**:323-332, 1955.

Unit 4

Clinical nursing

Chapter 13

Anesthesia and operative care

The elderly patient is no longer necessarily a poor surgical risk. Results from surgery are often excellent, provided that attention is paid to individual physical changes, that the patient is under the care of a skilled surgeon and anesthesiologist, and that he receives understanding nursing care. Recent advances in knowledge of physiology and increased skill in the medical management of such physical changes as endocrine imbalance, instability of electrolyte balance, and limited respiratory excursion have decreased the dangers of surgery. There is clear evidence, however, that the margin of safety in extensive operative procedures decreases with age. It has been found that with careful preoperative and operative care, patients over 60 years of age will survive major surgery such as thyroidectomy, mastectomy, and gastric resection as well as younger patients. The same is not true when the more extensive and time-consuming operations such as esophagectomy, pneumonectomy, or radical neck dissection are done. In these operations and in emergency surgery, which must be done without complete preparation, the operative mortality of patients over 60 has been found to be twice that of younger persons; the figures are even higher in some studies.[5] Particular skill and judgment on the part of persons caring for the geriatric surgical patient are needed in the period of preparation for surgery, during and immediately after anesthesia, and postoperatively.

PREOPERATIVE CARE

Emotional preparation and care

Optimism is essential. An attitude of mind that refuses to accept defeat, so valuable in all nursing, is doubly essential in dealing with the aged operative patient. Despite frequent reassurance, the aged patient (and often the younger one also) looks upon surgery as a most crucial episode in his life. For most people, no matter how old, the love of life is strong. Emotional response to an impending operation is determined by the patient's own personality and the circumstances of his particular illness. Some patients are truly resigned to any surgical eventuality and accept decisions for even extensive surgery with obvious calm. These patients tolerate anesthesia much better than the apprehensive patient. The patient who anticipates his operation with optimism may have surprisingly good results despite definite physical infirmities, whereas the one who is unduly apprehensive may have a stormy postoperative course despite few apparent physical handicaps. Some patients are truly fearful yet hide their fears under an outward appearance of calm. The nurse must be on the alert for any indications of the true emotional condition of the patient and must report pertinent information to the physician in charge. Some surgeons hesitate to operate upon patients in whom the will to live is gone.

It is now common practice for the anesthesiologist to visit the patient preoperatively to give him a feeling of confidence and reassurance, so important in his response to anesthesia and to the operation. Usually the surgeon visits the patient to discuss with him in detail the operation, the hoped-for outcome, and to answer any questions he may have. Many surgeons now believe that the patient must understand exactly what operation is contemplated, and that the patient must himself, if of sound mind, make the decision as to whether or not the operation will be done. This attitude of the surgeon toward the elderly patient as an independent person capable of making decisions should be duplicated by the nurse.

The nurse can help the patient in his initial adjustment by repeated explanations of his surroundings and of hospital regulations. It has been found that the less he is confronted by unfamiliar surroundings, the less likely he is to become confused postoperatively. The patient may be nervous and anxious about details of preparation or of the operative procedure he is facing; he may ask about the usual outcome and what his particular chances may be. Despite the fact that the surgeon has discussed his condition with him, he may ask many questions of the nurse that require careful answers. The nurse should also be considerate of special visitors whom the patient may have immediately prior to his operation. Careful attention to the delivery of messages adds a great deal to the comfort and emotional well-being of the patient at this time. The nurse must know the correct person in the hospital to whom the patient's request is referred if he wishes to have legal papers witnessed.

Physiologic changes and related care

The good operative record that has been achieved in recent years for aged patients is partly due to thorough appraisal of all physiologic changes and to careful preoperative preparation. This may be done in the hospital or at home, and most surgeons believe that preparation should be thorough but not unduly delayed, particularly when a condition such as cancer is known or suspected. After careful diagnostic study, effort is made to improve any conditions that may predispose to operative failure. The importance of accuracy in diagnostic tests is obvious. An electrocardiogram to test heart function, urea clearance and concentration tests to determine adequacy of the kidneys, and liver function tests may be done. Specific gravity of the urine and examination of the blood for nonprotein nitrogen may be ordered to check kidney function further, and tests for blood sugar and for response to the administration of glucose may be conducted. The test for excretion of 17-ketosteroids by obtaining both blood and urine samples after the administration of adrenocorticotrophic hormone is usually done routinely when major surgery is anticipated. The blood volume determination is considered imperative by many surgeons in order that an accurate check of blood loss and subsequent replacement can be carried out postoperatively.

Many of the tests, procedures, and examinations are expensive, time consuming, and disturbing to the patient in a variety of ways. The nurse has a responsibility to explain diagnostic and related procedures to the patient and to do her part in seeing that that they are carried out effectively so that delay and repetition are avoided.

It is important to evaluate the general physical condition of the patient for operation. Observations made by the nurse may assist the surgeon and the anesthesiologist in the selection of suitable anesthesia and operative procedure. Because of the dread of illness, surgery, and pain, and for other reasons, aged patients frequently do not give a complete medical history of the doctor. Later they may reveal pertinent information to the nurse. This must be recorded and related to the doctor. Sensitivity to drugs, "fainting spells," short periods of dizziness or of amnesia, and accidental injuries are examples of problems that may be significant and yet are forgotten or considered unimportant by the patient. Signs of cerebral clouding, disorientation, or confusion are important in determining the amount of surgery that can be done safely and the anesthesia to be chosen. These are most likely to be apparent during evening and night hours, and their occurrence in the hospital during the period of preparation for surgery must be reported in detail. Physiologic and pathologic changes that lessen vital reserves are often present and are potential sources of postoperative complications. The aged patient usually has a limited cardiac reserve even though no symptoms are conspicuous. Often the pulse is slow. The patient's pulse and blood pressure should be taken regularly (the blood pressure at least daily and the pulse every four hours) for several days preceding major surgery, and pulse volume should be noted carefully. Dyspnea upon exertion should be noted and reported. Intravenous barbiturate anesthesia is seldom used if the patient has dyspnea, regardless of what the electrocardiogram may show.

The elderly person often has impaired pulmonary function with decrease in vital capacity and a lowered inspiratory reserve. This presents real problems at operation since anoxia is the complication encountered most often during anesthesia. Poor pulmonary function also results in poor elimination of carbon dioxide and this problem, along with limitations of renal function and endocrine imbalance, leads to postoperative electrolyte imbalance. The doctor may do the simple test of asking the patient to hold his breath since the normal younger person can do so for up to fifty-five seconds without difficulty. It is extremely important that the elderly patient be protected from upper respiratory infection preoperatively and after surgery. Close family members should know this, and no one with an upper respiratory infection should be permitted near the patient.

Arterial changes that come with age affect the outcome of surgery. Arteriosclerosis lessens the flexibility of the vascular system and predisposes the patient to shock. The danger of hemorrhage is also accentuated by hardening of arteries since they do not collapse as readily and clotting is delayed at points where small vessels have been cut. Pronounced varicosities, particularly in the lower extremities, predispose to shock and for this reason the doctor may order that elastic stockings or bandages be applied to the patient's legs preoperatively. Cardiac response may be altered by certain drugs such as the ataractics, and for this reason any tranquilizing drugs that the patient may have been receiving usually are discontinued for two weeks before elective major surgery is undertaken.

Hormonal changes and deficiencies occur with age and must be considered when operations become necessary. Thyroid function is usually somewhat lower than in earlier years, and so is basal metabolic rate. There is an impairment of function in use of glucose reaching the bloodstream even when no real signs of diabetes are evident. The nurse should expect that intravenous solutions containing glucose will be ordered to be given more slowly than for the younger patient. The most pronounced endocrine changes occur in the gonadal function after the climacteric. Reduction of the output of testosterone in the elderly male patient tends to cause a negative nitrogen balance. It is abundantly clear that the elderly patient tolerates stress less well than the younger one, and it is believed that one cause is endocrine imbalance or deficiency; there is probably some impairment of function of the adrenal cortex and perhaps also of the pituitary gland, since the excretion of 17-ketosteroids is reduced in both sexes. Many patients now receive cortical hormones, and sudden withdrawal of these before the operation can result in serious hypotension. The nurse should get all the information she can concerning drugs the patient has been receiving and make her report to the doctor, as he may not have the complete list. Occasionally, the fact that the patient has been receiving a hormone regularly is overlooked when he is transferred within the hospital preceding surgery.

Malnutrition. Malnutrition is found often in elderly patients and particularly in those who have been chronically ill for a long time. Many times it will be necessary to improve the patient's nutritional health before surgery can be attempted. Vitamin C is often given in addition to that taken in food, since this vitamin is thought to benefit wound healing. Combined vitamins are often ordered. Some surgeons believe that a long-term, low-protein diet contributes to weakening of heart muscle as well as to liver damage and slowing of wound healing. Many elderly people have a low blood protein level caused by a diet that has been deficient in protein over a long period of time, and the doctor may wish his patient to receive at least 100 gm. of protein each day. This may be more than the patient has been used to taking and may be difficult for him to consume. The nurse should observe the patient's appetite and should attempt in every way to ensure an adequate protein intake for him. A variety of protein preparations to be given in liquid form are now available. Though not unpalatable, they are not always wholly acceptable to all patients, and an effort should be made to suit these necessary foods to the preferences of the individual. For example, one person may like the drink iced; another may prefer it mixed with chocolate or orange juice. If adequate protein cannot be taken by mouth, the protein hydrolysates may be given intravenously in a solution of 5 percent dextrose. Occasionally these solutions have a tendency to produce nausea, which further decreases the amount of food taken by mouth.

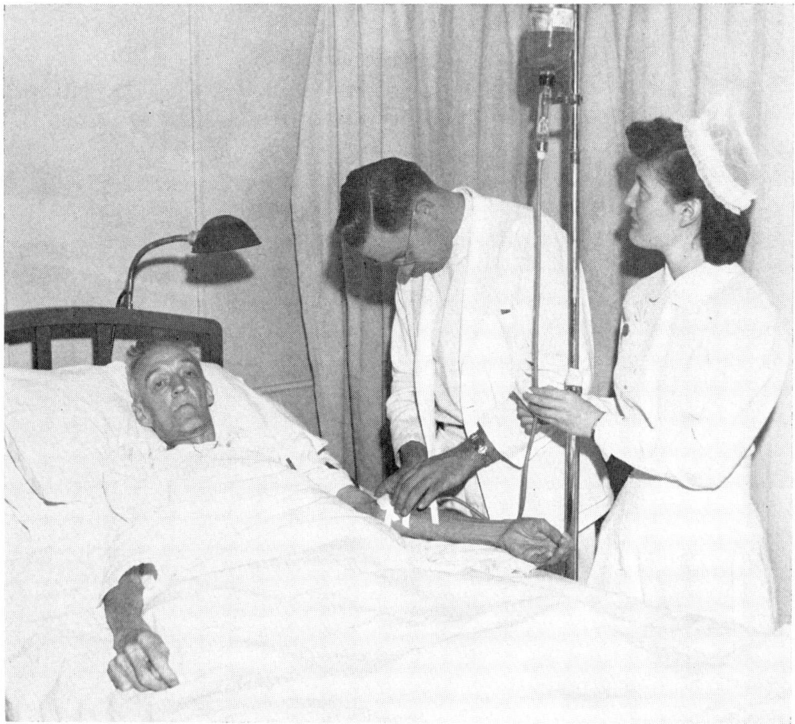

Figure 26. Teamwork and skill make hospital procedures easier to bear.

Blood transfusions may be given preoperatively when blood protein is low and for anemia, but they are expensive and there is the danger of transmitting to the patient the virus of infectious hepatitis or homologous serum hepatitis; therefore, they are generally used for this purpose only when other methods of increasing blood protein level have failed. Amino acids may be given intravenously, although most of the preparations in use cause pronounced nausea in some patients. Occasionally a small polyethylene catheter is passed through the nose into the duodenum and liquid feedings high in protein are fed to the patient during his sleeping hours.

Immediate preoperative care

Haste should be avoided in carrying out routine preoperative procedures. Older people cannot tolerate bustle and excitement. Delirium reactions may at times be a result of apprehension and bewilderment during the preoperative period. The patient needs a night of rest and unhurried preparation on the morning of surgery. The bath and enema should be given the night before unless the patient is accustomed to arising early in the morning. In many hospitals the patient is now sent to the operating room in his bed. He may be put to sleep while in bed, which lessens excitement and confusion.

Some anesthesiologists believe that elderly patients should be allowed to drink water up to within four hours of the operation and to have a liquid breakfast if surgery is delayed until the afternoon.[13] There seems to be no physiologic basis for the order, "Nothing by mouth after midnight." It is well known that elderly patients tolerate starvation less well than the middle-aged.

Anesthesiologists warn against too much emphasis being placed on the use of a hypnotic for a good night's sleep preoperatively. Preoperative preparation must begin earlier than the evening before operation. A large dose of sedation in the evening, followed by additional sedation in the morning, and this followed by an opiate may not be good for the aged patient. Barbiturates in small doses do have a value of lessening the amount of anesthesia that will be needed. The barbiturates may be ordered in small doses to be given for several days before surgery is done. It must be remembered, however, that barbiturates are prone to cause restlessness and other untoward reactions in the aged. Some physicians prefer to prescribe single doses of a barbiturate such as pentobarbital (Nembutal) whose effects are quickly dissipated. The barbiturate is then given about two hours before the preoperative opiate is to be administered.

Geriatric patients often need less sedation and less anesthesia because in senescence the vitality is lowered, the basal metabolic rate is reduced, and the rate of excretion of drugs is often decreased. Smaller doses of drugs are needed, and cumulative effects must be watched for closely. Tolerance for pain increases with age, and this is another reason why less sedation and anesthesia are needed. A noted surgeon has stated, "Age is its own anesthetist," and most nurses have seen this statement confirmed in the aged person who enters the hospital with peritonitis or another acute illness and yet appears to have relatively little pain.

Selection of preoperative medication and of anesthesia is usually made by an anesthesiologist in consultation with the surgeon. Choice of anesthesia is determined by the condition of the patient, the operation to be performed, and the personal preference of the anesthesiologist. Preanesthetic drugs must be administered exactly at the time specified. Authorities believe that the short-acting barbiturates should be administered two hours before anesthesia is to be given, and that the opiate hypodermic dose should be given not less than seventy-five minutes before; thus the peak effect of the drug will fall at the time of anesthesia induction. If administered later, it may cause an undesirable respiratory depression. Morphine or Demerol is usually given to secure maximum relaxation and to lessen metabolic activity. Some anesthesiologists prefer that atropine be given, feeling that it inhibits mucosal secretions. Atropine should be given at least thirty minutes before induction of anesthesia is started. Scopolamine is preferred over atropine by many anesthesiologists because of its synergistic action with morphine. It is not given if the patient has bronchial asthma since it may cause spasm of the bronchioles.

OPERATING ROOM CARE

Patients should be made as comfortable as possible on their way to the operating room. If a stretcher is used, rather than the bed, a pillow should be placed under the patient's head. Thoughtfulness is necessary in handling elderly patients. If the patient must remain on the stretcher for some time, the nurse should offer to help him change position since he may be afraid to move on the narrow stretcher. No patient, particularly the elderly one, should ever be left alone in the hall, the anesthesia room, or the operating room. Unfortunately, in many operating rooms today much moving of patients is done by orderlies, many of whom are unmindful of the individual sensitivity of the patient who is often covered by a hospital gown, open down the back, and an uncertain bath blanket. The patient may be moved from bed to stretcher or to operating table with little concern for his being kept covered. It is no wonder that the entire experience is often most upsetting to old and helpless patients.

Careful explanation should be made to the patient in moving him from the bed or stretcher to the operating table. Slow and distinct instructions as to the desired position on the table will make him feel less awkward and more comfortable. The older patient may need several pillows either for general comfort or to protect marked kyphosis of the back; a small pillow to support the lumbar curve of the spine may help to prevent postoperative back soreness and fatigue. Patience is needed in assisting older patients. The older patient may have a stiff knee, a lame hip, or some other infirmity that makes it hard for him to move easily to the table or to lie in the necessary position for long periods of time. Positions on the operating table such as the lithotomy and the kidney positions may reduce the chest capacity, which could lead to serious difficulties since it is imperative that respiratory embarrassment be avoided. They may also alter circulation and affect blood pressure or predispose the patient to thrombosis. If such a position must be used, it is imperative that the nursing staff have equipment available for immediate use and do their part so that the operative procedure may be completed as quickly as possible.

Restraints should never be used until after the patient is under anesthesia. The effect of tying the wrists to the table and strapping the knees is obvious. Wrist straps or other restraints that are applied after the patient is asleep must be carefully adjusted to avoid trauma or interference with circulation.

If the patient has been put to sleep while in his bed, it must be remembered that he is relaxed and helpless. He must be moved carefully, with support of body parts to protect him from strain on muscles and joints. The aged patient who is on the operating table for several hours should be moved at intervals if this is feasible. This helps to prevent joint and muscle strain and improves circulation. Unusual positions such as the lithotomy position may alter the circulating blood volume. For example, it has been found that there is a variation of 600 ml. in the blood volume in the leg with marked elevation and lowering of the limb.[13]

The decubitus ulcers that sometimes appear in older patients a few days after surgery may be the result of the patient's remaining on the operating table long enough and with enough pressure to result in necrosis of tissue over the bony sacrum. Sponge rubber should be placed under bony prominences if the procedure to be done is likely to require much time. Pressure areas during surgery occur most often on fracture tables when surgery of the hip is being done because of the small weight-bearing surface under the sacrum. Pressure areas may occur also on the perineum when fracture tables are used for such procedures as applying a cast to the hip. These can be prevented in most instances if areas of direct pressure are brought to the attention of the doctor by the nurse and sponge rubber is used for protection.

ANESTHESIA

There is a variety of anesthetizing agents; only a few can be mentioned here. The greatest danger in administration of anesthesia to an older patient is that hypoxia (inadequate oxygen) may occur; therefore the anesthesiologist selects the agent to be used with this in mind. Local and regional anesthesia are employed quite widely in geriatrics in order to avoid respiratory irritation and changes in blood pressure. Barbiturates are almost always given when local or regional anesthesia is used because they have the effect of combating the toxic effect of the anesthetizing drug.

Intravenous anesthesia is used with caution for the aged, though many skilled anesthesiologists believe that it is safe as an induction anesthetic or for surgery that demands a very short interval of anesthesia. It can be used safely in this way in many instances and may then be followed by some other anesthetic agent and oxygen. Certainly the patient is less disturbed by the insertion of an intravenous needle than he is by an anesthetic mask over his face for administration of an inhalation anesthetic. Thiopental sodium (Pentothal Sodium) is the drug most often used for intravenous anesthesia. It is not given if dyspnea or cardiac or respiratory embarrassment is present. Curare, which is not an anesthetic but which causes muscular relaxation, is quite widely used in combination with thiopental sodium.

Spinal anesthesia has been used extensively in the past, but authorities disagree about its present place in anesthesia for geriatric patients. The amount of anesthesia required and the location of the area to be operated upon partly determine whether it will be used. If a low sacral anesthesia is all that is necessary, the patient is relatively safe, but when sufficient amounts are given so that relaxation to the nipple line is secured, a drop in blood pressure is likely to occur, as well as respiratory depression. A drop in blood pressure for any interval of time is particularly dangerous to patients who have degenerative diseases of the blood vessels and the heart. A degenerative vascular lesion may be the site for formation of a thrombus and for emboli which may cause sudden death. Ephedrine may be given either before spinal anesthesia is started or during anesthesia if a fall in blood pressure occurs. The dosage must be individualized for each patient.

Inhalation anesthesia is considered relatively safe if it is administered by a skilled anesthesiologist. Anoxia is particularly dangerous to the elderly patient and must be guarded against both during anesthesia and in the immediate postoperative period. Cyclopropane has many advantages. For example, it is given in a mixture of pure oxygen; thus anoxia is not likely to occur. It seldom produces nausea, which often occurs following the use of ether. Its serious limitation is that it affects the conduction mechanism of the heart and is contraindicated when arrhythmia is present.

Ether is considered a relatively safe anesthetic agent, though it must sometimes be avoided because of its irritating effect upon the respiratory passages.

Nausea and decreased peristalsis also may follow its use. Renal function may be depressed by ether and shock may occur. Nitrous oxide is considered a safe anesthetic agent if given in a mixture containing enough oxygen. Its usefulness is limited because of its low potency as an anesthetizing agent. Halothane (Fluothane) is a nonexplosive and nonflammable anesthetic. It is a colorless, volatile liquid of very high potency that does not cause postoperative nausea. The recovery from this anesthetic is rapid, but its usefulness is limited because it affects the cardiovascular mechanism and may cause hypotension and bradycardia.

Muscle relaxants are often used in conjunction with anesthesia. The most widely used are *d*-tubocurarine chloride (curare), decamethonium bromide (Syncurine), and succinylcholine chloride (Anectine Chloride). These drugs are in no way analgesic but act only by relaxing the striated muscle. Overdose or an untoward reaction causes difficulty with respiration.

Refrigeration anesthesia, or hypothermia, can be used for elderly patients, and care is similar to that described for younger patients in current nursing texts.[17]

POSTANESTHESIA CARE

Careful observation of the patient following anesthesia is important. Ideally, the patient should be in a recovery room or an intensive care unit where any kind of equipment that might be needed is available for immediate use. The patient's blood pressure should be taken every fifteen minutes for the first few hours, and any failure of the blood pressure to stabilize must be reported to the surgeon at once. Even moderate hypotension may be tolerated poorly by the aged patient and may be followed by renal failure, cardiac failure, thrombophlebitis, or other complications. Hypotension can follow the use of several anesthetic agents, can result from a decreased output of adrenal cortical hormone, or may be caused in part by changes in position of the patient, as well as by blood loss, the trauma of operation, psychic factors, and many other causes.

The effect of muscle relaxants given intravenously should have worn off by the time the patient reaches the recovery room. The nurse should be on the alert for signs of delayed reaction, particularly involving the respiratory muscles. The physiologic antidote for curare is edrophonium chloride (Tensilon Chloride) and for Anectine is Tensilon Chloride or Prostigmin Bromide.

The two most important systems to check carefully after surgery are the cardiovascular and the respiratory systems. In addition to taking the blood pressure, the nurse must check the patient's pulse and report any significant changes in rate or volume.

An airway is almost always used when inhalation anesthesia has been given. The nurse should keep this in place until the patient shows signs of definite reaction or until it is removed by the doctor. Once an airway is removed from a sleeping patient, it is sometimes difficult to replace. Although the tongue cannot be really "swallowed," the relaxed tongue can fall back and obstruct passage of air unless the lower jaw is held forward. Some patients who have had plaster casts applied or have undergone special surgery that requires them to remain on their backs need to have the jaw kept forward until they have reacted from anesthesia fully. In most situations it is much better to turn the patient on his side with his neck extended so that the jaw may fall forward. Restlessness during the period of reacting should be reported, since it may be due to anoxia or to impending shock.

The older patient is a likely candidate for pneumonia or atelectasis. His lung expansion is decreased, and the elasticity of alveolar tissue is less than in youth. The acuteness of the gag reflex is diminished, so that he may aspirate mucus or vomitus. One study showed atelectasis to occur three times more frequently in the elderly than in younger adult patients.[10] A suction apparatus should be on hand when the patient returns from the operating room. The most careful technique is necessary in suctioning the aged patient to avoid trauma and the introduction of infection into the respiratory tract. All equipment should be sterilized before use, and separate catheters must be used for the nose and for the throat. When he awakens, the patient must be urged to cough frequently, and often the nurse can help by applying firm pressure over the incision while he does this. The pressure not only lessens pain but gives the patient a feeling of security that he will not damage the incision. Heavy covers, which may mechanically impede respiration and movements of the body (particularly the legs), should not be used.

Pain and tingling in the lower extremities can be caused by mechanical contact with adjacent nerves at the time of injection of spinal anesthesia or by the irritating effect of procaine solution, particularly if a concentration of over 5 percent has been used. Headache may occur and may be severe. If these symptoms appear, they should be reported to the surgeon promptly. It should be explained to the patient that any symptoms are usually temporary and should disappear in a relatively short time.

Because of impaired circulation and perhaps slower healing ability, the danger of sloughing and of wound infection is greater in age than in youth. The nurse must be constantly on the alert for signs of wound infection, such as pain in the wound, increase in temperature, and drainage from the wound. Peritonitis following abdominal surgery occurs fairly often in aged patients, and the mortality from this is high. Because the patient may have only minor complaints of pain when peritonitis is advanced, even the apparently minor signs and symptoms must be reported immediately.

Strain on muscles and joints may occur during operation and in the immediate postoperative period. Aged patients may complain of general aches and pains for several days following surgery. To lessen the effects of this strain and to prevent further strain, attention should be given to the bed position of the patient. If the patient is placed on his side, a pillow should be placed lengthwise between his legs so that there will be no strain on the upper hip joint, or the upper extremity may be flexed and supported at hip height on pillows. His body should be straight, and care should be taken to see that the under arm is not twisted or deprived of adequate circulation. The patient should have his position changed frequently during the period before he reacts thoroughly from the anesthesia.

Exercise and change of position are important in all postoperative patients, but imperative for elderly patients. The patient is usually instructed to do regular postoperative arm and leg exercises the day of surgery and becomes ambulatory the following day or even in the evening of the day on which extensive surgery has been done. Care must be taken, however, not to overtire the patient. The elderly patient needs a great deal of help when he gets up; early ambulation is helpful in the return to his normal vital capacity and thus restores oxygen intake to what it was preoperatively. It also helps to prevent pulmonary complications and may help to prevent vascular complications. As little sedation as possible is given, since the person who has had a large dose of sedation is less likely to move about. If the patient is in deep sleep, his position should be changed at least every hour. When he is awake, he must be urged to do deep breathing at regular intervals. So important is this to the safety of the patient that the nurse should remain at the bedside to be certain that it is really being done. Unless otherwise ordered by the surgeon, the patient is instructed to breathe deeply and to expand his rib cage three times each day—often every two hours. Voluntary deep breathing, which is so easy for younger persons, is often difficult for older ones. The nurse may have to carefully reinstruct the patient in how to breathe deeply and to repeat the instruction each time such an exercise is to be done. Rarely can she depend upon the very elderly patient to assume responsibility for performing this or any other exercise.

The older patient must be protected from chilling since his circulation is often poor. Warm bath blankets should be used instead of sheets for both the upper and lower covering of the postoperative bed. The patient must be protected from drafts when he gets up to sit in a chair, and it is often necessary to cover his legs with a bath blanket. A warm bathrobe is needed since the hospital gown is either open or loosely tied in the back, and the elderly patient. in most instances, has been used to warm covering over his back and shoulders.

Many older patients are extremely modest and resist ambulation or even sitting on the bedside unless adequately robed. Their reluctance to get out of bed may be less the result of physical causes than of the emotional distress of improper clothing. The nurse who remembers to close the patient's door or draw curtains while he goes through the awkward procedure of putting on a robe while in bed and of getting out of bed will often find that the aged patient gets up more readily and is happier.

Intravenous solutions are given to the surgical patient for several reasons. They are given to replace blood loss at operation, to maintain blood pressure and prevent or treat shock and shocklike reactions, maintain the fluid and electrolyte balance, and provide food when it cannot be taken by mouth. The nurse can be of invaluable assistance to the surgeon in checking the fluid intake and output carefully. The patient's safe progress often depends on the finest discrimination between too little fluid, with resultant dehydration, and too much fluid, with resultant threat of cardiac failure. Intake of sodium chloride is important. Most surgeons agree that 1,000 ml. of physiologic solution of sodium chloride is adequate for a twenty-four-hour period. Glucose and/or protein solutions in distilled water may be given in addition. Potassium may be added to solutions given intravenously. The nurse must be certain that the needed fluids are available, administered according to the surgeon's wishes and with a minimum of discomfort to the patient, and recorded accurately. Careful attention must always be taken in setting up solutions for intravenous administration in order that correct solutions are given.

Because there is danger of increasing the blood volume excessively and causing strain on the heart, some surgeons prefer that intravenous infusions be given slowly during a twenty-four hour period, rather than two or three times each day. When this is done, skillful nursing is needed so that the patient may be moved often and his other needs met without the misfortune of the needle slipping out of the vein. Puncturing of the veins for intravenous injection is a tedious procedure for the aged patient, who resents being repeatedly disturbed. Intravenous injections are usually started by the physician, but in some institutions they are started by the nurse. A simple detail such as inserting the needle well into the vein, where it is less likely to pierce the lumen of the vein and consequently have to be reinserted, adds greatly to the comfort of the patient. It is best to fasten the arm securely on an arm board since the patient is likely to nap at intervals during the day and may move his arm or forget that an intravenous injection is being given. Some elbow and shoulder movements must be permitted if the needle is to remain in the vein for several hours.

Protein needs must be met if the postoperative course is to be satisfactory. Many surgeons feel that the aged surgical patient should receive at least 100 gm. of protein daily and that even a few days of "nothing by mouth" may cause damage to the liver and result in poor healing of the wound unless adequate protein is given in some other way, such as transfusions of whole blood. The best route of administration is by mouth. When this is not possible, the intravenous route must be used. Some protein solutions are slightly more irritating than glucose solutions, and the danger of thrombus formation in the vein at the site of injection is greater. Complaints of pain at the site of injection and any swelling or discoloration should be reported to the surgeon immediately. Most patients have a tendency to rub any uncomfortable swelling at the site of injection. This should be discouraged because it increases the danger of an embolus being released into the blood stream. Patients who receive numerous infusions postoperatively need encouragement, particularly when the surgery is only palliative. Many times they hope that the operation will cure them immediately and are disappointed to find that subsequent treatment must continue for a long time or even indefinitely.

Although the method is seldom used at this time, the patient may be given fluids by means of hypodermoclysis. Usually the solution ordered contains no more than 2 to 5 percent of glucose and 0.87 percent of sodium chloride. Up to 3,000 ml. of fluid can be given daily in this fashion. It must be remembered that the aged person has less subcutaneous tissue and his circulation is often less effective; therefore the fluid may absorb less quickly than in the younger patient. Thus, it is necessary that the nurse watch for signs of pain and swelling at the site of injection. If the patient complains of pain during the hypodermoclysis, the physician should be notified. The doctor may order a small amount of procaine solution added to the fluid being given, which will anesthetize the site of injection and lessen discomfort, or he may wish the rate of flow to be reduced.

A careful record of the output of all aged surgical patients is important. Normally, as in other age groups, the urinary output should be roughly one third of the fluid intake, or about 1,000 ml. per day. If the patient is to receive limited fluids, the nurse must watch the output even more closely. The toxic effects of anesthesia may suddenly precipitate renal failure in the aged patient. Not only the quantity, but also the character of the urine must be watched for unusual cloudiness, sedimentation, or evidence of other abnormal constituents. These should be recorded and reported to the physician.

REFERENCES AND RELATED BIBLIOGRAPHY

1. Beecher, Henry K.: Pain, Surg. Clin. N. Amer. **43**:3:609-617, 1963.
2. Bradshaw, Howard H.: Surgical principles. In Johnson, Wingate M. (editor): The older patient, New York, 1960, Paul B. Hoeber, Inc., Medical Book Department of Harper & Row, Publishers.
3. Case, Thomas C.: The changing trend in surgery for the aged, J. Am. Geriatrics Soc. **10**:677-690, 1962.
4. Case, Thomas C., and Giery, R. A.: Surgery in patients between 80 and 100 years of age, J. Am. Geriatrics Soc. **12**:345-349, 1964.
5. Cole, Warren, and Mason, James H.: Surgical aspects. In Cowdry, E. V. (editor): The care of the geriatric patient, ed. 2, St. Louis, 1963, The C. V. Mosby Co.
6. Fishback, Frederick C.: Essentials of geriatric surgery. In Stieglitz, Edward J. (editor): Geriatric medicine, ed. 3, Philadelphia, 1964, J. B. Lippincott Co.
7. Gittler, Robert D., and Friedfield, Louis: Adrenocortical responsiveness in the aged, J. Am. Geriatrics Soc. **10**:153-159, 1962.
8. Glenn, Frank: Surgical care for the aged, J. Am. Geriatrics Soc. **10**:927-931, 1962.
9. Hanlon, C. Rollins: Preparation of geriatric patients for anesthesia and operation, J.A.M.A. **174**:1827-1829, 1960.
10. Hickey, Mary Catherine: Hypothermia, Amer. J. Nurs. **65**:116-122, 1965.
11. Klug, Thomas J., and McPherson, Richard C.: Postoperative complications in the elderly surgical patient, Am. J. Surg. **97**:713-717, 1959.
12. Litin, Edward M.: Mental reaction of trauma and hospitalization in the aged, J.A.M.A. **162**:1522-1524, 1956.
13. Lorhan, Paul H.: Anesthesia for the aged. In Cowdry, E. V. (editor): The care of the geriatric patient, ed. 2, St. Louis, 1963, The C. V. Mosby Co.
14. Parsons, W. H., Whitaker, H. T., and Hinton, J. K.: Major surgery in patients 70 years of age and over, Ann. Surg. **143**:845-854, 1956.
15. Rose, D. L., and others: Physical measures in the aged, J.A.M.A. **162**:1524-1526, 1956.
16. Scully, Harold F., and Martin, Stevens J.: Anesthetic management for geriatric patients, Amer. J. Nurs. **65**:110-112, 1965.
17. Shafer, Kathleen Newton, and others: Medical-surgical nursing, ed. 3, St. Louis, 1964, The C. V. Mosby Co.
18. Sherman, E. David, and Robillard, Eugène: Sensitivity to pain in relationship to age, J. Am. Geriatrics Soc. **12**:1037-1064, 1964.
19. Stahl, William M.: Major abdominal surgery in the aged patient, J. Am. Geriatrics Soc. **11**:770-780, 1963.
20. Wang, Kuo Chen, and Howland, William S.: Cardiac and pulmonary evaluations in elderly patients before elective surgical operation, J.A.M.A. **166**:993-997, 1959.

Chapter 14

Nursing in cardiac and renal disease

Heart disease is the first cause of death among the elderly. Statistics for 1963 show that 707,830 persons died of heart disease.[2] One third of these were 75 years of age or older. As the proportion of aged in the population increases, the number of deaths from cardiac disease will increase. At the present time cardiovascular diseases, including heart disease and cerebrovascular disease, account for over one half of the deaths from all causes for the total population of all ages. Approximately 1,000,000 out of an approximate total of 1,800,000 deaths were caused primarily by these disorders.[25]

In this short chapter no attempt will be made to discuss in detail the nursing care of patients with cardiac and renal disease and some of the special treatments they receive. Much of the care for elderly patients is the same as for the younger ones and is covered fully in current nursing texts on medical and surgical nursing.[17] Only the differences that pertain to care of the elderly will be mentioned here. Care of the older patient having heart surgery differs only in the aspects related to surgery, which are described in Chapter 13, Anesthesia and Operative Care.

CARDIAC DISEASE

Normal and pathologic changes merge and become difficult to differentiate in the age interval after 65 years. Certain changes that are considered pathologic in youth may be termed normal in old age. Age changes in the heart include dehydration, loss of ability for cellular replacement, and vascular degeneration. With age, the hearts of most people undergo some atrophy. Muscle fibers become smaller, fibrous tissue within the heart muscle increases, the coronary vessels become tortuous, and degeneration of elastic tissue occurs in all vessel walls. In old age the pulse rate usually is slowed but normally is regular in rate with a volume that appears even and consistent.

Heart disease in old age may not seem a distinct entity since other pathologic changes may be present to confuse the clinical picture. There may be generalized circulatory changes and renal impairment resulting from arteriosclerosis, or limitation of the respiratory function from emphysema, bronchiectasis, or other causes. These may make a failing cardiac system more apparent, or they may lead to symptoms that make the diagnosis of heart disease more difficult. Gallbladder disturbance, hiatus hernia, neuromuscular disorders, and many other conditions may further complicate the diagnosis.

Heart disease involving the coronary arteries is by far the most common disease of the heart in those over 45 years of age, and it is the main cause of disability and death in the elderly.[16] Angina pectoris is not a disease but a symptom complex indicating limitation of coronary blood flow. Myocardial infarction occurs when a coronary vessel narrowed by arteriosclerosis and atherosclerosis becomes obstructed, thereby cutting off nourishment to a portion of the heart muscle. Ischemic heart disease is the medical term that describes these conditions most accurately. Arteriosclerotic heart disease (sometimes called senile heart disease) is a term used most often to identify the gradually developing signs that can result in decompensation (heart failure), when the heart becomes unable to meet body requirements in the pumping of blood to the lungs and throughout the body. Coronary artery disease including "silent coronaries" or small, unnoticed myocardial infarctions that damage the heart muscle, generalized arteriosclerosis throughout the body with poor venous return of blood to the system, and poor lung function may be associated with arteriosclerotic heart disease. Enlargement of the heart may occur as the heart attempts to cope with other failing systems.

Prevention

Despite the spectacular surgical approaches to heart disease, the monitoring and emergency care of those hospitalized with myocardial infarction, and the part that nursing plays in new methods of treatment, it is quite possible that in the future the nurse's greatest contribution will be in the field of health teaching.

The epidemiological approach to heart disease has uncovered some strong hints that with very specific but not necessarily difficult changes in our way of life, we need not be a nation with one of the highest death rates from heart disease. In addition to the high death rate, there is a disturbingly high incidence of cardiac disease among men in the younger age group. Autopsies done on soldiers killed in the Korean War showed a very high incidence of advanced atheromatous changes in the blood vessels of young men in their early twenties. In 1963 the death rate from cardiovascular disease among men in the group from 45 to 54 years of age was more than twice the rate for women in the same age group. After the menopause women lose their advantage, and the increased incidence narrows the difference between the sexes.

In recent decades an enormous amount of scientific research and epidemiological investigation has been conducted in the search for the cause of coronary artery disease. Reports of studies and conclusions of investigators and of specialists in this field are numerous and should be read and studied with a critical eye and an unbiased viewpoint by nurses. Although there is definite agreement that the true cause of coronary artery disease has not yet been found, some facts have emerged that should alter health practice at the present time. Every nurse should be familiar with these. She should know what is recommended, should be an example of good health practices in this regard, and should teach these facts and practices to the public, regardless of what her professional area of nursing practice is. The nurse who is a full-time homemaker can contribute as much as the nurse engaged in public health nursing or in a hospital. Most of the health practices that are believed to contribute to prevention of myocardial artery disease are accepted as good practice for general health and have long been recommended.

Repeated studies have shown rather convincingly that the incidence of coronary artery disease is higher in those who have less regular exercise and who have a high standard of living, often with accompanying obesity. Contrary to popular opinion—or popular conversation at least—there is no evidence that physical work started in youth and carried on at an even pace throughout life ever hurt anyone providing there is no chronic heart condition, such as a congenital anomaly. The indications are that it is beneficial. Epidemiological studies conducted at various places throughout the world do not bear out what has also been a widely accepted presumption in the United States—that nervous tension contributed to the development of coronary artery disease. There is somewhat conflicting evidence on smoking and its effect (if any) on coronary artery disease. Because statistical reports from insurance companies show a higher incidence of coronary artery disease among smokers than among nonsmokers and because inhaled smoke is known to be injurious to poorly functioning peripheral blood vessels and harmful to the lungs, most cardiologists now discourage cigarette smoking. The American Heart Association has prepared a pamphlet for the use of physicians in helping their patients to stop smoking.

Habits in regard to regular exercise should be established in youth and carried on in the middle and later years of life. In an age where many people literally do not walk anywhere, it is difficult for many people in young adulthood or middle age to establish a practice of some daily exercise, such as a walk. Strange as it may seem, this is easier for the city dweller who can step from his apartment to the street than for the suburban dweller who must travel by car for most errands and who often cannot take a walk without being offered a ride or considered peculiar by his neighbors. Automobiles and trucks have become so numerous and so swift that in many parts of our country it is extremely dangerous for children to walk to school, and little provision for safe walking is made. The nurse cannot change some aspects of our technologic age, but she can stress constantly to all the need for regular physical exercise.

Statistics from insurance companies have demonstrated consistently for many years that obesity and long life were not compatible and that excessive weight gain after the age of 45 runs parallel with shortening of the life-span. At the present time there is study of the *kind* of overweight and its relationship to heart disease. There is some evidence that weight itself may be less important than the kind of weight. For example, one study[27] showed that persons in a somewhat primitive environment who were quite heavy with highly developed muscles from vigorous exercise had practically no coronary artery disease. There does seem to be some relationship between the obesity caused by the consumption of large amounts of saturated fats, with the deposition of fats throughout the body, and coronary artery disease. Although this relationship is unclear, it is certainly known that obesity places a strain on the heart and entire vascular system as well as upon the musculoskeletal system.

The time to learn to control weight is in early middle age. Concern for overweight in early adulthood and attention to diet so that weight is not gained is infinitely better than attempting weight reduction when obesity has developed. It is probable that too much attention in this country has been paid to undernutrition and that more should be paid to overnutrition. Nutrition, however, appears to be a subject of interest to many people, as demonstrated by the enormous sales of completely unscientific, popular books on nutrition and dieting. The nurse should stress the need to avoid fads and notions about dieting and to seek information from reliable sources, such as the family physician. Emphasis should be on eating a normal, well-balanced diet as outlined in Chapter 7, Nutrition, and in basic nutrition texts. When discussing weight reduction with an elderly person, the nurse should urge that medical supervision be sought. Usually, rapid weight loss is not recommended for the elderly. Management of obesity is discussed in Chapter 7, Nutrition.

There is now quite general agreement among cardiologists that some modifications in the usual diet of people in this country are advisable for persons who have signs that may mean heart disease is developing, such as high blood pressure, high cholesterol level in the blood, and obesity, and for those with known coronary artery disease. The American Heart Association has made similar recommendations. It is quite likely that within the near future these changes will be considered best for everyone as preventive measures. Teaching about them will then become an important responsibility of nurses. Changes in diet are concerned with the amount of fat, the kind of fat, and possibly the kind of carbohydrate. Studies from the United States Department of Agriculture show the increased consumption of fat in American diets over recent years. In 1910, the average American diet approximated; in grams: carbohydrate 450, protein 93, and fat 113, giving a total of 3,189 calories. In 1948, it had changed to carbohydrate 375, protein 90, and fat 130, giving a total of 3,030 calories, It was estimated that many businessmen have an average daily fat intake of 180 grams. It is now advocated by some leading nutritionists[13, 20] that the average diet should contain, in grams: carbohydrate 300, protein 90, and fat 70, giving a total of 2,200 calories. It is believed that fat should constitute only about 25 percent of the total calories and that this fat should be derived mainly from unsaturated fats. Recently there has been suspicion that the high consumption of refined sugars (sucrose) may not be nutritionally as good as eating more carbohydrate foods in their natural state, such as fresh fruits.

When encouraging people to make modifications in diet in line with recommendations for possible prevention of coronary artery disease, the nurse should be practical. Food practices are largely a matter of habit, and it is generally easier to make some modifications in the usual diet than to try to urge drastic changes and rigid curtailment. For example, marked improvement in diet—in line with what many investigators believe may be helpful—would be achieved simply if oil such as corn oil were used instead of lard or hydrogenated oils for frying and baking; if skim milk were used instead of whole milk; and if the family established the pattern of having fish or chicken sandwiches instead of the customary luncheon bologna or liverwurst and had fish, chicken, or other fowl and veal as dinner entrees once each week. The practice in some European countries of ending the meal with fresh fruit is excellent in that it provides a dessert low in calories and low in fat. It is also high in a desirable form of carbohydrate—from a dental standpoint if for no other reason.

The nurse can help the middle-aged person to understand and to carry out his physician's instructions. Regular physical examinations for persons over 40 years of age by a physician who has an interest in the aging person would help to control the development of conditions conducive to heart disease. Much can be done to prolong life within the limitations imposed by the physiologic and pathologic changes that may be developing. High blood pressure, for example, is very common in association with heart disease among the elderly. This is particularly so when the person has diabetes mellitus also. High blood pressure now responds in most instances to drugs that are available.

Heart disease is feared by most people. The nurse should bear this in mind as she questions people about symptoms and encourages them to seek medical care. Although their cause may prove trivial, the nurse should urge any person to see his doctor if the following occur: attacks of shortness of breath or unexpected dyspnea on exertion, feeling of pressure in the chest on awakening at night and a consciousness of heart action or discomfort, or discomfort resembling indigestion that is relieved by sitting up.[19] One study showed that of seventy-three patients who developed myocardial infarction, only fifteen had had no clinically recognizable signs or symptoms.[23] Pain, however, does not necessarily always occur. It was reported by only approximately half of the patients in the same study. Dyspnea upon exertion and particularly upon climbing up steep grades or upstairs is a significant sign, and any precordial discomfort related to exertion or to meals should be reported. A feeling of need to take a full deep breath at intervals in order to get enough air may be a sign of approaching coronary difficulty. On the other hand, it may be due to fear and nervous tension. The person may hold his breath unconsciously and thereby develop dyspnea. Medical investigation should be encouraged whenever a person complains of dyspnea so that the true cause can be determined. Nosebleeds in the older person are sometimes caused by hypertension and should be cause for a check with the physician.

Prevention in rehabilitation. The nurse's responsibility in the area of prevention includes helping to prevent permanent invalidism for those who have had myocardial infarctions. The potential each patient has for full normal participation in living varies with the individual patient and depends upon the recommendations made for him by his doctor. The nurse must know exactly what these recommendations are and use them as her guide in all aspects of her care of the patient in the convalescent phase of illness.

In addition to care of the individual patient, the nurse should contribute to education of the public in an area where again fact and fallacy are confused. It is widely believed, for example, that people who have had a myocardial infarction should cut down substantially on their work load and that exertion may produce another heart attack. This is believed in spite of the fact that several individuals prominent in public life have demonstrated otherwise. Many nurses themselves share these views, and they consciously or unconsciously contribute to the myth that an attack of coronary artery disease means the end of active, useful life.

It is believed that approximately three fourths of persons who have had myocardial infarctions can return to full employment. Many of these are in the late middle age or older age group, and many times the heart attack is considered by employers as a good time to have the worker wind up his business affairs and retire. This may be a disastrous experience for the older person both physically and emotionally, as well as a needless inconvenience to the employer.

It has been found that most jobs require less energy output than is within the capacity of the person who has marked cardiac limitation. In the categories designated by the American Heart Association this category means that it requires 2.5 calories or less per minute.[4] It is believed that exercise and work are good for most people following a myocardial infarction. Exercise appears to stimulate the development of collateral blood vessels in the heart and may have other benefits not yet understood. Exercise may have to be limited in some instances following a myocardial infarction, and often it is curtailed for the elderly person who has heart enlargement, generalized arteriosclerosis, and signs of impending cardiac decompensation. It should be repeated that before the nurse gives *any* counsel to *any* elderly person with heart disease, she must know the patient and she must know what the doctor's findings and recommendations are. The heart and its function are related so closely in every person's mind with life that one misplaced word or gesture of concern or apprehension on the part of the nurse may dampen the patient's spirit and delay rehabilitation.

General nursing

When a diagnosis of cardiac disease has been made and the patient is under medical care, the nurse may help to prevent progressive development of the disease. Often the patient needs help in setting up a plan so that medications will be taken as prescribed (see Chapter 12, Special Treatments). The nurse should discuss with the patient his method for assuring that medications are taken regularly, should learn what signs of toxicity or untoward reaction the doctor has suggested might occur, and should encourage him to report these signs at once. She should determine what plans he has made to have an adequate supply of medications on hand at all times.

Older people with heart disease usually are advised by their physicians to avoid large meals. Servings should be small and there can be added nourishment between meals if hunger is troublesome. A rest period after each meal gives an opportunity for relaxation and furthers digestion. The diet should be as prescribed by the doctor. Very often salt is limited in amount, and this deprivation is extremely difficult for some elderly persons to accept. By getting to know the patient, the nurse may motivate him to accept the necessary restrictions. For example, one patient may respond to a fairly complete explanation of the action of extra salt in the body and how it increases the burden upon the heart, while another person might respond to this discussion with fear and might be better persuaded by a discussion centered around the planning of palatable dishes that require little salt. Sometimes the doctor will permit the patient to have some greatly enjoyed food such as a slice of bacon once or twice a week, providing he avoids salt in other foods, and this simple measure enables him to cooperate more fully.

The counseling interview with the patient should include discussion of a plan of activity for the day that provides for regular rest periods. Provisions for shopping, care of the home, or other problems should be discussed. If the patient is attending the outpatient clinic in a fairly large community, a social case worker may be available and can often help the patient in planning for continued living in his home and community.

Diagnostic tests

The numerous tests and procedures that must be performed when a patient has signs of heart disease should be explained carefully. Blood pressure and pulse may be taken frequently and this may alarm older patients. Electrocardiograms are often useful in judging the amount of heart muscle damage that has occurred and the recovery that is taking place. Several tests, such as the transaminase test for myocardial infarction, involve the taking of blood. These tests and the nursing care involved are discussed in current nursing texts.[17] All procedures must be explained, since the patient may be frightened as when leads are applied for an electrocardiogram. Freedom from apprehension should be sought for the person with heart disease. Any apprehension or fear mentioned to the nurse should be reported to the doctor so that he may give additional reassurance.

Acute cardiac disease

An older person with acute cardiac disease may be treated in the hospital or in his home. Most physicians believe that the patient who becomes ill suddenly with a heart ailment should be moved to the hospital, where treatment not available for the home can be given if needed. The patient may not remain in the hospital long, however, and may progress quite as satisfactorily at home provided that family members are willing and able to care for him and that nurses are available to give needed care and to teach and supervise family members in giving care.

At the present time oxygen is not generally considered too important in the treatment of heart disease. Some physicians order oxygen primarily because they believe the cool air within the oxygen tent is conducive to rest, particularly during hot weather. Oxygen can be given in the home either by tent or, more simply, by nasal catheter or mask. When oxygen is used, the family must be cautioned regarding the danger of fire; candles used in religious rites, lighted cigarettes, and kerosene heaters and lamps are all sources of danger. Family members must be instructed to refrain from talking to the patient who is receiving oxygen by mask. When oxygen is used, its purpose must be thoroughly explained to the patient, since many patients still believe that its use is a last resort and therefore an indication that their chances for recovery are exceedingly poor.

Following an acute attack of heart disease, the patient must be kept quiet and in bed. Whether the patient is in the hospital or at home, visitors must be restricted. During the first few hours or first few days following an acute heart attack, the patient may be so frightened and so ill that he remains willingly in bed. On the other hand, he may be irrational and may attempt to get up. After a few days he may become restless and decide that no harm can come of his getting out of bed and going to the bathroom. In many instances the doctor permits a patient with cardiac decompensation to be out of bed for meals and to use the commode. He must be attended constantly if he shows any signs of being irrational or if he is disinclined to comply with the doctor's instructions.

It is most important that attempts be made to prevent thrombus formation with embolism by attention to bed exercise. During the time of acute illness, the doctor may prescribe passive exercises. If necessary, the nurse should ask for specific instructions for carrying out the exercises. Usually the procedure consists of taking each limb slowly through a complete range of joint motion five to ten times, and is repeated three times daily. The patient may have a tendency to attempt to do the moving actively. If absolute rest is ordered, the nurse must remind the patient to relax and to allow her to do the moving. Gradually, as his condition improves, he may be permitted to do the same exercises actively. Muscle setting or isometric exercises may be ordered by some physicians. These may be taught by the physical therapist or by the nurse if she is familiar with them. The contraction of the muscles even without joint movement compresses peripheral veins and aids the return of venous blood to the heart.

Diet and elimination are important in care of older persons with heart disease. Meals should be small, and foods that are likely to cause distention should be avoided. During the first few days after a myocardial infarction or if the patient is in acute congestive failure, the diet may consist of fluids and soft foods only. Most doctors do not favor rigid and incomplete diets, but prefer to prescribe easily digested soft or solid foods, with limited fluids. It has been found that in order to function at its best, a faulty myocardium must have a regular supply of glucose; small amounts of honey or glucose, taken every two hours, have been helpful in the treatment of acute heart failure in aged persons.[19]

Emphasis by some physicians is not so much on low fluid intake as upon low sodium intake, because the sodium ion passing into the tissues draws water to preserve a normal isotonic balance of tissue fluids. If the sodium ion is not present, the water alone will not leave the general circulation to enter the tissues, and edema will not occur. What is more, it is now believed that liberal amounts of water, harmless in the absence of sodium, are needed in the excretion of waste products. On the other hand, it is often more difficult in the long run to free patients of fluid accumulations when fluids are allowed liberally than when they are restricted.

It must be remembered that older people accept radical diets poorly. Many physicians feel that there is little to be gained by insisting that elderly patients follow a rigid diet, with the exception of the necessary restriction to a low salt content. Food low in salt is not readily acceptable to many people, and ways to make it attractive tax the resourcefulness of the dietitian and the nurse. So far, no safe and entirely satisfactory salt substitutes have been found.

When sodium chloride is restricted, the patient and his family should be cautioned against the use of sodium bicarbonate and soft drinks containing soda water, since these preparations will release the sodium ion and their use may result in fluid accumulation in the tissues. Many people think of sodium bicarbonate as an innocuous substance that can be taken liberally without medical consultation when gastric disturbance occurs and may not think to mention its use to the doctor or the nurse. If some gastric antacid is needed, the doctor may prescribe calcium carbonate, which will have no effect on the control of edema.

Other practices should be queried. One patient, for example, had edema that persisted until his practice of using snuff was discovered. Restriction in its use led to improvement in symptoms, since it was found to contain large amounts of sodium.

A period of rest should follow the taking of food. Pillows should be comfortably placed, the back rest should be lowered as much as is consistent with ease in breathing, the blinds should be lowered, and visitors should be restricted. This routine should be strictly adhered to both in the hospital and in the home and after all three meals of the day.

Drugs. Digitalis preparations and mercurial drugs are used extensively in treatment of cardiac disease with congestive heart failure. Most of the mercurial diuretics now in use have been proved to have no injurious effect upon the kidneys even when they are used over long periods of time. Preparations of mercury and theophylline administered intramuscularly in doses of 1 or 2 ml. and given daily or several times each week are effective in controlling edema. Because they can be taken by mouth, the newer synthetic drugs such as chlorothiazide (Diuril) are now prescribed very widely.

Weight. Many physicians depend on the weight record to indicate fluid retention and feel that it is a more dependable guide than the record of fluid intake and output. When a patient is receiving diuretics, his weight usually must be recorded daily. It is imperative that the nurse weigh the patient as often as is ordered and with as little physical exertion on his part as is possible. Movable scales that can be wheeled to the bedside are essential. Weighing of patients is a nursing responsibility that should be delegated to auxiliary personnel only when the nurse is absolutely certain that they have been thoroughly instructed in close observation of the patient for dizziness or uncertainty when being weighed and in accuracy in recording the patient's weight. Accidents can occur from the patient's becoming faint while standing on the scales and from insufficient care in assisting him in and out of bed.

Often an output record is requested by the physician since the volume of urine output is another guide to the effectiveness of diuretics.

Elimination. Constipation and straining with elimination must be avoided. Vigorous laxatives are not used, but a regular dose of mineral oil, the bulk laxatives such as those containing agar agar or psyllium seed, or other mild cathartic is usually ordered. Most physicians prefer that their patients take enough laxatives so that enemas are not needed, since expelling the enema may cause straining and fatigue. The use of enemas, rectal suppositories, and even rectal thermometers may not be permitted for the patient with acute cardiac disease, because it is believed that this may stimulate the vagus nerve and in turn may slow the heartbeat. The doctor may permit the patient to be out of bed to use the commode once or twice each day. This must not be construed by the nurse as an order that permits the patient to be out of bed at other times. There are indications, however, that moving to a commode once or twice a day consumes less energy than using a bedpan.

Straining at micturition must also be avoided. Assurance to the patient that there will be complete privacy when a bedpan or urinal is being used will prevent some of the voiding difficulties of bed patients. Elderly men who are troubled with prostatic hypertrophy may find it impossible to void in the reclining position. If this difficulty is encountered, the doctor must be notified. He may allow the patient to sit on the edge of the bed with feet on a chair to void or even to stand up. Insertion of a catheter in men patients is avoided because of the danger of its causing infection.

Bed posture. Attention to pillow arrangement and to bed posture is an important part of nursing of elderly cardiac patients. The cardiac patient may not be permitted out of bed. Because of his age he is likely to become stiff and tired after prolonged recumbency in the same position. His shoulders may become fatigued from the weight of his unsupported arms when he is in the sitting position. Pillow supports for the arms offer a welcome change as does also an overbed table against which he may rest for short periods. If an ice bag is used, it should be fastened to the head of the bed, since it is extremely difficult for the patient to hold it in place. If the left arm and shoulder continue to be painful or stiff as a result of anginal symptoms or if other stiffness should occur, physical therapy may be used. Physical therapy can be given at the patient's bedside when it is impossible to move him to the department of physical medicine for treatment.

Convalescence. Since the convalescent period following acute cardiac illness is quite long, it is important that dependence upon sedatives be avoided. Phenobarbital is sometimes used in small doses during the day and as a somnifacient, but it should be avoided if the patient can possibly sleep without any drug. The importance of a warm drink at the hour of sleep, a thorough backrub, a cheerful word, and the provision of adequate bedcovers and suitable ventilation cannot be overemphasized in nursing care for the patient with heart disease.

The patient may have no pain and may become restless and impatient with the restriction of activity prescribed for him. He must be taught to live within the limit of his cardiac capacity when he returns to his family group and to society. He is happiest when he is kept quietly employed so that he will not brood over things he cannot do and will not worry unnecessarily over situations that may never develop. For instance, the patient often becomes depressed and obsessed with the fear that he is "through" and is no longer of any use to his family. Simple reassurance does not usually give him consolation for long, but psychotherapy may be of value, and occupational therapy until he is able to resume some really constructive and remunerative activity is of inestimable value in maintaining mental well-being.

Ischemic heart disease—angina pectoris and myocardial infarction

The common name for ischemic heart disease is coronary artery disease and it is by this name that it is known to the laity. By far the most common form of heart disease in persons over 45 years of age is that which affects the coronary vessels supplying nutrition and oxygen to the heart muscle.

Coronary artery disease is only one manifestation of a pathologic process in which there is degeneration of the arteries, with involvement of the intima and later of other blood vessel layers. The intima thickens, and cells become loaded with fat. This tissue may then further degenerate, and cholesterol crystals appear and finally combine with calcium salts to form calcified plaques. This condition is termed *atherosclerosis* and occurs most often in large vessels. Partial occlusion of the blood vessel results from this narrowing of the vessel lumen. In addition, the roughened inner lining of the blood vessels becomes a likely site for the formation of a clot, which may partially or completely occlude the vessel. The media and outer layers of the artery may become involved and become hardened with an additional calcium deposit; this can be seen in blood vessels when x-ray examination is made (see Figure 28). This is termed *arteriosclerosis.* Both conditions often occur together, and the terms are sometimes used interchangeably.

Coronary artery disease is not exclusively a disease of late middle life and old age. Many persons have atherosclerotic changes of blood vessels in their thirties, particularly if there is hypertension. The specific cause is obscure. Heredity seems to be a factor in the development and the degree of atheromatous change. It is rare in women before the menopause, but after the menopause the incidence in women rises to become almost half that of men.

The part that cholesterol plays in the development and progress of atherosclerosis and in the development of a myocardial infarction is not clear. Neither is it known what other factors may determine the development of a myocardial infarction. For example, interest in recent years has focused on the coagulability of the blood as a possible factor, since it is known that the coagulation time has been found to increase shortly after the ingestion of a meal high in fat. The possible effect of certain carbohydrates in the production of substances in the blood that may contribute to infarction are also being studied at this time.

Myocardial damage with associated congestive heart failure may accompany chronic pathology of the coronary vessels, or may follow a partial coronary occlusion in which nutrition to the heart muscle has been restricted. Hypertension and generalized arteriosclerosis are more frequently associated with coronary disease in the aged than in younger persons. It is known that many elderly persons have suffered from one or more so-called "silent coronaries" that gave no pronounced symptoms yet damaged the heart muscle.[23]

Angina pectoris is not a disease but a symptom complex that occurs in many persons who have cardiac ischemia or inadequate supply of oxygen to the heart muscle. The first warning is often a vague discomfort usually under the sternum and may appear after a large meal. This may be confused with indigestion and is often treated by the patient with sodium bicarbonate or a laxative. From the feeling of pressure and discomfort under the sternum, symptoms may progress to a precordial pain radiating down the left arm. This usually is brought on by exertion and diminishes with rest. Walking uphill in cold weather or against a strong wind may aggravate symptoms. The most common cause is exercise, although many times anginal pain may be brought on by emotional tensions. Anginal pain usually indicates serious myocardial ischemia; especially is this true if it occurs during the night caused, supposedly, by the prone posture. The best medical treatment for angina pectoris has not changed for decades. Rest at the first sign of pain is always recommended. Nitroglycerin tablets, 0.4 mg. ($\frac{1}{150}$ gr.), placed under the tongue at the first sign of pain are still considered the best drug available. Amyl nitrite perles, which are to be broken and the drug inhaled at the onset of pain and discomfort, may also be prescribed. These drugs have a vasodilating effect that may relax the coronary vessels sufficiently to permit enough blood to flow through the partly occluded vessels to relieve the pain. Because they lower blood pressure and may, therefore, predispose to development of myocardial infarction, their use is now advised with caution. Some physicians recommend the use of slower acting vasodilators such as alcohol at regular intervals.[15] Alcohol dilates blood vessels and ordinarily is a safe medication in the hands of the laity. It may be given immediately when an attack of coronary artery disease seems imminent.

If early signs of narrowing of the lumen of the coronary vessels go unheeded, a complete obstruction of a vessel may occur and may cause sudden death. When occlusion is almost complete, a thrombus may form, and the portion of heart muscle supplied by the vessel may be denied all nutrient supply except what may be brought by collateral vessels. The term myocardial infarction is used to designate the area of ischemic muscle beyond the occlusion and thrombosis and is the preferable term to describe this kind of heart lesion. The severity of the attack will depend upon the extent of the area of heart muscle deprived of blood supply and the efficiency of the collateral circulation. The coronary arteries have many collateral vessels. If this were not so, death from acute coronary occlusion and resultant myocardial infarction would be more frequent than it is. Evidence at autopsies shows that many patients have had silent infarcts that gave few or no symptoms but caused scarring of areas of heart muscle. Thrombosis in a coronary vessel and subsequent infarction may occur when there is no exertion, such as during sleep.

The classic symptoms of acute myocardial infarction are quite definite. There is excruciating pain that may radiate down the left arm and may spread to the entire chest and abdomen and into the neck. The pulse may be weak and irregular, the skin is moist and pale or cyanotic, and the blood pressure is low. Within a few hours the polymorphonuclear blood cell count increases, the temperature may become elevated, and the sedimentation rate increases. Partial or complete anuria may occasionally follow a sudden, marked drop in blood pressure. Cardiac arrhythmias may occur and may lead to death from fibrillation.

Continued state of shock and arrhythmias that do not yield to emergency treatment are indicative of a guarded prognosis.

Immediate treatment consists of giving 50 to 100 mg. of meperidine hydrochloride immediately and moving the patient, if possible, to a hospital. Complete rest, oxygen, drugs to produce dilation of blood vessels, and anticoagulants may be ordered. The patient should be attended constantly since he is in extreme distress and is fearful of death. *l*-Norepinephrine (Levarterenol, Levophed) is the drug most often given for profound shock. Theophylline ethylenediamine (Aminophylline) is often given intravenously or by mouth for its diuretic and vasodilatory effect. Papaverine hydrochloride may be used to produce dilation of blood vessels, and heparin, bishydroxycoumarin (Dicumarol), and warfarin (Coumadin) may be given to deter coagulation of the blood. The nursing care related to the use of these drugs is discussed in current texts on medical and surgical nursing.[17]

Armchair care is the term used to designate a plan whereby the patient with an acute myocardial infarction is placed in a chair for long periods. It is believed by those who prescribe this treatment that the upright position prevents "pooling" of blood in the pulmonary vessels and thereby lessens the work load of the heart. When this treatment is ordered, the patient must be lifted very carefully to the chair and not permitted any more activity than if he were in bed.

Though it is the policy in many clinics to mobilize cardiac patients much earlier than was done in the past, it is still quite generally believed that a person who has had a myocardial infarction should be treated with rest for a long period of time, usually four to six weeks. The nurse should be particularly alert for sudden changes in the patient and should guard him from activity in the time interval from eleven to sixteen days after the acute attack. During this time the area of heart muscle to which the blood supply is restricted undergoes certain changes and is replaced by scar tissue. It is soft and likely to rupture if any strain is placed upon it, such as overexertion, which would increase the pulse rate or pulse pressure.

A myocardial infarction does not necessarily mean that there will be a marked shortening of life. With care the patient may expect to live at least from five to ten years, and some patients have lived longer than twenty-five years. The length of time will depend a good deal upon the way a person lives after acute illness is over. When he is considered completely recovered from the acute attack, he should look upon himself as a well person, not an invalid. He should accept certain limitations which will permit him to live normally with his particular heart condition. A person who has had a myocardial infarction should have nine to ten hours of sleep each night. He should relax for a short period after each meal, he should arise slowly in the morning, dress deliberately, and prepare for the day leisurely. He should eat less at meals and in consequence lose weight if he has been overweight. He should not experiment to see how much he is still able to do. Questions regarding activity, such as whether he can play golf or tennis and dance, should always be referred to his physician for decision. Usually if the patient can tolerate alcohol in moderate amounts, he should take some regularly. In all the details of his daily living he must be made to see the wisdom of following his doctor's instructions accurately.

Generalized arteriosclerotic heart disease with congestive failure

As has been mentioned earlier, arteriosclerotic heart disease may follow partial occlusion of coronary vessels, with resultant poor nutrition to cardiac muscle and impaired cardiac capacity. However, in this disease there is usually generalized arteriosclerosis, increased blood pressure, and renal impairment. Many patients with arteriosclerotic heart disease also have mild diabetes. Many are overweight. Cardiac failure, heart failure, and cardiac insufficiency are terms also used. All signs and symptoms occur because the heart is no longer able to meet body requirements in pumping blood to the lungs from the right ventricle and to the body from the left ventricle.

Early signs of arteriosclerotic heart disease with congestive failure are those of cardiac decompensation. Symptoms often develop slowly. The patient may have difficulty in sleeping when he lies flat. He may waken during the night feeling vaguely uncomfortable and finally fall asleep when he is propped by several pillows. He may then notice dyspnea on exertion. He may have to pause for breath when walking, when carrying a rather heavy package, and after climbing a flight of stairs. Other symptoms may be pallor and a general fatigue, which often becomes so marked that it is difficult for an older person to prepare meals and carry on the activities of daily living. Ankle edema and general edema of the abdomen, sacral region, and other parts of the body may then occur and are due to failure of the right side of the heart. Pulmonary congestion from accumulation of fluid in the lungs due to left-sided or left ventricular failure may be the final precipitating symptom that brings the patient to the doctor.

Congestive heart failure with decompensation can often be prevented in aged patients with arteriosclerotic heart disease if they are treated early before symptoms become pronounced. Education in the importance of avoiding obesity and in cutting down the work load of the heart as its capacity declines would do much to control the disease. An extremely important aspect of care is to initiate treatment before decompensation has progressed far, since the aged patient cannot withstand the results of impaired circulation without some penalty. Mental disease, vascular disease, and many other conditions may appear and may be secondary to the inadequate blood supply to parts of the body.

Treatment for arteriosclerotic heart disease with congestive failure consists of physical and mental rest. Oxygen is given in an attempt to meet the requirements of the body tissues, a low-sodium diet to control edema is prescribed, diuretics to remove excess fluid are administered, supportive measures to prevent attendant complications are instituted, and digitalis to strengthen the heart muscle is given. Digitalis leaf remains the best preparation for routine digitalization and maintenance of patients requiring digitalis. But one of the quick-acting glycosides or a preparation like digitoxin, which can be given intravenously when oral administration is not possible, should be available for emergency use.

Lanatoside C (Cedilanid), a glycoside of digitalis, is given intravenously in emergencies. Usually 0.8 mg. is given as the first dose. After the pulse has been carefully noted for half an hour, an additional 0.4 mg. is given, and this is repeated in one half to one hour if the pulse rate and rhythm have not yet approached normal. Because the effect of this drug is dissipated in twenty-four to seventy-two hours, one of the digitalis preparations is usually ordered also. This is so that digitalization can be maintained, without repeated intravenous injections of the quick-acting drug. Diuretic drugs usually are given.

A patient with congestive heart failure may be allowed to be out of bed for short intervals. The nurse must have definite orders regarding the patient's rest and activity. Sometimes he does not need the absolute rest that is necessary during the healing period following myocardial infarction. He is likely to develop pulmonary congestion and thrombosis of the peripheral blood vessels if he is kept constantly in bed. The patient should be placed in a comfortable chair with arm supports from which he cannot readily slip; usually a footstool adds to his comfort. While sitting up, the patient must be observed closely for signs of dyspnea and fatigue and changes in pulse or skin color.

If the patient must remain in bed, passive or active exercises should be done regularly under the direction of the physician. The older person's skin breaks down easily because it is thin and suffers from restricted blood supply; edema and poor tissue nutrition are factors that predispose to a breakdown of the skin. The nurse should have a regular schedule for back care and change of position for the patient lest this essential part of care be neglected for long periods during the day. Pillows must be arranged so that support to the entire back is provided and crowding of abdominal viscera against the diaphragm is avoided. Sometimes the patient may be comfortable with the head of the bed raised on shock blocks. This prevents pressure of abdominal organs against the diaphragm, which so often occurs when the patient is placed in high Fowler's position.

It is usually helpful to have the nurse from the public health nursing agency visit the patient restricted to his home. She may give the mercurial diuretic and thus spare the patient the expense and exertion of a regular trip to the hospital or the doctor's office. The nurse can check the patient's weight and help him or his family with problems connected with diet. A salt-free diet is usually difficult for the family to prepare, and the nurse can often make useful suggestions. Sauces prepared from a tomato base with liberal amounts of a variety of herbs may help to make low-salt food more palatable. She can give the patient encouragement in following his diet by pointing out to him that he feels much better than he did (if this is true) and that there are things he can now do that would not be possible were he to continue with his accustomed free use of salt.

Fortunately for the patient there has been a swing away from the rigid, severe salt-free regimen advocated a few years ago. It is now believed that excess salt contributes to edema and is contraindicated, but that too little salt can cause trouble, particularly in elderly patients.[18] The nurse can clarify instructions regarding rest and activity that may not be clear to the patient or to his family, and she can be of great assistance to the physician in reporting the patient's condition at regular intervals.

The patient with heart disease needs encouragement. He fears death and

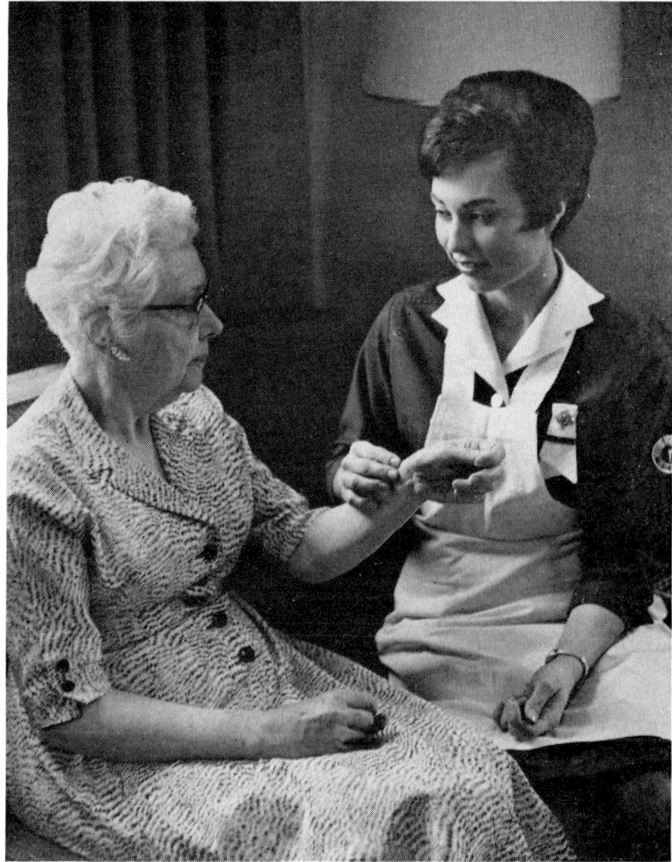

Figure 27. The patient is spared unnecessary trips for medical supervision when the nurse visits her regularly and reports to the physician. (Photograph by Harold Ferman.)

worries excessively. He must be told that if he follows his doctor's directions accurately and lives within his cardiac reserve, he need not live in daily fear of cardiac failure. Many persons who have needed specific treatment for mild cardiac decompensation may be able to carry on with outside work and lead relatively normal lives simply by resting more on weekends, going to bed early, and eliminating a few inconspicuous but energy-consuming tasks about their homes. A tempered pace with some curtailment of vigorous activity and of situations conducive to heart strain do not mean in any sense that the patient should become an invalid.

RENAL DISEASE

Renal disease, which in the older person is often due to chronic and progressive degenerative changes, is fairly common in the aged. In 1961 nonspecific chronic renal disease and nephrosclerosis accounted for 11,500 deaths. Degenerative changes may progress for years before the kidney reserves become exhausted and symptoms appear. Acute infections involving the kidneys may occur, but are rare in the aged, whereas most persons who have chronic glomerular or interstitial nephritis in their younger life do not survive to old age.

Classification of disease of the kidneys is not consistent, and theories as to the exact etiology of kidneys disease are conflicting and uncertain. The name nephrosclerosis has been used by some authorities to designate kidney disease that is definitely related to vascular impairment characteristic of aging; others use the term nephrosclerosis to signify renal disease accompanied by hypertension, including the malignant hypertension of young people.

It is impossible, at the present time, to provide the nurse with a clear-cut explanation of renal changes and renal disease in age. A few facts, however, seem to be fairly definitely established. The kidneys do decrease in size with age; some of the glomeruli have been worn out or destroyed and have been replaced with scar tissue; therefore fewer functioning units remain. The kidney uses more oxygen than any other organ in proportion to its weight and during rest uses 9 percent of the total body consumption.[22] Obviously, the oxygen deprivation that occurs from anemia, surgical shock, or other causes may be disastrous. Generalized arteriosclerosis results in reduced blood supply (oxygen) to the entire organ and consequently lowers the effectiveness of the kidney itself. A smaller volume of blood may be brought to the functioning units of the kidney, and the output of waste products will be decreased commensurately. This may be because of cardiac limitations, obstruction of blood vessels, low blood pressure, or other causes. The glomeruli and tubules of the aged person are more susceptible to damage from toxins and similar irritants than are those of younger persons.

Degenerative changes in the kidneys that occur in age cannot be prevented. The nurse can help to avoid renal failure in the patient by prevention of factors that may overtax kidney function. Infections must be guarded against since the effect of toxins produced, plus the increase in metabolic rate, may precipitate renal failure. The elderly patient responds unfavorably to toxicity of medication; the nurse must observe him closely for signs of cumulative effect of drugs, as well as for the earliest signs of reaction to their toxic qualities.

Large amounts of urine of low specific gravity may be excreted as a result of the kidney's inability to concentrate the urine. The most common sign of renal decompensation is the output of quantities of urine of low specific gravity as the kidneys continue a losing battle in their futile effort to excrete waste products as fast as they accumulate. The nurse should observe the urinalysis record on the patient's chart at intervals. A low fixed specific gravity gives an excellent clue to the presence of renal limitations. Edema is often entirely absent in the nephropathy of old age. The general appearance of the patient may give no hint of his actual renal limitations; frequency and nocturia may be the only obvious signs of approaching or incipient renal failure. Mental confusion may be the first sign, and this is fairly common in kidney disease in old age. Pallor is consistently present in kidney disease.

Edema may occur and is most often seen in renal disease that is accompanied by arteriosclerotic cardiac failure with decompensation. Edema is usually treated with a diet that is low in sodium chloride, but adequate in protein to replace blood and tissue deficiencies, and generous or high in fluids. Digitalis preparations are often given, and the xanthine diuretics such as theobromine may be ordered. Large amounts of plain water by mouth or distilled water by vein are usually ordered.

Renal failure in an older person does not necessarily mean death. It is extremely serious, however, and few persons survive many repetitions of renal decompensation. If it is possible with medical treatment to induce the remaining glomeruli to improve their function and to reduce overtaxing the resources of the kidney, it may be possible to prolong life for months or even longer. Peritoneal dialysis and other measures used in attempts to compensate for failing kidney function are discussed in current medical and nursing texts.[1, 17]

The terminal stage of nephropathy in older people is uremia. Mental confusion is often the first and most pronounced sign. In many patients severe retinal damage occurs and may lead to complete blindness. Halitosis, nausea, vomiting, headache, tremor, and convulsions frequently occur. Nursing for these patients includes prevention of accidents and careful bathing of the skin. Deodorants must often be used about the room of the person who lingers in uremic coma since the body releases an odor that is most distressing to those around the patient. The patient's mouth may require attention as often as every hour. A well-equipped tray will facilitate this important nursing measure. Prevention of pressure areas by frequent changes of position and attention to the careful cleansing and massage of the skin are beneficial.

REFERENCES AND RELATED BIBLIOGRAPHY

1. Beeson, Paul B., and McDermott, Walsh (editors): Cecil-Loeb textbook of medicine, ed. 11, Philadelphia, 1963, W. B. Saunders Co.
2. Bureau of the Census: Statistical Abstracts of the U.S., 1965, ed. 86, Washington, D. C., 1965, U. S. Government Printing Office.
3. Christakis, George, and others: Crete; a study in the metabolic epidemiology of coronary heart disease, Amer. J. Cardiol. **15**:320-332, 1965.
4. Cross, Joseph C.: Back to work after myocardial infarction, Amer. J. Nurs. **61**:58-61, 1962.
5. Dawber, Thomas R., Moore, F. E., and Mann, G. U.: Coronary heart disease in the Framingham study, part 2, Am. J. Pub. Health **47**:4-24, 1957.
6. Dawber, Thomas R., and Kannel, William B.: Coronary heart disease as an epidemiological entity, Am. J. Pub. Health **53**:433-437, 1963.
7. Griep, Arthur H., and Sister De Paul: Angina pectoris, Amer. J. Nurs. **62**:72-75, 1965.
8. Grollman, Arthur: Abnormalities in blood pressure associated with age. In Johnson, Wingate M. (editor): The older patient, New York, 1960, Paul B. Hoeber, Inc., Medical Book Department of Harper & Row, Publishers.
9. Harrison, T. R., and others (editors): Principles of internal medicine, ed. 4, New York, 1962, McGraw-Hill Book Company.
10. Hollazy, John O.: Epidemiology of coronary heart disease; national differences and the role of physical activity, J. Am. Geriatrics Soc. **11**:718-725, 1963.
11. Kinch, Sandra H., and others: Risk factors in ischemic heart disease, Am. J. Pub. Health **53**:438-442, 1963.
12. Krug, Elsie E.: Pharmacology in nursing, ed. 9, St. Louis, 1963, The C. V. Mosby Co.
13. McGavack, Thomas Hodge: Modification and treatment of atherosclerosis by a dietary regimen, J. Am. Geriatrics Soc. **11**:707-717, 1963.
14. Modell, Walter, and others: Handbook of cardiology for nurses, ed. 4, New York, 1963, Springer Publishing Co., Inc.
15. Priest, Walter S.: Angina pectoris, myocardial infarction and acute coronary failure. In

Stieglitz, Edward J. (editor): Geriatric medicine, ed. 3, Philadelphia, 1954, J. B. Lippincott Co.

16. Sawyer, C. Glenn, and Headley, Robert N.: Disease of the heart. In Johnson, Wingate M. (editor): The older patient, New York, 1960, Paul B. Hoeber, Inc., Medical Book Department of Harper & Row, Publishers.
17. Shafer, Kathleen Newton, and others: Medical-surgical nursing, ed. 3, St. Louis, 1964, The C. V. Mosby Co.
18. Sharpe, George, and Stieglitz, Edward J.: Cardiac decompensation. In Stieglitz, Edward J. (editor): Geriatric medicine, ed. 3, Philadelphia, 1954. J. B. Lippincott Co.
19. Sprague, Howard B.: The normal senile heart. In Stieglitz, Edward J. (editor): Geriatric medicine, ed. 3, Philadelphia, 1954, J. B. Lippincott Co.
20. Stare, Frederick J.: Overnutrition, Am. J. Pub. Health **53**:1795-1802, 1963.
21. Steiner, A., Howard, E. J., and Akguan, S.: Importance of dietary cholesterol in man, J.A.M.A. **181**:186-190, 1962.
22. Stieglitz, Edward J.: The nephritides. In Stieglitz, Edward J. (editor): Geriatric medicine, ed. 3, Philadelphia, 1954, J. B. Lippincott Co.
23. Stokes, Joseph, III, and Dawber, Thomas R.: "The silent coronary"; the frequency and clinical characteristics of unrecognized myocardial infarctions in the Framingham study, Ann. Int. Med. **50**:1359-1369, 1959.
24. Health, Education and Welfare Trends, ed. 1963, Washington, D. C., 1963, U. S. Government Printing Office.
25. U. S. Department of Health, Education and Welfare; Monthly vital statistics, Nov., 1964.
26. White, P. D.: The role of exercise in the aged, J.A.M.A. **165**:70-71, 1957.
27. Whyte, H. Malcolm: Behind the adipose curtain; studies in Australia and New Guinea relating to obesity and coronary heart disease, Amer. J. Cardiol. **15**:66-80, 1965.
28. Wolff, Ilse S., and others: The patient with myocardial infarction, Amer. J. Nurs. **64**: C-3–C-32, 1964.

Chapter 15

Nursing in peripheral vascular disease

Though peripheral vascular disease is an inclusive term meaning disease of any blood vessels outside the heart, this section will discuss only a few of the many diseases of arteries and veins of the lower extremities that are commonly seen in the aged. General measures for prevention of complications and care of vascular changes will be considered before nursing in a few of the more common diseases is described.

PHYSICAL CHANGES IN BLOOD VESSELS

Aging is accompanied by several distinct changes in the blood vessels. These changes begin in childhood and progress with individual variation throughout the life of the individual. It is not known with certainty at this time whether changes in blood vessels are nonpathologic and simply occur with the passage of time and with use, or whether they are pathologic and produced by stress, faulty nutrition, trauma, or other causes.

Arteriosclerosis is common. In this condition there is involvement of the middle layer of the arterial wall with thinning, loss of elasticity, and sometimes the deposition of metabolic substances containing calcium. The smaller arteries farther away from the body trunk usually are affected more than the large vessels close to the heart. Arteriosclerosis accounts for the firm and sometimes almost crisp quality of the radial pulse in some elderly people. It is what lessens the ability of a severed vessel to collapse and support a clot, thus predisposing the elderly patient to hemorrhage, and it is the cause of the loss of the pinkish skin color by middle age and the increasing sallowness of the skin in old age.

Atherosclerosis is also common among elderly people. In this condition, which involves more extensively the large vessels as they leave the heart, there is involvement primarily of the intima, or inner layer, of the arterial wall, with deposition on its surface of atheromatous material (plaques) containing cholesterol and sometimes calcium. These deposits produce a roughness on the vessel lining that is believed to predispose to the formation of clots when and if conditions are favorable, and which in turn may lead eventually to complete occlusion of the artery. Arteriosclerosis and atherosclerosis may occur together in varying degrees in a single artery. Many times the term arteriosclerosis is used to denote both kinds of deterioration of the arteries.

Veins throughout the body change with age. They lose some of their elasticity and strength and the valves become less effective in preventing stasis of blood within the vein. These circumstances may well be affected by the loss of subcutaneous tissue and fat that help to support superficial veins and by loss of muscle strength and tone that help to return venous blood to the heart. Reduction in the amount of active physical exercise taken has a pronounced effect in lowering the efficiency of the venous return of blood to the heart.

SIGNS AND SYMPTOMS OF DISEASE

Signs and symptoms of disease may or may not follow when the usual changes of age occur in blood vessels. Their appearance will depend upon whether or not there is adequate blood supplied to the tissues to meet nutritional needs and enough returned to prevent stasis and to remove waste products. Blood pressure will affect this and is, in turn, affected by the rate and force of the heartbeat, the resistance within the arterial walls, and the pressure within the tissues.

Certain specific signs that may indicate the presence of peripheral vascular disease include pain, color changes, skin temperature changes, changes in the size of the part (edema or atrophy), and the presence of trophic changes or infection.

Pain of any nature is important. Pain occurs in ischemia of leg muscles from arteriosclerotic changes, in the neuritis that accompanies ischemia, in impending gangrene, in deep or superficial venous thrombosis, and in infection. The patient often attributes pain to fallen arches, joint stiffness, age, or other causes. His assumption may be correct, but it is imperative that the judgment of the physician be obtained.

Skin color, skin temperature, and size of the limb can be noted by the nurse when she is giving a bath, getting the patient out of bed, or doing other nursing functions. For example, are the feet waxy and white on elevation or rubric on dependency, as in arterial inadequacy? Are they bluish and swollen as sometimes occurs in venous inefficiency? Are the feet cold? Is the foot colder than the leg? Are the two feet and legs the same color and the same relative temperature? If the patient complains of cold feet and if the feet are cold to touch and blanch quickly on elevation, the arterial supply is probably diminished. The size of the two legs should be compared since atrophy of the muscles, often most apparent in the calf of the leg, may follow arterial insufficiency. Edema of the foot and leg should be noted since edema often occurs with deep venous thrombosis, although the possibility of its being of cardiac, nephritic, or malnutritional origin must not be overlooked. Observation by the nurse is exceedingly important since the patient may not have observed his extremities carefully.

The condition of the skin and nails may suggest inadequacy of arterial circulation. Dryness and thickening of the nails and dry, thin, scaling skin are evidences of poor circulation. These so-called trophic changes of the extremities are often the site of definite tissue breakdown such as varicose ulcers or gangrene.

Vascular disease frequently involves the whole organism to some extent, though signs and symptoms may be more apparent in the lower extremities. The nurse must observe her patient closely for general symptoms such as pallor, generalized edema, drowsiness, sensitivity to chilling, memory disturbances, or any other abnormal findings that should be called to the physician's attention.

PREVENTION OF COMPLICATIONS AND TEACHING THE PATIENT

General hygienic habits in regard to foot care need attention. In the hospital the patient's feet should be carefully inspected on admission and observed regularly thereafter. Appearance of any skin disease, such as apparent dermatophytosis, should be reported. Innumerable cases of gangrene of the toes or foot and also of varicose ulcers in persons with vascular impairment have followed fungus infections, which are commonly associated with poor hygiene.

So dangerous are vascular diseases to the health, happiness, and even the lives of older people that no time should be wasted, if symptoms occur, in having them see a physician at once. Authorities in this field of medicine feel that more important than the most skillful treatment of advanced vascular disease is its prevention and its control in early stages. Some aspects of prevention must be emphasized long before old age is reached. For example, varicosity of veins is often increased by obesity and by poor posture. Occupational practices in which the person stands for hours without walking or moving about also predisposes to varicose veins in the legs since there is little muscle stimulation to aid in the return flow of blood.

Most patients with either suspected or diagnosed vascular disease would benefit from a routine for the care of the lower extremities. It often becomes the responsibility of the nurse, working under the direction of the physician, to teach this care. The aim of all teaching is to give the patient the information he needs in order to prevent complications from the vascular disease yet disturb as little as possible his mode of living.

The nurse must know the diagnosis of the patient's disease, the physician's wishes in regard to immediate care, and his long-term plans for care. She must begin instructing the patient as soon as the diagnosis is made since he may have sight, hearing, or memory defects, and repetition may be necessary. She must endeavor to make her teaching practical and adaptable to the conditions under which her patient has to live. She must herself be optimistic about the outcome for the patient. Patients who follow such instructions carefully may have many years of comfort and freedom from symptoms.

Certain essential points of general care are taught the patient by his physician, but may need reemphasis by the nurse. It is absolutely mandatory in any occlusive arterial disease that tobacco be avoided completely. This may be one of the most drastic privations for the older patient with long-established habits of smoking. So definite, however, has the relationship been found between tobacco smoking and arteriospasm in any kind of arterial disease that many physicians feel that it is practically useless to treat the patient unless he will honestly attempt to give up smoking. Constant reiteration by the doctor and the nurse of their faith in the patient's comprehension and ability to follow instructions may yield better results than attempts at strict discipline. Unless there are contraindications, alcohol should be encouraged in moderate amounts since it has a vasodilatory effect and is particularly helpful in conditions in which arteriospasm is present. Rest is important as is also moderate exercise, within the limitations of the disease, as prescribed by the physician. Obesity should be avoided. The diet should be high in protein, minerals, and vitamins. The patient should avoid patent remedies and mechanical devices that are widely advertised and purport to improve circulation. This applies especially to diathermy and other heating equipment to be operated by the patient. Results from treatment in vascular disease are not always too encouraging, and the patient is likely to become restless and to search for a quick cure. The nurse, therefore, has an obligation to help the patient understand the fallacy in constantly shopping around.

The patient must be instructed about his shoes, stockings, and garters. Shoes should be of leather in order to give good support to the feet. It is poor economy to purchase cheap, poorly made shoes since they are harmful and sometimes really dangerous to persons whose feet and peripheral circulation are not normal. Rubber-soled and canvas shoes are poor since they become misshapen and particularly because they retard evaporation and thus encourage the development of fungus infections. The shoe should extend about one half inch beyond the first or second toe, whichever is the longer; it should be wide enough to prevent pressure on the sides of the foot. If bunions have developed, a wider shoe must be worn to prevent pressure on the bunions. The inner last of the shoe should be straight, and the arch of the shoe should support the longitudinal arch of the foot. Shoelaces that are tied too tightly may cause injurious pressure on blood vessels and are not necessary if shoes fit properly. Elastic shoelaces that can be adjusted to be quite loose are now available and may be suitable for some patients who tend to have slight foot edema at the end of the day. New shoes should be broken in gradually, and old shoes should be kept until the new pair is completely comfortable. Every patient should possess at least two pairs of shoes and avoid wearing the same pair day after day. It is advisable to air shoes after use and to use shoe trees. If shoes become wet, shoe trees should be inserted or the shoes should be stuffed with paper while they dry. Otherwise they may become misshapen and possibly injure the feet.

It is necessary for the patient to wear light-colored socks and stockings and to change them daily. The dye from dark socks may be irritating to the skin. Wool socks may be dried on a frame to prevent shrinkage since tight socks or stockings may interfere with circulation to the toes. A simple inexpensive frame for drying socks can be made by hand from a lightweight metal clothes hanger.

Stretch or support hose are now prescribed widely for both men and women who have vascular difficulties. They are often ordered for the person who must stand much of the time at work and whose ability to walk is limited for any reason. They may be ordered to be worn during surgery, when the hospitalized patient is first permitted up after a period of bed rest, and in a wide variety of other circumstances. Support hose should be worn only if prescribed by the physician, who usually measures the patient and orders hose that are large enough and have enough stretch to fit comfortably while giving the desired pressure on the peripheral vessels. The physician decides whether or not the hose should extend above the knee; those coming above the knee are most often ordered. Elastic stockings should be removed and laundered daily. The extremity should be observed for signs of excessive pressure at any point. Occasionally, hose that do not have a full foot are ordered, and signs of pressure may appear at the toes or in the instep or heel. These should be reported to the physician.

A garter belt or a well-fitting corset is best for supporting the stockings. Rolled garters, rolled hose, and elastic-topped hose or socks are avoided since they will further interfere with an already impaired circulatory mechanism. When venous disease is or has been present, girdles and even snug pantie girdles should be avoided since they provide sufficient pressure to impair venous circulation and in the presence of severe occlusive arterial disease may interfere with superficial collateral blood flow.

Foot hygiene must be planned with each patient or with the persons responsible for his care. It is useless to teach the patient the need for washing his feet each day when there is no provision for this to be carried out. A family member or neighbor should perform this necessity if the patient cannot see sufficiently well, cannot reach his feet, or cannot understand or follow instructions.

The feet should be bathed daily in warm water. The temperature of the water should be taken and should be between 35° and 37° C. (95° to 98.6° F.). The patient should be instructed to buy a bath thermometer, and care should be taken that he understands what the correct temperature should be and how to read the thermometer correctly. A small amount of nonmedicated soap should be used. The skin should be patted dry with a soft towel, and particular attention should be paid to the skin between the toes. Some physicians feel that fungus infections would be practically unknown if the feet were kept dry. Desenex powder is widely used, but other powders such as boric acid, talcum, and thymol iodide are quite satisfactory. Lumps of powder should not be allowed to accumulate between the toes. Small pieces of lamb's wool or cotton may be placed between the toes if the patient perspires freely. If he is employed, he should rest for a few minutes with the shoes off and the feet at heart level during the noon hour and again on returning home from work.

Toes and nails need special care. Lanolin is useful as a lubricant to massage toes, bases of nails, and other dry or calloused areas on the feet. No attempt should be made to cut hard and thickened nails until the feet have been soaked, and then nails should be cut straight across. It is well for someone else in the family to cut the patient's toenails, and, if they are greatly thickened, a podiatrist may be needed. The patient must be cautioned not to go about the house in bare feet and thereby run the danger of injuring his feet. Feet should be examined frequently for signs of calluses, abrasions, or infections, and any lesion should be treated at once by a physician.

Warmth is important for a person with vascular disease. The patient should be taught to keep his entire body warm. Long underwear is often advisable, also fur-lined slippers, fur-lined coats, and extra sweaters. Woolen socks with bedroom slippers will help to prevent chilling of feet and ankles when the patient sits about in the evening. The patient at home may be tempted to place his feet on the radiator or on the oven door, which is dangerous since sensation may be diminished and burning can occur very easily. Heat applied locally increases the local metabolism; therefore the circulatory demands of the part are increased, and often more harm than good is done. Patients with circulatory disturbances must avoid the use of a hot-water bottle, light cradle, heating pad, or any other form of local heat to the lower extremities.

Contrast baths, quite popular in the past, are seldom prescribed. There seems to be little logical reason for their use since the heat increases metabolism and therefore increases the need for blood supply, and the cold may produce arteriospasm and thus increase pain and yield no benefit. Tub baths, however, used with proper supervision can often be helpful. The value of the tub bath (the temperature of which should be 35° to 37.8° C., or 95° to 100° F.) is that the blood vessels of the entire lower extremities and the lower trunk are dilated. About twelve inches of water should be used. The water should be carefully tested with a thermometer, and the patient should remain in the bath approximately thirty minutes unless this period proves too weakening.

Circulation to the lower extremities may also be improved by the application of heat to the abdomen. The result of this is not increased metabolism in the feet, but improved circulation from reflex action of heat that causes a dilation of blood vessels of the lower extremities. The patient must be cautioned not to apply heat to the lower extremities.

There are some general measures that may be employed for improvement of circulation. The patient may be taught to alternate rest with exercise, to avoid standing for long intervals, and to avoid sitting with the knees bent or with the legs crossed. He may be taught to elevate the feet to heart level at intervals, keeping the knees straight to avoid pressure on blood vessels under the knees. Instructions vary according to the type of vascular disease. If the insufficiency is arterial, the feet should not be kept elevated above the heart level, whereas if venous involvement is present, elevation above the heart and even above head level may be prescribed for periods of time in order to drain the congested veins of the legs.

Special exercises (Buerger-Allen) may be used to improve circulation in arterial insufficiency. These exercises must always be prescribed by the physician. The exercises consist of elevating the feet until they blanch, lowering them until redness appears, then resting the legs at heart level for a few minutes with the body flat, and repeating the procedure a prescribed number of times. Two minutes up, two minutes down, and three to five minutes flat is often ordered, but this would vary with each patient and would depend on changes in foot color. Exercises are usually repeated five to ten times, three times a day. If the nurse is asked to supervise this exercise, she should know the purpose of the exercise and should not permit the feet to remain elevated longer than it takes to produce whiteness. In the hospital the overbed table covered with a pillow may be used to elevate the feet. At home, while lying on the sofa, the patient may raise his feet against the wall or over the arm of the sofa.

Certain exercises should be done by all patients unless they are definitely contraindicated by infection or impending gangrene. The toes should be wiggled within the shoes several times during each day if the patient is up and about. The foot should be stretched down, in, and up, ten times twice each day. The toes should be curled while doing these movements. Sitting in a well-fitting rocking chair and gently rocking from time to time aids circulation and also helps to maintain joint mobility.

Certain danger signs in vascular disease should not be emphasized in the mind of the patient enough to cause undue apprehension. Nevertheless, he should realize that they are significant and should report them to his physician. Pain upon walking (intermittent claudication) is found in arterial insufficiency and is the result of inability of the sclerosed arteries when exercise is taken to meet the increased circulatory demands of the extremities. Intermittent claudication is characteristic in that it always disappears spontaneously when exercise is stopped, only to recur on further exertion.

Night cramps occur in arterial insufficiency. The patient with this difficulty is usually instructed to elevate the head of the bed about ten inches by using shock blocks, to place a hot-water bottle on the abdomen, and to eliminate the pressure of bed covers by placing a bolster or footboard at the foot of the bed, to use extra bedcovers and loose wool socks, and to take small amounts of alcohol if he is accustomed to its use. Night cramps are thought to be caused by diminished arterial supply because of the flat position in bed and are relieved when the extremities are lowered. However, the patient should not sit on the side of the bed since this may cause chilling, and bending the knees will interfere with circulation.

Generalized arteriosclerosis

Definitive medical and nursing care becomes necessary when the limitations of arterial supply increase more rapidly than is compatible with normal metabolic processes. Arteriosclerosis obliterans is the most common arterial disease in age and is due either to closure of arteries from sclerosis and atheromatous changes or to the formation of a clot in the vessel narrowed by these changes. Many older people with arterial disease also have diabetes mellitus.

There are several means by which the arterial supply may be evaluated. Oscillometric tests are performed to determine arterial pulsation at various levels. Surface temperature studies may be done, in which case it is necessary that the patient be in a warm room for one hour prior to the test. Reflex vasodilation tests may be taken. Arteriography and x-ray examination are helpful in revealing calcification in arteries (see Figure 28). Calcification can, however, be present when function is quite satisfactory. One test alone is not conclusive; therefore the nurse should anticipate that a variety of tests will be made and should prepare the patient for each procedure.

The patient with pronounced arterial insufficiency is put to bed, and the feet are kept below heart level by use of shock blocks to raise the head of the bed about eight inches. Buerger-Allen exercises may be ordered. Tub baths with water at a constant temperature of 37.8° C. (100° F.) for thirty to forty minutes once or twice each day may be ordered. It is advisable to keep the entire room

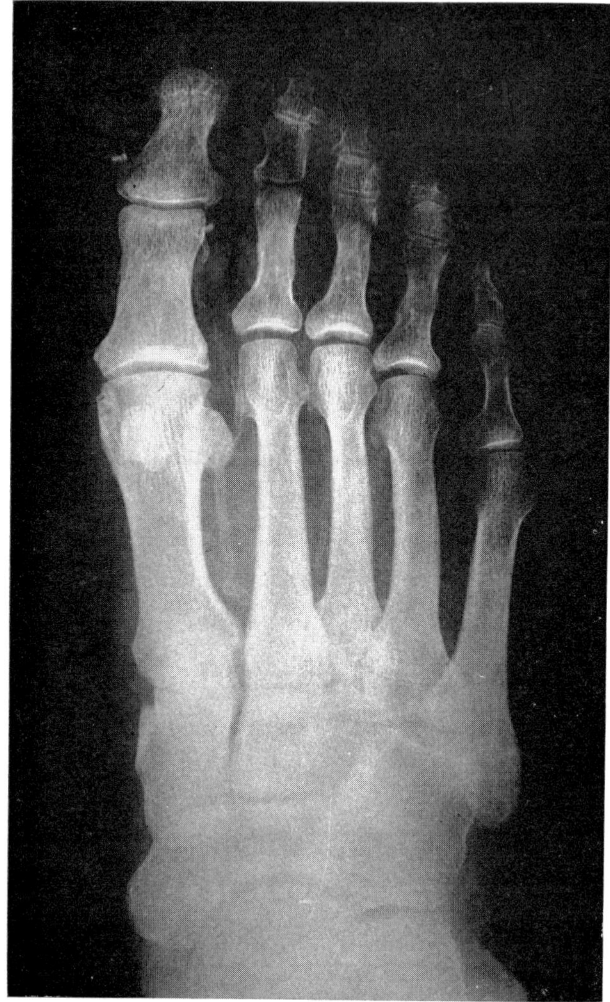

Figure 28. Calcification in the artery passing between the first and second metatarsal bones and to the terminal phalanx of the great toe can be clearly observed.

warm and to avoid the use of a cradle with light bulbs or of any other local heat except woolen socks.

Patients with arterial disease may have excruciating pain. The patient's bed should be placed in a protected part of the room, and the nurse must be careful not to jar it when making it or in working about the ward. A cradle or a footboard may be used to protect the feet from the pressure of covers. Quiet is important since the patient often sleeps poorly. The patient who is depressed and in pain is grateful for any attention and is often better off in a ward where there are distractions. Sedatives are used for sleep, but narcotic drugs are to be avoided since the disease is often chronic, and there is danger of addiction to drugs.

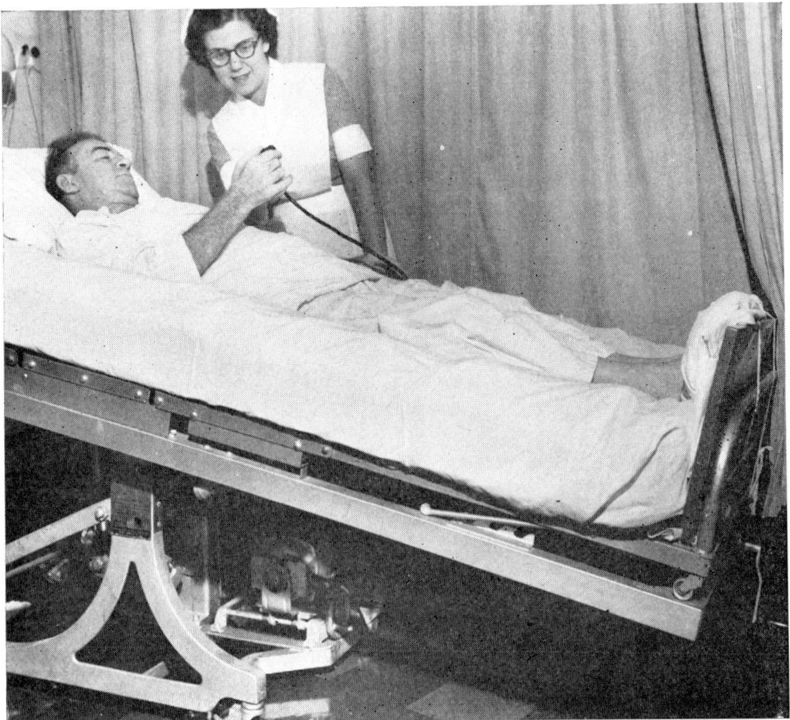

Figure 29. The patient learns to operate the oscillating bed. Note the pillow for protection of sensitive feet.

The oscillating bed is often used for patients with arterial disease. The mechanics of such a bed are simple. The patient may have difficulty in accustoming himself to the constant motion of the bed, and during the first day it is well to let him have the cord where he can reach it and turn the current off for a few minutes if he feels this necessary. The bed should be oiled and checked for function each week when it is in use, and it should operate without any disturbing sound or vibration. Some patients whose feet are exquisitely sensitive complain that, particularly during sleep, they slide down until their feet are against the foot of the bed as the foot tilts downward, and this causes pain and awakens them. It is often helpful to use a block or box protected with a soft pillow tied to the foot of the bed, so the patient's feet may rest against it as he tilts downward.

Measures may be taken to produce a generalized vasodilation and thereby improve circulation to the involved limb. Hot fluids by mouth, heat to the abdomen for its reflex action, and warm baths may be used. Alcohol may be ordered in dosages of 30 to 60 ml. (1 to 2 oz.) every four hours for its vasodilating effect. Papaverine, one of the alkaloids of opium, in a dosage of 30 to 60 mg. (½ to 1 gr.), or one of several available sympatholytic drugs such as tolazoline hydrochloride (Priscoline Hydrochloride) or phentolamine hydrochloride (Regitine Hydrochloride) may be given for the same effect. Some physicians, however, have reservations about the use of these drugs, believing that the lowering of blood pressure that they produce may lessen the flow of blood through a partially occluded artery and do more harm than the good derived from increase of blood flow through collateral or other vessels. Since hypotension may lead to faintness, the ambulatory patient should be advised to lie down at once if he feels faint or dizzy and to contact his doctor before he takes more of the drug. Usually the doctor requests that the patient's blood pressure be taken routinely when these drugs are being used, and the nurse should also take it if any signs of lowering of blood pressure occur.

In selected cases a sympathetic ganglionectomy is performed to produce a permanent vasodilation of blood vessels. Advanced age is no longer considered a prohibitive factor in considering this operation if the general health of the patient is satisfactory. Following this operation, the patient should be helped to learn how to control sudden drop in blood pressure when changing to a sitting or a standing position. Further details of nursing care are discussed in current nursing texts.[16]

The patient with arterial disease needs good general nursing care. Progress is often slow and discouraging. Special measures must be taken to see that pressure areas do not develop, particularly on the heels. If it is available, an air mattress is helpful. Position in bed must be observed not only for pressure over bony prominences but for occlusion of superficial vessels and body alignment. Position should be changed frequently so that deformities do not develop or circulatory stasis does not occur. Bed exercises are important to prevent contractures and help to preserve muscle tone. Permitting and encouraging self-help activities is equally important and effective. Occupational therapy is extremely useful in helping the patient to stay relatively content while in the hospital and is particularly helpful to the patient who is trying to overcome the desire to smoke. In the home, recreational activities and performance of simple, useful household tasks help reduce the patient's irritability at being unable to get about.

Arterial aneurysm and arterial occlusion

Aneurysms are enlargements of a portion of the artery due to weakness of the arterial wall. Arterial aneurysms in the elderly usually occur in those who have pronounced arteriosclerosis. Any artery may be involved, but the popliteal artery at a point just before it divides into the two main arteries of the lower leg is such a common site that a physical examination of the elderly patient now includes careful palpation of this area (see Figure 30). Some aneurysms can be detected only after radiopaque dyes have been injected and roentgenograms taken. Others can be felt as soft pulsating masses. The efficiency of the arterial system distal to the aneurysm is decreased. Clots may form within aneurysms, and rupture may occur with severe bleeding into surrounding tissues.

Signs and symptoms of sudden arterial occlusion are dramatic, with severe pain at the site of the occlusion and immediate pallor of the extremity distal to the occlusion. Fainting, nausea, palpitation, and complete shock may follow. The limb beyond the occlusion may become cold, and cyanosis with signs of

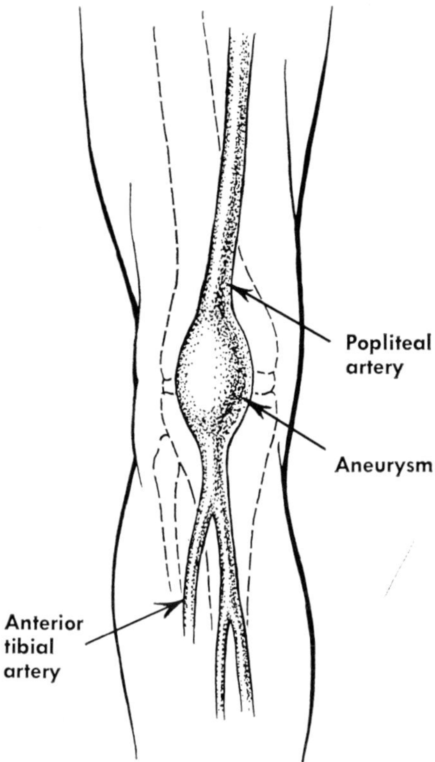

Figure 30. Schematic drawing showing posterior view of the knee with aneurysm in the popliteal artery.

approaching gangrene may appear. Any of these signs indicates the need for immediate medical attention.

Arterial occlusion usually produces acute symptoms, although occasionally, if the condition has developed gradually in a small artery, collateral vessels may have developed and taken over full function of the artery in conveying blood to the extremity so that no symptoms appear. Occlusion may result from arteriosclerotic changes and from atheromatous lesions on the inner wall of the lumen of the artery. Emboli floating in the bloodstream after breaking away from a vascular lesion in a larger artery or from a valve of the heart may obstruct the lumen, especially at its bifurcation into smaller vessels.

Surgery usually is the preferred method of treatment for arterial aneurysms that are producing symptoms and for acute arterial occlusion. The type of operation depends upon the patient and his general condition, and upon the kind and extent of his vascular difficulty. The aneurysm and affected portion of an artery may be resected and a graft of plastic material used to replace it. It may be removed with a bypass graft inserted above and below the lesion. Some surgeons now believe that these operations should be done as elective operations on elderly patients before acute symptoms appear.[6] Others believe that early grafting slows the development of collateral vessels while the life of a graft may have limitations.[1]

An occluded artery may be opened surgically and a thrombus removed (embolectomy), or the diseased portion of the artery containing the occlusion may be resected and a graft used. There are many modifications of these procedures involving grafts or redirection of arteries. These may or may not be emergency operations, depending upon the severity of the symptoms. If symptoms are severe and a complete occlusion has occurred, embolectomies usually are done as quickly as possible before inflammation and infection have occurred at the site of the occlusion. A lumbar sympathectomy may be done also if the lower extremities are involved.

Patients who are treated surgically for arterial disease may have, both preoperatively and postoperatively, all the conservative measures that have been described to further circulation. After surgery the patient must be watched extremely carefully for significant changes. Blood pressure is checked at frequent intervals for several hours and should be compared with the patient's normal blood pressure preoperatively, since lowering of the blood pressure may predispose to new thrombus formation at the site of operation or elsewhere. Hemorrhage is watched for since blood vessels not used before the operation, and not ligated during the operation, may now function. The limb is watched for changes in color, temperature, and sensation that might indicate the development of a new thrombus at the operative site. Usually the patient receives heparin and Dicumarol postoperatively. Fibrinolysin may be injected into a thrombus preoperatively to attempt to soften and dissolve the clot. It has also been inserted by slow drip into the operative site if formation of a thrombus threatens. Use of this substance is still experimental and is described in medical publications.[5]

It is not unusual for the elderly patient who has an acute arterial occlusion and who escapes gangrene of the entire limb to have a small area to which collateral circulation has not been adequate and for which emergency measures have not been successful in providing enough blood supply. This area becomes necrotic. The treatment and nursing care of the patient with this difficulty is similar to that for the patient who has arterial limitations and also that described later in this chapter for the patient who has a varicose ulcer. Because of the generally poor circulation of the patient, these lesions heal with discouraging slowness. Yet steady progress often depends upon faithful adherence to simple measures such as exercises, posture changes, warm baths, protection from infection, and correct diet. The patient often finds it extremely tiresome and difficult to adhere to the prescribed regimen. Continued interest and encouragement on the part of the nurse helps the patient to continue the necessary treatments.

Thrombophlebitis

Thrombophlebitis is the occurrence of a clot or thrombus in a venous channel, with accompanying inflammation, and may occur in both superficial and deep veins.

Prevention of thrombophlebitis is important since emboli can easily occur from the site of a thrombus formation, with fatal results. Superficial thrombophlebitis accompanied by pain and tenderness commonly follows operative procedures in persons with varicose veins. It is imperative that older people with varicose veins have the limbs raised above heart level for a few minutes every two hours postoperatively to drain the veins of the leg until such time as the patient can do this for himself. Deep thrombosis often manifests itself as a pain in the calf of the leg, particularly upon dorsiflexion of the foot. It follows immobilization associated with surgery or other illnesses, infections in the vein, and other causes. It is possible that some cases of thrombophlebitis can be prevented by early mobilization of elderly patients and by detailed attention to bed exercises for patients who cannot be mobilized. Despite early mobilization, however, the incidence of postoperative thrombophlebitis has not been reduced. It is believed that this may be only statistically true, because operations are now being performed on patients who are older and whose condition is less good than formerly was thought necessary. The nurse must be alert for signs and symptoms of thrombosis in all patients. At the first complaint of pain in the legs, the patient should be put to bed, and the doctor should be notified.

Treatment for superficial venous thrombosis may include immediate ligation of the vein at the femoral juncture, supportive measures, and early mobilization. The preferred treatment of deep venous thrombosis is usually conservative. Heparin and Dicumarol are used with or without ligation in involvement of both deep and superficial veins, and the dosage and care in regard to their use are the same as for coronary artery disease. Occasionally a patient is maintained on small doses of Dicumarol indefinitely, particularly if he has had repeated attacks of thrombophlebitis. This will mean weekly visits to the hospital or private physician for prothrombin level determinations. Such trips may be difficult for older persons unless transportation difficulties can be solved. On the other hand, it may be a life-preserving procedure.

Rest and moist heat are often prescribed for thrombophlebitis. Warm moist packs to the entire extremity are exceedingly helpful. They should be kept warm by the use of hot-water bottles, but the temperature of the water must be taken and must not be over 40.5° C. (105° F.). The nurse should be certain that she understands the physician's wishes regarding immediate care. Many physicians believe the limb should be elevated at 30 degrees from the horizontal to help prevent edema. A few believe that the limb should be flat to lessen danger of a loosened thrombus being carried into the circulation. Physicians differ, too, regarding the amount of activity for the patient. Some favor complete immobilization for fear a thrombus loosen and produce an embolism. Others believe that the clot is sufficiently adherent to the inflamed blood vessel wall that its dislodgement is not likely and that moving about is helpful in improving general circulation and preventing a further stasis of blood in the veins. Infarcts to the lungs may complicate thrombophlebitis. Sudden coughing, respiratory difficulty, or hemoptysis must be reported at once. The patient is kept absolutely quiet.

As soon as edema and inflammation in the limb have subsided, mobilization is started. An elastic stocking, preferably made to measure, must be provided in time to be used as soon as the patient gets up. The most satisfactory length is one inch below the bend of the knee joint. The lighter nylon stockings are not firm enough to be satisfactory. The patient, or some family member, must be taught how to apply the bandage or stocking before the patient leaves the hospital. The bandage is applied to the entire foot, except the heel, and to the leg; it should be smooth and snug, but must not be so tight that it interferes with arterial circulation. Since the bandage is difficult for the average patient to apply, a stocking is most often used. The stocking is removed and reapplied once during the day, then removed for sleep, but applied in the morning before the patient gets out of bed. After a month to six weeks the stocking is removed for one-half-hour to one-hour periods, which are gradually increased until no evidence of edema appears on walking and normal exertion. It often requires three to twelve months for this to be achieved. Two stockings or bandages for each affected limb are required before the patient is dismissed from the hospital in order that one may be used while the other is being laundered.

The patient who has had thrombophlebitis should be taught to follow the instructions outlined in the beginning of this section and to return for observation to the clinic, the hospital, or the doctor's office as instructed by his physician.

Varicose veins and ulcers

Varicose veins are among man's most common ailments, and many older people are troubled with them. They are presumably due to valvular defects in the veins, to pressure of venous blood on the lower venous system from assumption of the erect posture, to hereditary weakness of veins, to obesity, and to other contributory factors. In older people, varicose veins may be the result in part of loss of strength and elasticity of venous vessel walls, as well as to decreased exercise. The veins may be large and tortuous, and there may be dull pain and chronic leg fatigue. Dizziness on arising after lying is sometimes observed and is thought to be the result of localization of an appreciable percentage of blood volume in the lower limbs and diminished blood supply to the brain.

Control of symptoms by rest, elevation of the limb, and use of an elastic stocking or bandage are preferred methods of treatment. In elderly persons, sclerosing solutions are likely to cause thrombosis elsewhere and are used only rarely as adjuncts to obliterative surgery of the veins. Hemorrhages are rare, but the stasis that accompanies varicose veins results in gradual replacement of fatty tissue by a fibrous tissue that may be firm, discolored, and nonresistant to infection.

Ulcerative lesions occur frequently in older persons who have varicose veins, particularly in those who also have diabetes mellitus and are overweight. The treatment must depend primarily on reducing venous stasis so that the most important step is frequently the ligation or obliteration of the varicose veins that drain from the ulcerated area. Active exercise, especially rapid walking, may be advised if arterial blood supply is adequate. Treatment of varicose ulcers may include adequate diet, antibiotics, and sometimes sulfonamides, and it is often tedious and unsatisfactory. Local treatment may be in the form of warm compresses, soaks using potassium permanganate solution 1:6,000, Dakin's solution dressings, ultraviolet light, ointments such as scarlet red or cod-liver oil, and occasionally excision followed by skin grafting. Thiersch's, thick-split, and pedicle grafts are used but are not always satisfactory since they may break down when activity is resumed. Occasionally cancer develops in old, unhealed, neglected ulcers.

The Unna paste boot was formerly more widely used in the treatment of varicose ulcers than at present. It is applied in the clinic or the doctor's office and is changed at intervals of about ten days or two weeks. It provides a smooth, protective, supportive, gentle pressure to the extremity. The paste preparation comes in a package with instructions for melting over a water bath. Newer preparations come ready for immediate use and consist of gauze impregnated with melted paste. Usually the limb is shaved, and open lesions are covered with a small dressing. The limb is elevated for about three minutes to drain venous blood before the boot is applied. The toes are usually left uncovered, and paste is applied, alternating with three-inch gauze bandage, until three layers of paste and three of bandage have been applied. The limb is supported in an elevated position for about twenty minutes during the drying process. If the lesion is such that the limb will not be used actively, it is important that the position of the foot be so well placed that no tightening of the Achilles tendon or other abnormality will interfere with walking when it is permitted. Sometimes severe infections develop under these boots. Signs or symptoms such as pain, odor, drainage, or signs of elevation of temperature must be reported to the doctor at once.

Elevation of the extremity, use of an oscillating bed, and exercises may also be used. The time required to heal varicose ulcers may be out of all proportion to the size of the lesion, and the patient may become discouraged and fretful. Occupational therapy should be used. Attention must be paid to the prevention of deformities and preservation of muscle tone so that activity will not be hampered when healing finally takes place. The patient should have routine exercises for the noninvolved extremities.

When healing is finally achieved, the patient is usually instructed to use an elastic stocking in an attempt to prevent stretching of the skin over the ulcer, general venous enlargement, and edema. Ulcers can recur. The patient should avoid gaining weight and should have a definite schedule of living that includes regular rest periods during which the legs are elevated. Pruritus may occur, and the patient must be cautioned not to scratch or otherwise irritate the skin and not to use strong, unprescribed salves or home remedies. If any signs of recurrence appear, the doctor or the clinic should be notified.

Gangrene and amputation

If gangrene due to impaired circulation, infection, or trauma has developed, amputation may be necessary. The patient then needs the greatest care and consideration. For the aged person, weary, discouraged, and in pain, the news that he must have a foot or a leg amputated comes as a terrific shock. He may feel that his freedom and independence and probably his very existence are

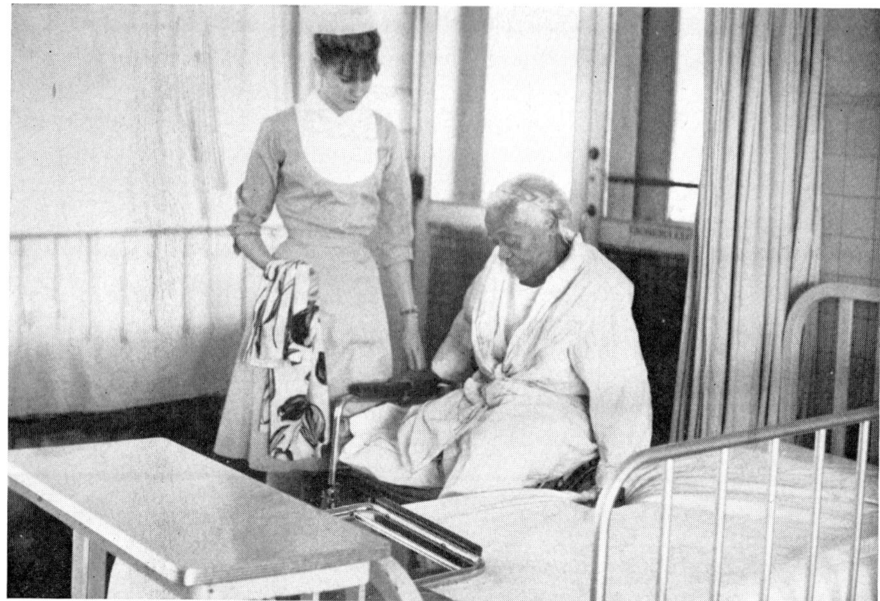

Figure 31. If both legs must be amputated, the nurse can help the patient achieve a degree of self-sufficiency beyond the patient's expectations. (Courtesy American Journal of Nursing.)

approaching an end. He feels sure that amputation of one limb means that the other limb will be lost within a relatively short time. Nothing could be farther from actual fact since in many instances, with good care and attention to instructions, the elderly patient who has had an amputation may live many useful and relatively happy years and undergo no further surgery.

The nurse's attitude must be a positive one. She must ask herself how she can help her particular patient to use his remaining capacities and how she can foster his feeling of independence and self-sufficiency. There is no reason for the average person who has had an amputation to be helpless and confined to a wheelchair for his remaining life, regardless of his age. An over-bed bar is invaluable in that it enables the patient to move about, raise himself, and shift his position for relief of pressure. If his condition permits, the patient should be taught to lift his body from the bed while in the face-lying position by pushing with his hands upon the bed and straightening his elbows. A less difficult yet effective method of strengthening the muscles necessary for crutch walking is sitting in bed with sandbags or blocks beside the hips. The patient must place his hands on the blocks and push down, raising his hips off the bed. This can be done in a wheelchair or sturdy armchair by pushing on the arms of the chair. This is of psychic benefit, in addition to being a good way to strengthen the muscles of the arms and the shoulders. Exercises that are done preoperatively will depend upon the individual patient, but it is often possible to have him do some exercises before surgery, and thus he is better prepared for rehabilitation after the operation.

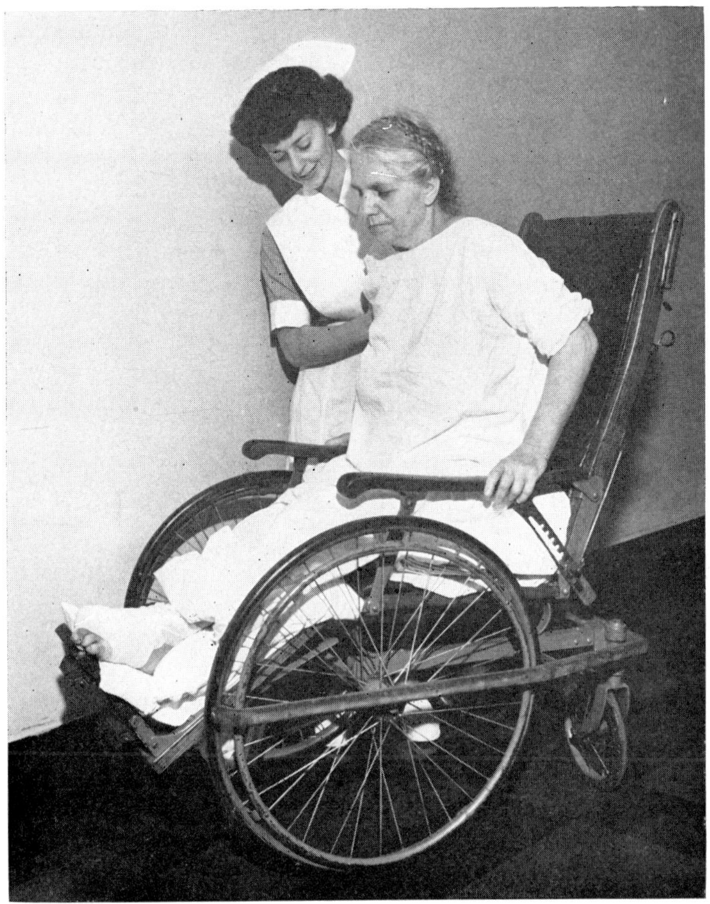

Figure 32. When she is in a wheelchair, the patient can exercise to strengthen her arms and shoulders in preparation for crutch walking.

After surgery, the nurse watches for specific complications such as hemorrhage, infection, complaints of phantom limb pain, and necrosis of tissue about the incision. She has the patient perform exercises to help prepare him for ambulation. These exercises are directed toward strengthening the extensor muscles of the arms, trunk, and lower extremities. The tendency for flexion contracture to develop at the hip joint can be prevented by having the patient lie on the abdomen several times each day, beginning the day after operation, and, while he is in this position, have him hyperextend the stump several times. This will also strengthen the muscles that will eventually be used when he walks with an artificial limb.

If the amputation is above the knee, abduction and outward rotation contractures of the hip must also be prevented. If permitted, the patient should lie on the side of the amputation part of the time. When he is in the back-lying position the stump should be held in neutral rotation and normal alignment by a firm trochanter roll. A satisfactory trochanter roll can be made by using a folded bath blanket rolled firmly outward to produce the desired internal rotation of the entire lower limb.

Crutch walking. Crutches should be measured to fit the patient. A method of measuring length is to have the patient lie on his back with his arms at his sides. The measure is then taken from the axilla to a point six inches out from the heel, allowing three fourths of an inch for the rubber crutch tips. Another satisfactory method is to have the patient lie flat in bed wearing the shoe that he will wear when he walks with crutches and measure from the axilla to the end of the heel of the shoe. The hand supports should be measured from the axilla to the palm of the hand, with slight flexion of the elbow. This enables the patient to extend his elbow and to bear the weight on the palms of the hands when the crutches are in use. Even with careful measurements, alterations may have to be made after crutches have been used for a short time.

Before attempting to walk with crutches, the patient should stand at the bedside or against the wall and practice balancing and shifting his weight while using the crutches to help to support himself. Prior to crutch walking, the patient can be helped to achieve good standing balance by using a walkerette or by standing between two chairs (weighted with sandbags on the seats) or by using parallel bars in the physical therapy department or on the ward. Portable parallel bars are becoming more prevalent in chronic care facilities and are now part of the regular equipment on the floors of general hospitals. Learning to balance on one leg, particularly after an above-knee amputation, requires considerable practice. If this precedes using crutches, the difficult coordination and more tricky balance using crutches may be mastered more easily.

In all crutch-walking instruction it is necessary to emphasize rhythm in walking and to try at all times to establish a normal walking pattern. The patient is urged to take small steps and is reminded not to watch his feet but to concentrate on rhythm, balance, and good posture. Crutches should be held about ten inches from the side of the foot when walking is first attempted. As the patient becomes more skilled in walking, the crutches are brought nearer to the body and therefore may need to be adjusted in length. It is important that they do not press against the superficial radial nerve in the axilla since crutch paralysis may result. They should be fitted so that two fingers can be placed between the axilla and the crutch when it is in place. The patient is taught to bear his weight on the palms of his hands and not to slump on the bar of the crutches; the bar of the crutch seldom needs any padding. If padding is used it should be the smooth-finish sponge-rubber type available commercially. This is less likely than bandage to catch on clothing if the patient should fall.

If a physical therapist is available, correct crutch-walking patterns should be taught and supervised by her. In the absence of such help, the nurse must take the responsibility for teaching the patient to walk with them. Even before the patient is fitted with a prosthesis, he needs to get about with crutches. He will use the swing-through gait in which both crutches advance together. This is a simple, fast gait that gives little muscular exercise to the lower extremity, but its excellent for rapid maneuvers such as are needed in crossing streets. When he begins to walk with either his artificial limb or a temporary pylon, the patient uses this same gait, in which his artificial limb and both crutches move forward together, alternating with his normal limb. From this gait, using two crutches, he should progress to the use of only one crutch and finally to a cane. The crutch or cane should be held in the hand opposite the amputation since in normal gait, the left hand swings forward with a step of the right foot, and vice versa. Holding the single cane or crutch on the same side as the amputation will result in an awkward, unrhythmic, and poorly balanced gait.

In addition to teaching her patient to manage crutches, the nurse must assist him in becoming as self-sufficient as possible in other ways. Such simple daily activities as getting out of bed, in and out of a chair, in and out of the bathtub, and on and off the toilet seat present real difficulties to the new amputee. He must be taught to bring his good leg well under him before shifting his weight, as when rising from a chair to the standing position. By doing this he will avoid the danger of losing his balance that comes with the sudden shift in his center of gravity.

Care of the amputation stump and the prosthesis. The artificial limb is fitted by the surgeon and the limb fitter, but it is the responsibility of the nurse to teach the patient and his family the care of his stump and which signs should be reported when he begins to use his prosthesis. The patient is likely to have difficulty if he continues to use an artificial limb that is causing pressure on the stump end or in any part of the extremity. He must be urged to report any signs of skin irritation on the stump and about the groin if amputation is at the level of the thigh. The stump should be washed daily and powdered lightly; in hot weather, gentle massage with alcohol may be added to the daily routine. Some patients are more comfortable if the artificial limb is removed early in the evening since this allows free circulation of air to the stump for a longer period. The amputee must at all times have at least two stump socks; this permits him to have a fresh sock daily. He is taught to wash his sock daily in a mild soap, to rinse it well, and to dry it over a wire stretcher to prevent shrinkage.

Adjusting to a prosthesis is not easy. One way to minimize difficulties in the adjustment is to tell the patient early that it will take him some time to become accustomed to an artificial limb and to use it effectively, and that he must not become discouraged at small reverses and annoyances that will occur. Often the patient will be tempted to give up and simply stay in bed or in a wheelchair; the family, in an effort to be kind, may permit him to do this and may wait upon him. The patient may accept this, but he may become irritable and demanding, since subconsciously he will resent his helplessness. The family, in turn, eventually may become impatient as worry subsides, and an unfortunate family situation can develop.

After an artificial limb has been fitted, it is necessary that the patient have the assistance of the physical therapist or the nurse in either a treatment center or the patient's own home. Most patients should be under observation for many months since the recovery may begin well, but, after what seems to be a good adjustment, the amputee may become discouraged and lay the artificial limb aside. It is extremely important that the home to which the patient will be returning be visited by the nurse in advance of his dismissal from the hospital so that the steps toward rehabilitation that were started in the hospital will be continued. If it should happen that an older person at home is equipped with an artificial limb but is not taught how to use it, the nurse in the community should initiate steps to help him and to obtain rehabilitative services that are available.

A person who has had an amputation may become so engrossed in the care of his stump and the management of his prosthesis that he completely forgets the care of his other foot. Exercises and other measures to keep the arterial supply to the remaining limb as adequate as possible must be carried on while the patient is in the hospital, and he should be warned that the instructions of the physician must be followed meticulously when he leaves the hospital.

REFERENCES AND RELATED BIBLIOGRAPHY

1. Abramson, David I.: An approach to better circulation in the extremities, J. Am. Geriatrics Soc. **10**:605-617, 1962.
2. Allen, Edgar V., Barker, Nelson W., and Hines, Edgar A., Jr.: Peripheral vascular diseases, ed. 3, Philadelphia, 1962, W. B. Saunders Co.
3. Beeson, Paul B., and McDermott, Walsh (editors): Cecil-Loeb textbook of medicine, ed. 11, Philadelphia, 1963, W. B. Saunders Co.
4. Bradby, Robert L.: Amputation in the aged, J. Am. Geriatrics Soc. **8**:901-902, 1960.
5. Cliffton, Eugene E., and others: Symposium on fibrinolysin, Amer. J. Cardiol. **6**:367-563, 1960.
6. Crawford, E. Stanley, and others: Peripheral arteriosclerotic aneurysm, J. Am. Geriatrics Soc. **9**:1-15, 1961.
7. Davis, Loyal (editor): Christopher's textbook of surgery, ed. 7, Philadelphia, 1963, W. B. Saunders Co.
8. DeTakats, Geza: Vascular surgery, Philadelphia, 1959, W. B. Saunders Co.
9. Greeley, Paul W.: Plastic surgical repair of chronic leg ulcers, Geriatrics **8**:527-533, 1953.
10. Green, Harold D.: Diseases of the blood vessels. In Johnson, Wingate M. (editor): The older patient, New York, 1960, Paul B. Hoeber, Inc., Medical Book Department of Harper & Row, Publishers.
11. Knocke, Lazelle: Crutch walking, Amer. J. Nurs. **61**:70-73, 1961.
12. Krause, G. Lynn, and Vetter, Frances C.: Varicose veins, diagnosis and treatment and nursing care, Amer. J. Nurs. **53**:70-72, 1953.
13. Krug, Elsie E.: Pharmacology in nursing, ed. 9, St. Louis, 1963, The C. V. Mosby Co.
15. Linton, Robert R.: Venous thrombosis, pulmonary embolism and varicose veins, J.A.M.A. **183**:198-201, 1963.
16. Shafer, Kathleen Newton, and others: Medical-surgical nursing, ed. 3, St. Louis, 1964, The C. V. Mosby Co.
17. Wright, Irving S.: The treatment of thrombophlebitis, J.A.M.A. **183**:194-198, 1963.

Chapter 16

Nursing in neurologic disorders

The nervous system often suffers extensively in old age. Disorders may be part of normal aging, or they may be pathologic; at present it is often impossible to say which is their fundamental cause. Many changes may follow arteriosclerosis and circulatory impairment since it is well known that nerve tissue functions best when it is well supplied with normal blood. Some elderly people find that upon suddenly arising from a lying position they become faint. This may be due to impairment of venous return from the lower extremities that results in insufficient blood to supply the brain, to narrowing of vessel lumina that results in decreased blood flow, or to impaired heart action. Some older people are unable to lie flat in bed without suffering headache, dizziness, and confusion. This is thought to be due in some instances to impaired venous return in intracranial vessels, with resultant congestion of blood. Impaired nutrition may cause some neurologic change in age. Neurologic changes particularly in the extremities are known to respond in many instances to adequate diet with high intake of vitamins.

Some aspects of general nursing in neurologic disease are common to almost all clinical entities. These will be considered before a few of the diseases and the surgical procedures common in old age are described.

GENERAL NURSING

Loss of function. Some loss of motor function is common in neurologic disease. This may occur suddenly, as in some forms of cerebral thrombosis, or be slow in onset, as in Parkinson's disease. The ability to move about at will is precious to every human being. Regardless of the rate of its occurrence, loss of the ability to function independently is phychologically traumatizing to everyone. The patient needs constant reassurance from the nurse, who he knows is aware of what is possible for him, of her faith in his ability to do certain things for himself. The nurse must have good judgment in deciding what he may safely do without assistance. She must know activity that is dangerous and that which may end in frustration for each particular patient. To the neurologic disease itself are added other changes that are considered characteristic of age. Fatigue, joint stiffness, and general debility may be present to further hamper the ability of the aged neurologic patient to move about freely.

Physical facilities should be arranged so that the patient can do much for himself. Rails along the hallways, firm locks to the castors on the bed and bedside table, a handrail on the bathtub; all these help the patient to get about even though his movements are uncertain. He may be able to feed himself if food is cut up, if a large spoon is provided, and if a second napkin is used so that the thought of spilling food on the bed or clothing will not be disturbing. Sometimes closing the door of the patient's room so that his clumsy handling of utensils will go unnoticed adds to his self-control. Covered containers of fluids with an opening for insertion of a straw may make it possible for the bed patient to help himself to a drink without spilling (Chapter 11, Rehabilitation).

The patient who has limitation of motion from neurologic damage but whose condition is not a progressive one needs assurance that this is true. The doctor must give this reassurance, but his explanation may need repetition by the nurse. One elderly lady who had neurologic damage from pernicious anemia but whose condition was under good medical control worried herself almost to distraction with the fear that she would become progressively worse despite treatment. She had watched with tenseness another person suffering from a completely different disease progress to complete helplessness and was convinced that this was to be her fate. If assurance of arrest of disease or improvement cannot be given, then the patient must be given encouragement in getting about as long as is possible.

The patient needs honest and thoughtful preparation for procedures that may be done and that he fears may lead to some temporary or permanent paralysis. Even a spinal puncture is feared by the patient who already has some impairment of locomotion. He may have heard tales of paralysis following this procedure and must be assured that it cannot possibly increase his motor disability. It must be remembered that the elderly patient of today grew up in an era when, in many instances, the hospital was a place where one went only to die. Naturally, he may not have the confidence in the hospital that many younger people have developed.

The patient who has limitation of physical ability and cannot get about is often extremely sensitive and insecure. A little of the primitive fear that links inability to move about fast and freely with failure to survive may remain. This may be present despite the fact that the patient now lives in a civilized culture in which the social machinery for protection of the less fortunate members is highly developed.

The nurse must protect the patient from close scrutiny of strangers or disinterested people. In the hospital it may be the cleaning attendant who asks why a certain patient "gets that silly expression" when she talks. In the home it may be curious neighbors who speculate as to the nature of her ailment every time Mrs. X walks by with that particular hitch to her gait. The nurse can help her patient a great deal by making him feel that she is interested in him as a person and not merely in the physical ailment that has caused his limitation. On the other hand, she may find that the patient turns to her as someone whom he can tell how he feels about his neurologic involvement and what it really means to him. Listening attentively to his problems is an essential part of neurologic nursing.

Personality changes. Personality changes occur frequently in neurologic disease. The nurse must observe her patient for personality changes of any nature and report them accurately. Organic changes produced by the disease may cause personality change. Irritability due to frustration in attempts to get about and anxiety over general increasing helplessness add to the picture. In addition, emotional reactions to numerous other restrictions of age are present. The patient may suddenly be impulsive and irritable or sullen without apparent cause.

Emotional reactions must be dealt with calmly and quietly by the nurse. It is useless to argue with the patient or try to talk him out of his fears. A word of encouragement, a turning of the conversation to other topics, and an introduction to some diversional activity are helpful. The patient's childhood or his productive years may be safe topics of conversation since they usually contain happy memories and are removed from disturbing thoughts of the present.

Accidents. The neurologic patient must be protected from situations that may

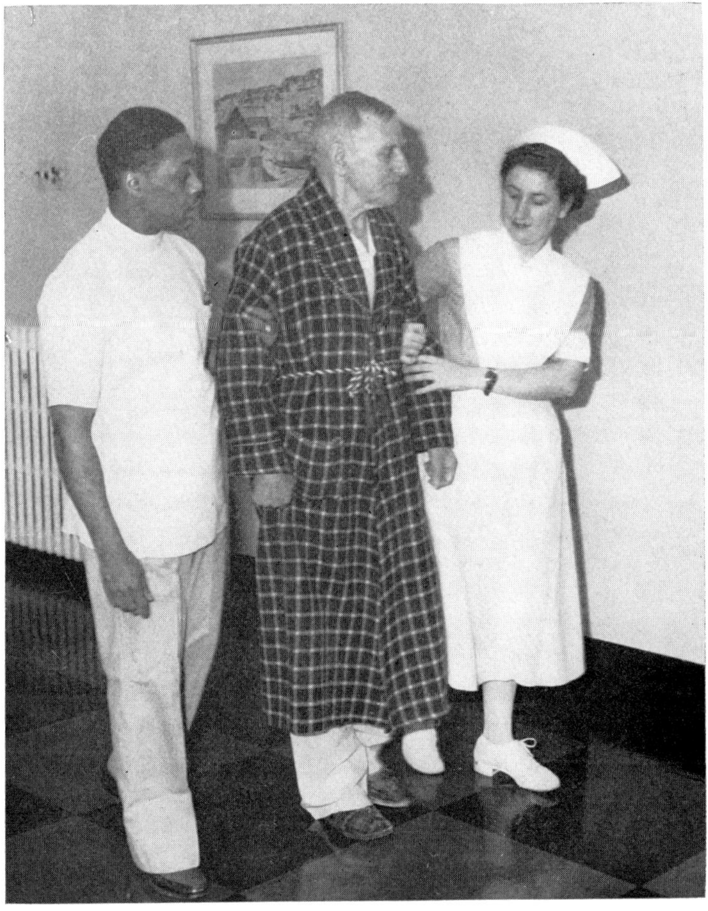

Figure 33. Accidents can be prevented when the orderly and the nurse assist the patient whose gait is unsteady.

result in accidents. Neuromuscular control as well as sensory function may be impaired, the aged bone structures are easily traumatized, and visual impairment may further predispose the patient to accidents.

The nurse must watch the patient carefully and analytically in order to determine his limitations and the particular accident precautions that should be taken. Unnecessary and self-evident precautions will only irritate the patient since the elderly person resents even more keenly than the younger one any enforced restrictions of his freedom of movement. Side rails should be used almost routinely at night if symptoms of neuromuscular involvement are present and a high hospital bed is used. Patients may accept the restriction of side rails more readily if it is explained to them that side rails are useful to hold onto when raising oneself to a sitting position and when turning over in bed. The patient should have assistance in getting out of the high hospital bed until it is certain that he is able to handle himself safely. If they are provided, footstools should have a broad base and be equipped with nonskid rubber tips. The patient must be accompanied when he first attempts to walk and until stability is evident. A walker or walkerette is useful for the neurologic patient since it permits him to be up when he might otherwise be confined to bed or to a chair.

Contractures. Patients with neurologic disease are likely to develop contractures and deformities. Failure to keep good alignment when in a rest position and to move at regular intervals may result in deformity. Parts that are paralyzed must be put through the normal range of joint motion each day so that the range will not become limited. The nurse can determine how limited patient's range of motion is by comparison with her own normal range of movement. The elderly patient may have slight limitation and yet be considered normal, and he may have another disease such as arthritis which may limit his range of joint motion. Some levels of joint motion cannot be achieved with the patient in the supine (back-lying) position and require that he lie prone at least once each day.

If the patient is conscious and rational, the nurse can teach him to help himself in order to prevent deformities. In the home much can be done to prevent the progress of deformity in neurologic disease by adapting equipment to the condition. For example, a comfortable arrangement may be made whereby the patient may stand supported by a walker for short intervals during the day. A walker may be rented in many communities, and often homemade devices fashioned out of wood are very satisfactory. Standing for even a few minutes each day will prevent the development of contractures at the hips, which occur from prolonged sitting. A railing may be put on the outside steps so that an unsteady person may be able to walk and get outdoor exercise in an erect position.

Pressure areas. When nerve supply to a part of the body is disturbed, it is deprived of adequate nutrition. Both arterial and venous efficiency are impaired by loss of muscle function. Consequently the skin breaks down easily, and pressure areas are difficult to cure in the person who has neurologic involvement. The neurologic patient must be reminded to change his position frequently if he is able to do so. If he cannot do this himself, he must be turned. Most normal persons move frequently during normal sleep. Occasionally, after a person has taken a nap when he was very tired, pressure areas may be noted on the skin.

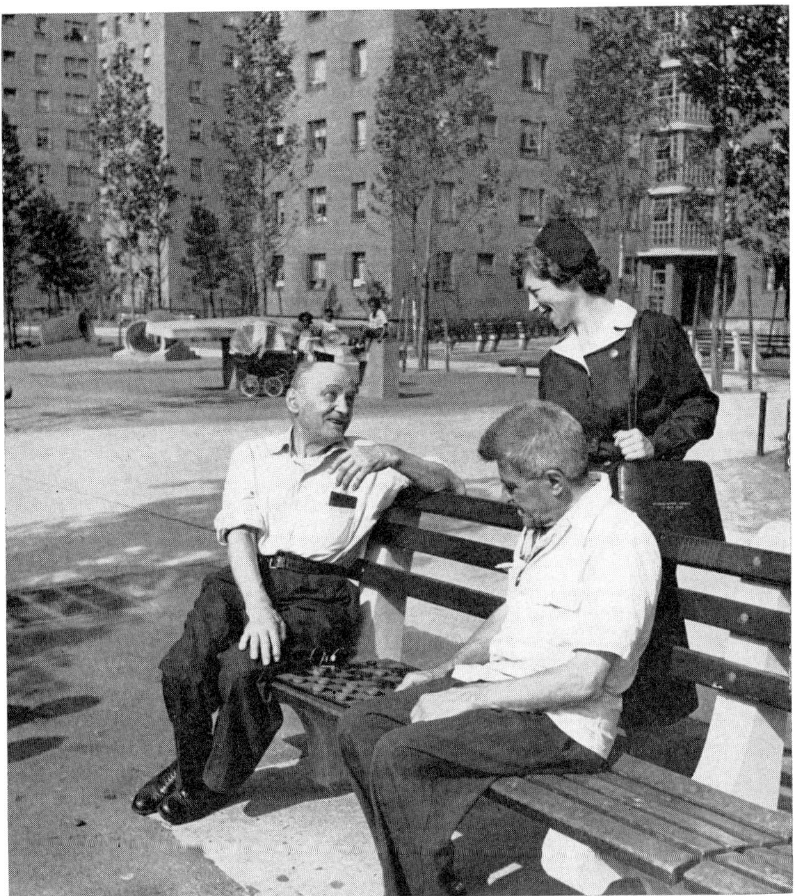

Figure 34. The nurse sees the results of her efforts in helping the patient through a difficult adjustment to a period of limited activity. (Courtesy Visiting Nurse Service of New York; photograph by Hazel Kingsbury.)

These are because sleep has been so sound that movement was less frequent than usual. To a much greater extent this happens in the paralyzed patient who has no relief except when he is turned by others. The patient with sensory involvement may feel no discomfort and may not ask to be moved, or he may be unconscious. No more important responsibility rests with the nurse caring for the neurologic patient than to change his position often. Light massage to the dependent areas should be given each time the patient is turned. Regular turning and gentle massage should be supplemented by an air mattress, sponge, or sheepskin under the bony prominences, and the skin should be kept clean and dry. Meticulous attention must be given to these aspects of care when a patient is unconscious or comatose.

Patient in his home. The nurse is often called upon to help with planning for the care of the aged neurologic patient in his home. The family that cares for a member who is difficult and demanding should plan so that the emotional life of all will be safeguarded. Sometimes it is possible to take the patient to a recreation center for periods of the day so that he may visit with contemporaries. It may be possible to employ someone for a certain number of hours each day to take care of the old person. One family, for example, hired a schoolboy to take an aged and rather irresponsible uncle fishing, a sport that he enjoyed but was unable to engage in alone. Members of the family should arrange to have nights out, even if it requires employing the services of a sitter. This entails expense and planning, but is essential if the family group is to remain normal and happy.

Anyone who cares for a difficult and demanding older person should have a regular vacation even if arrangements can be made for only a few days' absence. Sheldon,[18] in his study of old people in England, found that younger members burdened with the complete care of an older person were unhappy, frustrated, and discouraged. This was particularly true if their future seemed to hold no prospect of relief for even a brief period of time. A further discussion of how to help family members care for the patient at home is found in Chapter 10, Care in the Patient's Own Home.

DISORDERS

Paralysis agitans

Paralysis agitans, or Parkinson's disease, is a disease of the central nervous system that does not involve the pyramidal tract or the lower motor neurons. The so-called parkinsonian syndrome or typical clinical picture may follow acute epidemic encephalitis or drug poisoning. In the aged it is often associated with arteriosclerosis. Multiple small thrombi may occur in the basal ganglia and cause deterioration of this part of the brain tissue.

Parkinson's disease is more common in men than in women and occurs most frequently in the mid-fifties. It begins with a faint tremor that progresses gradually. Further symptoms are muscle rigidity, a masklike appearance to the face,

Table 3. Death rates per 100,000 from paralysis agitans (Parkinson's disease)*
White persons by sex and age. United States, 1959-62† and 1949-52

Age period (years)	*Average annual death rate*				*Percent change*	
	White males		*White females*		*White males*	*White females*
	1959-62	*1949-52*	*1959-62*	*1949-52*		
All ages‡	1.5	1.5	1.1	1.1	—	—
45 and over‡	5.5	5.6	3.9	3.9	− 2	—
45-54	0.5	0.6	0.3	0.4	−17	−25
55-64	2.7	3.4	2.0	2.4	−21	−17
65-74	14.0	13.8	9.1	9.2	+ 1	− 1
75-84	26.6	24.6	20.3	17.5	+ 8	+16
85 and over	21.9	15.4	19.1	14.9	+42	+28

*Courtesy Metropolitan Life Insurance Co.
†Excludes New Jersey in 1962.
‡Adjusted on basis of age distribution of total population, United States, 1940.

slowed monotonous speech, drooling, and difficulty in swallowing. There is a characteristic shuffling gait. The patient tends to walk on his toes, taking small steps and increasing his rate of motion. The trunk is slanted forward, the arms are held rigidly at the sides and do not swing as in a normal rhythmic gait. Neuromuscular control may be lost to the point where the patient is unable to stop his propulsive gait until an obstruction is met, and finally, until he is unable to walk at all. The skin is moist, the appetite may increase, and defective judgment and emotional instability may appear, though intelligence is usually normal. All signs and symptoms increase with excitement and frustration.

Treatment for Parkinson's disease in the elderly is only palliative. Surgical treatment and use of heat and cold as used for some younger patients are seldom attempted. Drugs that produce relaxation, such as atropine sulfate and its related drugs (hyoscine and stramonium), are widely used. It must be remembered that a tolerance is built up for these drugs; dosages may become large in advanced stages before any therapeutic effect is obtained. A synthetic atropine-like preparation, trihexyphenidyl hydrochloride (Artane Hydrochloride) appears to be useful. This drug is given by mouth. Bromides are sometimes ordered, but it must be remembered that the capacity to excrete may be reduced in age, and cumulative reactions may occur—particularly in persons who require treatment over a long period of time. Physical measures such as warm baths and massage give only limited physical relief but are often of marked psychic benefit.

Attention must be paid to an adequate intake of food. When symptoms become marked, it is necessary to take care that the patient does not choke when eating. Good nutrition, attention to posture, and plenty of fresh air will aid in improvement of general health and may possibly slow the progress of the disease. Rush and bustle should be avoided since they interfere with the patient's ability to handle himself effectively. The tremor of Parkinson's disease is increased when excitement occurs or when the patient is under tension. A quiet, unstimulating environment helps the patient to carry on normal activity.

The patient should continue his occupation as long as he is able. Most physicians give this advice to their patients unless their occupation is such that continued participation is dangerous. The patient should reduce his regular work gradually while building up some hobbies and interests in which he may engage as the condition progresses. Relatives of the patient must be given a complete understanding of the condition so that they may intelligently assist in the family adjustment that will eventually be necessary. Such problems as danger of accidents, personality changes, and progressing helplessness must be anticipated. In the hospital and in the home the nurse must help the patient and his family in planning his program so that he will be able to help himself. Such simple devices as a heavy rope fastened to the foot of the bed on which the patient may pull when he wishes to raise himself to a sitting position help to keep him active for a longer time.

Tremor

Tremor, often called senile tremor, is believed to be caused by very slight degeneration of basal ganglia. It is characterized by a fine tremor that is much more rapid than that of Parkinson's disease and that may involve only part of the body. It is common in the face. Trembling of the lower jaw may give the casual observer the impression that the victim of the disease is mumbling to himself or is about to cry. Senile tremor ceases with sleep, but is visibly increased by nervousness and emotional tension.

Cerebrovascular accidents

Cerebrovascular accidents as a cause of death rose from seventh place in 1900 to third place in 1944, where they have remained to the present time. Shock, hemiplegia, and stroke are names commonly used to designate cerebrovascular accidents, which have several causes.

Cerebrovascular accident may be caused by the rupture of a blood vessel within the brain so that pressure develops from blood flowing outside the vessel but within the cranial cavity; the portion of the brain that the ruptured artery supplies normally is deprived of blood supply. Persons who develop this trouble usually have severe arteriosclerosis and also have high blood pressure. Rupture of a cerebral vessel, however, accounts for only a small percentage of cerebrovascular accidents sustained by the elderly.

An embolus arising from a defective heart valve or from a thrombus somewhere in the body may obstruct an artery in the brain and cause a cerebrovascular accident. In most instances the embolus lodges in an artery that is already defective because of generalized arteriosclerosis and atherosclerosis.

By far the most common cause of cerebrovascular accident in the elderly in cerebrothrombosis. This lesion accounts for approximately 90 percent of all cerebrovascular accidents in this age group.[4] Thrombosis may be partial or complete, may involve either large or small vessels, or may occur in one or several vessels at the same time. Individuals in whom this occurs usually have arteriosclerosis and often have marked atherosclerotic changes in cerebral vessels. The blood pressure may not be increased at the time of the accident or even prior to its occurrence. In fact, many more individuals suffer cerebrovascular thrombosis during sleeping hours than during times of stress and excitement.

The nurse should realize that high blood pressure is not always indicative of early death and/or of extreme danger of cerebrovascular accident in the older person. This is apparent if the anatomy and pathology are understood. For example, high blood pressure may contribute to cerebral hemorrhage if the vessels are already damaged by vascular disease, whereas sudden lowering of blood pressure may permit thrombosis to occur in an artery already narrowed by arteriosclerotic changes.

Prevention of cerebrovascular accident in older people is difficult because it is not medically possible at the present time to control the development of atherosclerosis and arteriosclerosis. Perhaps the most important contribution the nurse can make is encouraging all middle-aged persons to have periodic physical checkups. For it is at this age that the first signs of obesity, elevation of blood pressure, and resultant heart damage may yield best to medical treatment. The nurse should also know the signs that may indicate impending cerebrovascular difficulty and if any of them occur urge a person who is not under medical care to see his doctor. In 1964, the National Stroke Congress listed the following as suggestive of impending stroke:[2]

1. Intermittent unilateral temporal or occipital headache that, if untreated, becomes persistent
2. Recurrent lightheadedness
3. Vertigo
4. Syncope accompanied by pallor and postural slump but no convulsion—particularly when experienced by a person over 30 years of age
5. Fall or "drop attack" with no loss of consciousness but associated with transient tonelessness of all extremities
6. Blurring of vision of both eyes
7. Transient monocular blindness
8. Transient paresthesia—unilateral or bilateral
9. Transient ataxia
10. Transient dysphasia
11. Transient disorientation
12. Serious impairment of memory
13. Convulsion (in a person over 45)
14. Behavioral changes noted by family or others
15. Transient cranial nerve palsies

In addition, nosebleeds in an older person should always be reason for a medical examination. The cause may be found to be trivial or it may be associated with high blood pressure.

Regardless of which accident occurs, the brain tissue is deprived of blood supply, and, in consequence, varying amounts of paralysis or hemiplegia follow immediately or gradually over a period of hours or even days. Since cerebral thrombosis is the most common cerebrovascular accident in older people, it will be considered in some detail.

Patient with multiple small thrombi. The patient with repeated thrombi in small blood vessels may not suffer complete paralysis or hemiplegia but may have numerous, small, barely perceptible strokes. There may be brief paralysis, with or without loss of consciousness. There may be periods of dizziness, staring into space, nausea, vomiting, and emotional instability. The patient with this trouble becomes a burden to himself and to his family. In the words of Alvarez, "the patient feels terrible," and no amount of reassurance or attempting to minimize his complaints can make him feel any differently.[1] This is often difficult for persons around him to understand. Perhaps the greatest contribution of the nurse to the comfort of the patient is to guide the patient's family to an understanding of this fact. The condition is progressive, and one attack is likely to follow another. On the other hand, the patient may have long periods of useful life between attacks and may appear to recover almost entirely.

Safe, simple, and satisfying activities must be permitted so that the patient is quietly stimulated. Gardening may be an excellent occupation. Working with the soil and making things grow yield satisfaction to persons who enjoy it. Light carpentry work, toymaking, rugmaking, and knitting are safe and useful occupations.

As the condition progresses, precautions for the safety of the patient must be taken. He then is likely to wander about the house at night, arise to cook breakfast in the middle of the night, develop a voracious and uncontrolled appetite, go on spending sprees, drive the family car, and in various ways disrupt and worry the household.

The patient who suffers from multiple small thrombi in the brain may live for years, and his presence should disrupt the family living as little as can possibly be managed. The patient needs thoughtful attention in order that his remaining years may be as happy and comfortable as possible. Despite his limitations, he should be treated as an adult and not as a child. Relatives must reach an acceptance of a program that will cause them no regrets when the older person has died, either in recriminations of not having done enough for him or in feelings of bitterness for the years of their own lives that were sacrificed. Much is now being written on this difficult subject that the nurse should know of and help to make available to family members.[20]

Patient with acute cerebral thrombosis. In contrast to the picture created when many small thrombi occur, a thrombus formation may involve a large vessel, and complete paralysis of a part of the body may occur suddenly or gradually. The clinical picture presented is then very similar to that which occurs following cerebral hemorrhage. Usually one half of the body is involved. The patient may suddenly fall and lapse into unconsciousness. There are times when this condition is confused with the coma of diabetes. The face may be flushed, and a puffiness often occurs, particularly on the paralyzed side. Respiration may be deep and labored, and the patient may be incontinent.

Little can be done immediately following a cerebrovascular accident except to keep the patient quiet. A physician must be called at once. The patient should be turned onto his side so that breathing is facilitated. No attempts should be made to remove his clothing or put him to bed until he has been seen by the doctor. The head may be elevated about 20 degrees on a pillow, and care should be taken that there is no sharp bend in the neck that might cause pressure on the blood vessels and interfere with the circulation of blood to the brain. For several reasons many patients with cerebrovascular accidents are often not hospitalized, and the public health nurse is often called upon after the doctor has made his diagnosis and recommended care in the patient's home. Nursing for the patient in the hospital or in the home does not differ, except that in the hospital a careful record of blood pressure is kept and more often oxygen is given, although oxygen can be administered in the home. Dicumarol and Heparin may be given if the patient is in the hospital and if it is certain that the cause of his illness is thrombosis and not hemorrhage. The details of nursing care when Heparin and Dicumarol are used are discussed in Chapter 14, Nursing in Cardiac and Renal Disease.

Rest and quiet are important. Pulse and respirations are checked closely. Slowing of pulse and respirations and deepening of the coma are signs of poor prognosis. No attempt should be made to rouse the patient from coma, though respiratory and circulatory stimulants may be given if prescribed by the physician.

The patient's eye on the affected side must be protected since the lids usually fail to close properly. Irrigations of boric acid solution or physiologic solution of sodium chloride followed by drops of sterile mineral or castor oil are used. Sterile petroleum jelly may be used, and an eye pad may be taped gently over the closed eye. If a pad is used, it must be changed daily, and the eye must be cleansed and examined carefully.

Mouth care is difficult since often the patient is unable to retain fluid and is likely to choke if it is introduced into the mouth. A good flashlight and padded tongue blades are essential in order that good mouth care may be given. Care of the mouth should be given several times each day, and special attention must be paid to the paralyzed side of the mouth and tongue. An Asepto syringe equipped with several inches of rubber at the tip is useful in irrigating the mouth. The patient's face should be turned to the side and forward in order that fluid may be extruded and not flow to the throat and cause choking or aspiration.

The patient must be moved often to avoid danger of circulatory stasis and hypostatic pneumonia. Care must be taken to see that the weight of the body is not borne for long intervals on the paralyzed side or on the back. Pillows should support the uppermost limbs when the patient is lying on his side. This will prevent strain on joints at the shoulder and hip and also allow freer respiratory movement of the chest. It is possible for the patient with hemiplegia to suffer complete dislocation of the hip joint from lack of support to the limb when he is placed on his unaffected side and the flaccid thigh is allowed to fall forward and downward. The patient may be turned to a face-lying or partial face-lying position, with pillows again being used to maintain good anatomic alignment. This is a good position for the semicomatose patient since the danger of aspiration of mucus in the throat is lessened.

If the patient survives the first few days, he may begin to regain consciousness, and some of the paralysis may disappear. It is then that the greatest understanding from the persons who attend him is needed. He may awaken to the realization that he cannot talk, that he is drooling, that he cannot move a hand or a leg or, if he can move them, the motions are shaky and uncertain. This is a terrific shock to any person. It is here that the nurse's active part in rehabilitation begins, and she must, by her quiet assurance, make the patient feel that his progress toward recovery and self-sufficiency has begun and will be continuous. If the patient is right handed and has had involvement of his right side, it means that his speech center may be involved since the speech center lies in the left hemisphere of the brain of right-handed persons. In order to be able to communicate, the patient then faces the difficulty of having to learn to write with his left hand, in addition to being partially speechless or incoherent. The nurse should try to anticipate her patient's needs and should make every effort to understand his indistinct speech since his repeated attempts to make himself understood only augment his misery and frustration. Usually, if there is partial ability to speak at the time of return to consciousness, there is a likelihood that speech will improve, and the patient is heartened by the knowledge of this fact.

If the patient is conscious, it is helpful to demonstrate to him and his family that he is able to think and to respond, such as in the use of a call bell. If he is unable to speak, the nurse should try to determine if he can understand and respond appropriately to questions or directions. Instructions to nod the head for "yes" and to shake it for "no"—the almost universal nonverbal signs—will establish whether or not the patient comprehends when spoken to. If his comprehension of the spoken word is questionable, he and his family need assurance that gestures, object recognition, and other means will effect communication. It is important to assure the family that the patient's needs can and will be met, and, above all, that his inability to speak or to respond appropriately to verbal directions does not mean that his mental processes are damaged. The nurse should speak directly to the patient even though he may not seem to understand all she says. Although he may not understand fully, her tone of voice may give him reassurance.

Administration of food and fluids to patients following a cerebrovascular accident requires nursing art. Fluids may be restricted for the first few days in an effort to prevent edema to the brain; then regular diet and regular fluid intake are desirable. Patience and persistence are necessary in supplying food and fluids to these patients. The nurse must make the patient feel that the problem is not discouraging and that time spent in assisting him to eat is well spent. He may encounter so much difficulty in getting food and fluids beyond his partially paralyzed mouth and throat that without encouragement the effort may not seem worthwhile. Turning the patient to his back or to his unaffected side often spares him the annoyance and embarrassment of having food spill from the affected side of his mouth. Foods that may cause choking, such as mashed potatoes, stringy meats, and semicooked vegetables must be avoided. Food may collect in the affected side of the mouth and be dislodged only with difficulty; slight pressure against the cheek of the affected side while chewing and swallowing often will prevent this.

An irrigation of the mouth at the conclusion of eating will prevent accumulation of food and subsequent poor mouth hygiene. As soon as possible the patient should help to feed himself, even if he must learn to do this left handed, since the helplessness of having to be fed by others is not conducive to good emotional health.

Urinary output should be noted carefully and recorded for several days after a cerebrovascular accident has occurred. Retention of urine may occur, but it is more likely that the patient will be incontinent. The person who is incontinent rarely empties his bladder completely, therefore residual retention occurs. If incontinence of urine does occur, the patient must be reassured and told that control of excretory function will probably improve day by day as a regular regimen is followed to reestablish his habit patterns.

Constipation and impactions develop readily in patients following a cerebrovascular accident. These can be prevented. As soon as possible the patient's intake of nutritious, laxative food and fluids to the amount of 2,000 ml. per day should be established. His pre-illness habit patterns of urination and bowel evacuation should be reestablished. This may take persistence and patience but usually can be accomplished. Occasionally accidents may occur if the person cannot be taken to the commode at the accustomed times. The patient should be helped to see that these have no serious implications.

It is nearly impossible for the bladder or rectum to empty completely when a bedpan must be used. A retraining regimen usually is most successful when the patient gets out of bed and onto a commode as soon as the doctor permits him to sit up. The nurse should not hesitate to ask the doctor if the patient may use the commode. Sometimes the doctor will permit the patient to use the commode once a day for bowel elimination even though he wants the patient to remain in bed the rest of the time.

Fecal impactions should be prevented. Daily palpation of the abdomen may reveal intestinal masses or bladder distention. Elimination must be noted carefully since diarrhea may develop around an impaction so that the impaction may go unnoticed for several days. Small daily doses of cathartics may be ordered, and an enema may be given every other day. Massage to the abdomen may be helpful in starting peristalsis, but is done only when ordered by the physician. Warm oil retention enemas are sometimes given regularly in an attempt to prevent impactions and are also given after impaction has occurred. Mineral oil by mouth is often ordered as a lubricant since straining should be avoided. The patient needs assistance in getting on and off the bedpan. Side rails which he can hold in order to turn himself for placement of a bedpan are very helpful. Lifting the hips even when a trapeze is used should be avoided because it requires more exertion than most elderly persons with a cerebrovascular accident should expend at that time.

The length of time the patient remains in bed will depend entirely on the type of accident he suffered and the judgment of his physician in regard to early mobilization. The trend is toward early mobilization of the patient with cerebral thrombosis, sometimes within a few days.

Return of motor impulses and consequently return of function is evidenced by a tightening and spasticity of the part affected. This often begins to appear from the second day to the second week after the accident. It is significant for the future use of the affected part, but presents new nursing difficulties. Flexor and adductor muscles become very active. The arm may be held tightly adducted against the body. The affected lower limb may be adducted to the midline, or even beyond it. The heel cord may shorten. In the upper limb, flexor muscles draw the elbow into the bent position, which we see so often in persons on the street; the wrist may be flexed and bent under and the fingers may be tightly curled.

Persistent nursing effort must be directed toward not letting any portion of the body remain in a position of flexion long enough for muscle shortening to occur and for joint changes to take place that may interfere with free use of the part. If the patient is lying on his back, a pillow can be used to help keep the upper extremity abducted away from the body. It is well to bandage the pillow to the top of the bed since otherwise the patient may merely slide down in bed and receive no benefit from it. A roll of one or two washcloths placed in the hand reduces the tight finger flexion and helps hold the wrist in extension. If the finger flexion is severe, the doctor may wish to use a splint to keep the fingers and wrist in extension. A firm box at the foot of the bed holds the foot at right angles and prevents contracture in the drop-foot position.

Range of joint motion should be preserved, and passive exercises are often started early. The nurse needs no order to put her patient's limbs through complete range-of-joint motion passively once or twice each day, but passive exercise in which the limb is to be moved, a definite number of times should be done only when an order has been given by the doctor. If no order is written, the nurse should consult the physician on the amount of passive exercise he wishes his patient to receive. Passive exercise to affected parts stimulates circulation and may help to re-establish neuromuscular pathways. No difficulty is encountered with these procedures until tightening of the muscles, particularly the flexors, begins to appear. Then other physical measures are needed, and the patient's treatment should be under the direction of the physical therapist. Heat and massage may be used if prescribed by the physician.

Much difficulty in the care of patients with cerebrovascular accidents might be prevented if the nurse started early to counteract the tendency to maintain a position of flexion. Often the services of a physical therapist are not available, and the total responsibility rests with the nurse. Perhaps the best reminder in regard to this contingency is that every minute counts. The nurse must not miss one opportunity to take a moment from her busy day in the hospital to move the patient's limbs back to the correct position. In the home she must teach the necessity for this same careful attention on the part of family members who are caring for the patient. One of the most common contractures and one that interferes most with rehabilitation efforts is a flexion contracture of the knee joint. A continued position of flexion of the knee and the use of pillows under the knee must not be permitted. Tightening of the heel cord with dorsiflexion of the foot must also be guarded against. Occasionally these positions of flexion are sought by the patient because of discomfort from pressure on the heel and ankle malleolus or some other area that has not been protected adequately from pressure. The patient may be taught to help with his own improvement, such as using the unaffected hand to help straighten out the flexed fingers of the affected side. He can move the affected arm into a position where the weight of gravity will straighten the elbow. He often needs help in performing abduction of the shoulder.

Active exercise to the affected side may be started early. This is ordered by the physician and, in the hospital, may be directed by the physical therapist. Under the guidance of the physical therapist, the nurse may supervise exercises while the patient is in the hospital, and she or the physical therapist may teach the family when the patient is to return home. Occupational therapy, such as knitting with heavy yarn or playing chess or checkers, gives the patient an opportunity to use his involved hand. Combing the back of the hair and washing the back of the neck give opportunity to rotate the shoulder outwardly. Propelling a wheelchair can give good exercise in extending the elbow. All these activities need supervision. The patient may do them and yet use only part of the range of motion that is possible for him and thus receive little benefit from them. Fatigue must be avoided. The elderly patient may be so anxious to become able to care for himself that he worries, tries too hard, and becomes exhausted and discouraged.

Before standing or walking, the patient may practice raising himself up in bed or may sit on the side of the bed, hold firmly to an over-bed table with his good hand for support, and press his feet on the floor or a stool. It is well to put his shoes on for this exercise since it improves the patient's morale, and in addition the paralyzed foot is kept in good position.

Some patients have persistent flaccid paralysis of the upper extremity. When sitting or standing the weight of the arm may tend to dislocate the shoulder. It is safe practice to put an arm sling on the patient before he stands or walks. While he is sitting, the arm, if not in a sling, should be supported on a chair arm, table, or pillows. The doctor should be consulted about the continuing need for the use of a sling. Some patients do well without a sling if they put their affected hand in a jacket, robe, or trouser pocket.

Teaching the patient good sitting and standing balance is very important and should precede teaching him to walk. Before taking steps, the patient should be encouraged to spend a few minutes getting his balance. Many older persons, especially following a stroke, lose their sense of vertical position. If this loss is great it may be unsafe for them to try to walk alone, especially in dimly lighted rooms. Such patients should not go to the bathroom at night but should use a commode at the bedside.

Some physicians prescribe fairly long periods of rest following a cerebrovascular accident. Others begin many activities early. Each new activity must be explained in detail to the patient because he is still unaccustomed to his clumsy, uncooperative extremities and becomes easily discouraged. Careful, detailed instructions as to how to hold and support himself will save him much embarrassment and confusion.

Motivation is undoubtedly the single most important ingredient in rehabilitation. Continued encouragement by the doctor, the nurse, the physical therapist, and all other workers is essential. Special measures must sometimes be taken for the "neglected" patient who may have come to assume that his situation is hopeless. If he has recovered hand function and overcome incontinence, it is likely that he can learn to care for himself.

The unaffected part of the body also needs attention in order to prevent contractures and preserve muscle strength. The patient will depend a good deal on his unaffected arm and leg when he begins to move about. Even while he is in bed, he should exercise his good arm and use it in all normal positions. The unaffected leg should be in a position of slight internal rotation most of the time while the patient is in bed. The knee should be bent several times each day, and exercises to strengthen the quadriceps should be performed. The quadriceps is the most important muscle to ensure stability to the knee joint in walking. One of the best exercises for strengthening the quadriceps is to have the patient straighten the knee against some resistance when he is sitting either on the edge of the bed or in a chair. A bucket of sand may be used, with care to protect the skin of the lower leg against pressure from the handle of the bucket. In the home, an ordinary cooking pan with a bucket handle may be used,

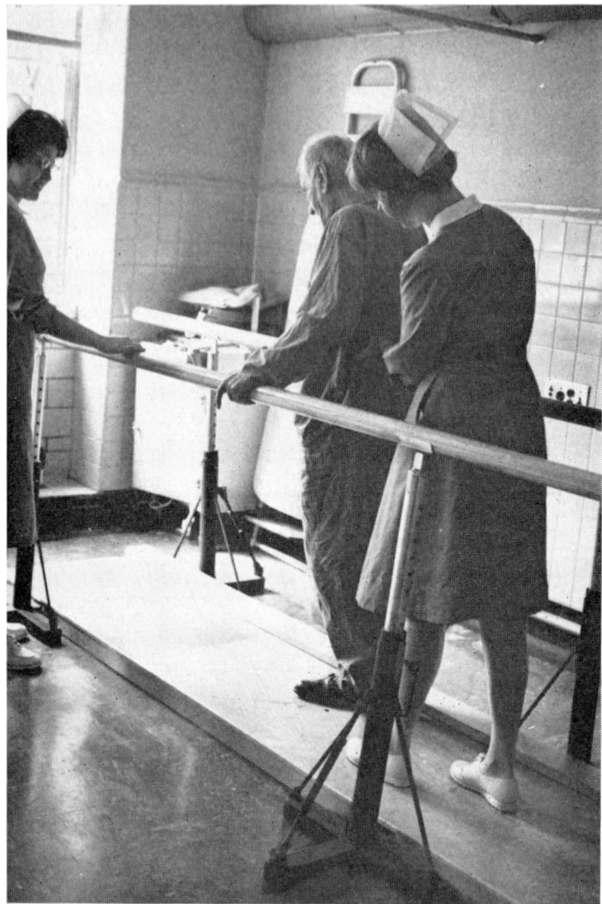

Figure 35. Learning to stand and balance between parallel bars is excellent preparation for walking. Safe, sturdy bars can be made for use in the home or nursing home at very little cost. (Courtesy American Journal of Nursing; photograph by Robert Goldstein.)

or a bag partly filled with sand can be suspended over the ankle with part of the sand on either side.

If preparation for walking has been adequate, the patient usually needs only one crutch when he begins to walk, and from that he progresses to the use of a cane. The crutch must be of the correct length so that pressure in the axilla is avoided and weight is borne on the palm of the hand (Chapter 15). The nurse remains close to the patient to allay his fear of falling when he first begins to walk. Good walking patterns must be established early because incorrect patterns are difficult, and sometimes impossible, to change. A side-to-side or sideways shuffle should be watched for and avoided. The patient should begin by leaning rather heavily upon the crutch or cane and lifting his body sufficiently to bring the leg and foot straight forward, with the toes pointing straight ahead, and effort should be made to avoid turning the foot and leg inward.

Special provisions may be necessary for the care of the person after a cerebrovascular accident. These are determined greatly by his own circumstances, the amount of recovery he obtains, and the guidance he is given in the early stages of his illness. For example, despite all effort, he may never be able to manipulate stairs. The social worker and the public health nurse are indispensable in helping to make the home situation one in which the patient may live with a moderate amount of self-sufficiency and independence. Family members often need a great deal of help in assisting the patient to accept his illness both physically and emotionally. They, too, must make adjustment to actual circumstances. Almost all patients who have had a cerebrovascular accident need health supervision for an extended period of time. The booklet *Strike Back at Stroke*[22] is extremely useful in teaching patients and their families.

A coordinated approach must be used in assisting the patient and his family to prepare for his homecoming, and a single set of realistic guides should be prepared. It is most helpful to all concerned if a group conference can be held in preparation for the patient's leaving the hospital. The nurse who has cared for the patient during his acute illness, the physical therapist, the public health nurse who will follow his progress and treat him in his home, the social worker, and the patient and/or a responsible family member should be present, as well as the physician, if this is possible. It is essential that the capacities and resources of the family to follow a recommended regimen of care be realistically appraised, and in this connection the contribution of the social case worker is essential. The patient's energy reserve must also be appraised realistically. The nurse who observes the patient during all hours of the day can often gauge not only his capacity for activity and his need for rest, but also the optimal times of day and duration for the performance of activities that require considerable energy expenditure. In addition, the family often needs help in actual scheduling of activities to fit the accustomed pattern of the patient in the hospital and his energy needs and also to fit their own way of life and the other obligations they may have.

Continuity and coordination of care must be planned for and enforced if the patient's progress is to be constantly forward and if the use of personnel and facilities is to be to the best advantage of everyone. The nurse can be a major influence in this if she will. She should, if necessary, take the initiative to be sure that transfers from one care facility to another or to home are planned, and that all information necessary for continuity of care is communicated correctly and to the right individuals and agencies.

It is not uncommon for cerebrovascular accidents to recur. Yet the patient may go for years with no further difficulty and may eventually die of some other cause. The physician usually explains this to the patient and to his family. The nurse must know what explanation he has given and must sometimes help in its interpretation to the family. Some patients may curtail activity to such a point that they secure no enjoyment in living and still have recurrences, whereas others may be active and escape further accidents for many years.

Trigeminal neuralgia (*tic douloureux*)

Trigeminal neuralgia is a disease of unknown cause. It occurs in late middle life and old age and affects women more often than men.

The most important symptom of the disease is pain, which usually comes on in acute paroxysms confined to one side of the face. Pain may be initiated by chilling, heat or cold, eating, pressure, or other irritating influences. Characteristic is a trigger zone in which the lightest touch or motion of a certain small area of the face will stimulate an attack. Pain may at first be blamed on a tooth, on sinus trouble, or on emotional tension.

The patient with trigeminal neuralgia requires thoughtful nursing care. He may not eat because chewing will bring on an attack; he may avoid exposure and contact of any sort that he may think will precipitate an attack of pain and as a result of such prevention may become malnourished, unhappy, and introspective.

In the hospital the patient needs rest and quiet. He should be placed where doctors, nurses, and other personnel will not constantly come into his room, ask about his condition, and expect an answer. He should be given a paper and pencil so that he may write if talking is painful. Diet should be high in calories and should be served at a temperature that the patient believes is least likely to bring on a paroxysm of pain. Liquid diet is often preferred. So exquisitely sensitive is the area to stimuli of any kind that the usual details of hygiene such as combing the hair and brushing the teeth may have to be omitted. Shaving may be impossible for male patients.

Trigeminal neuralgia does not yield permanently to medical treatment. Attacks can, however, be reduced in frequency in some patients by giving large doses of vasodilating agents, including histamine, nicotine, and carbon dioxide. The patient may have long periods without pain, but sooner or later the condition returns. Nicotinic acid and thiamine chloride in large doses appear to give relief in some instances. Alcohol injections are sometimes used but their effects are temporary. Procaine hydrochloride may be injected into the trigger zone, affording some relief. Mild analgesics have little or no effect, and there is real danger of addiction if narcotics are used. The only treatment known so far to give permanent relief is resection of the sensory roots of the trigeminal nerve.

The trigeminal nerve consists of three branches that supply the forehead, eye, cheek, lips, tongue, and chin of each side of the face. The most common operation for trigeminal neuralgia is resection of the sensory portion of the second and third branches, which supply the lower eyelid, nose, cheek, mouth, and chin. A small window is made in the bone of the temporal region, and the nerves are cut as they leave the dura or outer covering of the brain. Most patients welcome surgery as a means of relief from the excruciating pain. They must be prepared, however, for the numb sensation they will experience on return from surgery.

The patient is observed postoperatively for signs of increased intracranial pressure such as headache, vomiting, slowed pulse, and drowsiness. His position must be changed frequently until he is fully awake and able to take personal responsibility for moving about in bed. Mental confusion postoperatively is fairly common in older patients and is thought to be due to alteration in general circulation and to the unaccustomed environment. Confusion may be prevented in some instances by getting the patient out of bed soon after the operation. Care must be taken to prevent accidents, particularly if one eye has been temporarily protected with a dressing. If the first root of the nerve has been sectioned, the eye on the affected side must be cared for with irrigations and sterile oil. Often a patch or shield is used for a few days.

The patient needs reassurance following surgery. Though he is greatly relieved and happy about the outcome of his operation, he often cannot quite believe that he will no longer have pain. He may have become so accustomed to guarding his actions that he finds it difficult to realize that he can now talk, eat, and carry on other normal activities. Because of the loss of sensation, the patient may have the feeling that asymmetry of his face exists. Sometimes it takes time for him to accept the fact that he does not look different even though he has lost feeling in the side of the face. It is often helpful to give the patient a mirror so that he can see that his face is entirely normal in appearance.

The patient or persons responsible for his care must be taught to prevent injury to the part of his face in which sensation is now absent. Delicate nerve endings in the cornea of the eye may no longer be present, and excessive dryness and injury may go unnoticed. The patient may be instructed to consciously blink the eye frequently, to avoid rubbing it, and perhaps to continue use of mineral oil in the eye. Occasionally, particularly during windy weather, the physician may advise the patient to use glasses to protect the eye from dust particles. Lesions on the side of the face may go unnoticed. It is well to teach the patient to inspect the side of the face and the inside of the mouth at least once each day. Infection, toothache, and lesions of the mucous membrane will no longer cause pain.

Brain tumors

Brain tumors are not common in older people; 80 percent of all tumors of the brain occur in persons under 40 years of age, and only 7 percent in those over 50 years of age. Metastatic tumors comprise 5 to 10 percent of all brain tumors, and a fair number of these occur in the older age group. In spite of the low incidence of primary brain tumors in the elderly, they are important because they can often be removed surgically if diagnosed early. Some patients who cannot be completely cured can be aided substantially by surgery. Unfortunately, early diagnosis is not always made. Tumors in older persons may be in the frontal lobe and may cause personality change, forgetfulness, and headache. Symptoms may be attributed to arteriosclerosis, with the result that nothing is done until the lesion is far advanced, and surgical removal may then be impossible. It must be remembered that no classic signs are present in all persons with brain tumors, though visual disturbance, headache, vomiting, personality change, and sensory and motor changes are a few of the most common signs. It is important that the nurse be able to recognize signs of possible intracranial pressure in the elderly patient and direct him to competent medical care.

INTRACTABLE PAIN

Rhizotomy and cordotomy. It is possible in many instances to alleviate pain surgically even when it may be impossible to cure disease or prolong life for an extended period of time. Perhaps nothing is more demoralizing to the individual than constant pain, which not only affects the patient but also upsets everyone around him. Rhizotomy and cordotomy are surgical procedures in which the sensory nerve or nerve pathways are cut, and the sensations of pain and temperature are eliminated. (In a rhizotomy the sense of touch is also destroyed.) Pain-relieving procedures are often performed when patients are suffering severe pain from carcinoma that has undergone metastasis. These operations may be of benefit to persons of any age, provided that their general condition is fairly good at the time of operation. The operation does not in any way slow the progress of the malignant growth, but is often followed by most gratifying results. The patient feels better, his morale improves, and his appetite and nutrition improve. He may live in relative comfort for many months.

The patient's family must understand the purpose of the operation so that they will know what to expect. They should know that the operation often enables the ill person to actually participate in family life a little longer and that the more they can accept him as a normal member, the happier the patient will be.

The surgical approach for rhizotomy and cordotomy procedures is through a longitudinal incision on the back to one side of the spinous processes of the vertebrae. In the rhizotomy procedure, the sensory roots of the spinal nerves are severed as they emerge from the spinal canal and before they meet the motor root to form the main nerves leaving the spinal column. In the cordotomy procedure, that portion of the cord carrying the sensory fibers to the brain is severed at the appropriate level (see Figure 36). One limitation of the cordotomy procedure is that pain above the level of the nipple cannot be controlled be-

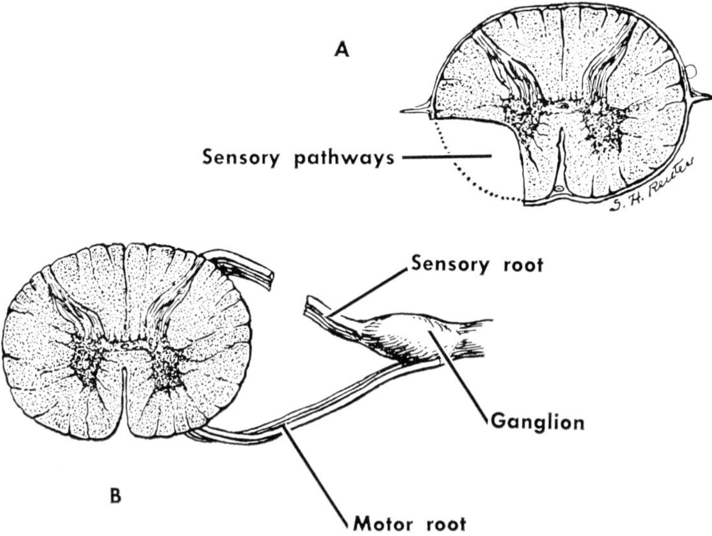

Figure 36. Cordotomy and rhizotomy. **A,** Cordotomy—incision is made through that portion of the cord carrying pain and temperature pathways; **B,** rhizotomy—a section of the sensory root is removed.

cause pathways cannot be cut high enough without danger of injury to the respiratory centers. The rhizotomy is a simpler procedure because there is less danger of disturbing nerve fibers that control vital functions. It does have limitations in that when metastasis is widespread many nerve roots must be severed to secure relief of pain, and this requires a large surgical wound. Shock and other postoperative complications can occur. The cordotomy operation requires a relatively small incision, and the danger of shock is not so great. However, trauma or pressure to adjacent nerve pathways during the operation may cause respiratory embarrassment, partial bladder paralysis, and other complications that may seriously interfere with a satisfactory outcome of the operation. These symptoms may be temporary because of edema at the site of surgery, and, if this is so, they often clear up within a few days. If he is to have a cordotomy, the patient should be told that he may experience temporary difficulty in voiding following surgery so that he will not be unnecessarily concerned by this annoyance if it should occur.

Preoperatively the nurse should prepare the patient for the loss of sensation that will follow the operation. This has been explained by the surgeon, but still the unique sensation comes as a shock to many patients. To many who have been in intense pain, the sudden loss of sensation is a distinct relief. To others it represents a peculiar and rather frightening situation to which they must adjust. The patient should know that following a rhizotomy the sensation will be similar to that after procaine has been injected. He should know that following a cordotomy he will still feel the presence of bedcovers against his skin, but that the feeling of pain will no longer be present if injury to the skin should occur.

The nurse must observe the patient postoperatively for special signs of complications of neurosurgery such as paralysis, impairment of motor function, and abnormal sense perception. She must watch the dressings for signs of hemorrhage and be certain that they are securely in place so that infection will not occur. Very careful recording of intake and output is necessary, as well as careful observation for bladder distention. Constipation may also follow this procedure so that daily elimination must be checked carefully.

Pneumonia develops easily after surgical procedures for intractable pain. Postoperative breathing exercises must be encouraged, and any difficulty in respiration or color change must be noted and reported immediately. The patient must be urged to cough and raise sputum at regular intervals since the acuteness of the pharyngeal reflexes diminishes with age, and the patient is likely to aspirate secretions into the lungs. If respiratory difficulty is encountered, oxygen may be ordered.

The patient may lie in one position for long periods without experiencing discomfort, and pressure areas develop quickly. Often the patient has poor nutrition, and this adds to the danger of development of decubitus ulcers. If the patient is quite helpless, a Stryker frame is helpful in making it possible to turn him with a minimum of handling. A turning sheet should be kept under the patient since he can be turned more easily by using the sheet than in almost any other fashion. Family members who are responsible for care of the patient at home should be taught why it is necessary to move him frequently. If he is able to help himself, they must realize that it is better for him to do so than to be waited on entirely by them. The patient and his family must be warned of the danger of accidents when sensation is no longer present. Hot-water bottles, for example, may cause burns without the patient's knowledge and must never be used if accidents are to be prevented. The general care of patients undergoing neurosurgery is discussed in medical and surgical nursing texts.[17]

REFERENCES AND RELATED BIBLIOGRAPHY

1. Alvarez, Walter C.: Cerebral arteriosclerosis; with little strokes that cause slow death, Amer. J. Nurs. **47**:169-170, 1947.
2. Anderson, Helen C.: Stroke; some nursing responsibilities, Cardiov. Nurs. **1**:1-5, 1965.
3. Beeson, Paul B., and McDermott, Walsh (editors): Cecil-Loeb textbook of medicine, ed. 11, Philadelphia, 1963, W. B. Saunders Co.
4. Camp, Carl D.: Organic diseases of the brain, spinal cord and peripheral nerves. In Stieglitz, Edward J. (editor): Geriatric medicine, ed. 3, Philadelphia, 1954, J. B. Lippincott Co.
5. Davis, Loyal (editor): Christopher's textbook of surgery, ed. 7, Philadelphia, 1960, W. B. Saunders Co.
6. Goda, Sidney: Communicating with the aphasic or dysarthric patient, Amer. J. Nurs. **63**:80-84, 1963.
7. Goldfarb, Alvin I.: Responsibilities to our aged, Amer. J. Nurs. **64**:78-82, 1964.
8. Harrison, T. R., and others (editors): Principles of internal medicine, ed. 4, New York, 1962, McGraw-Hill Book Company.
9. Hulicka, Irene M.: Fostering self-respect in aged patients, Amer. J. Nurs. **64**:84-89, 1964.
10. Hurd, Georgina Greene: Teaching the hemiplegic self care, Amer. J. Nurs. **62**:64-68, 1962.
11. Magee, Kenneth R., and Elliott, Alta: Parkinson's disease; neurologic management and nursing care, Amer. J. Nurs. **55**:814-818, 1955.
12. Moser, Doris: An understanding approach to the aphasic patient, Amer. J. Nurs. **61**:52-55, 1961.
13. Mullan, John F., and Van Schoick, Mildred R.: Intractable pain, Amer. J. Nurs. **58**:228-230, 1958.
14. Netsky, Martin G.: Diseases of the nervous system in the aged patient. In Johnson, Wingate M. (editor): The older patient, New York, 1960, Paul B. Hoeber, Inc., Medical Book Department of Harper & Row, Publishers.
15. Peszczynski, Mieczyslaw: The rehabilitation potential of the late adult hemiplegic, Amer. J. Nurs. **63**:111-114, 1963.
16. Schlesinger, Edward B., and Haber, Martha C.: Trigeminal neuralgia and nursing care of the patient with trigeminal neuralgia, Amer. J. Nurs. **58**:853-858, 1958.
17. Shafer, Kathleen Newton, and others: Medical-surgical nursing, ed. 3, St. Louis, 1964, The C. V. Mosby Co.
18. Sheldon, J. H.: Social medicine of old age, London, 1948, Oxford University Press for the Nuffield Foundation.
19. Smith, Genevieve Waples: Care of the patient with a stroke; a handbook for the patient, family and the nurse, New York, 1959, Springer Publishing Co., Inc.
20. Stern, Edith M., and Ross, Mabel: You and your aging parents, New York, 1952, A. A. Wyn, Inc., Publishers.
21. Turner, Gwendolyn E.: The cerebral vascular accident patient, Nurs. Outlook **8**:326-330, 1960.
22. U. S. Department of Health, Education and Welfare, Chronic Disease Program of the Division of Special Health Services: Strike back at stroke, Washington, D. C., 1958, U.S. Government Printing Office, Public Health Service Publication No. 596.

Chapter 17

Nursing in psychiatric illness

GENERAL PSYCHIATRIC NURSING

Adequate care for the mentally ill is one of the most serious medical and nursing problems of our times. Although total census of patients in mental hospitals has dropped gradually from a high of 633,504 in 1955 to 522,554 in 1964,[3] mental hospitals are still crowded, and many of them lack adequate facilities and services to give good care to all their patients. *Hospitals, Guide Issue,* August 1, 1965, reported 357,508 admissions to nonfederal mental hospitals for the year ending September 30, 1964. Approximately 26 percent of these were persons 65 years of age and older. Use of the ataractic (tranquilizer) drugs, wider use of electric shock therapy in the older age group, and intensive use of other psychiatric treatment has made some discharges possible. Group psychotherapy for selected patients has resulted in remarkable improvement in some instances.[14] A most pressing problem at present is the lack of suitable facilities for patients who could be discharged from the hospital if such facilities were available. Many interesting experiments are now being conducted both in methods of treatment and in housing, and as a result of these studies, the geriatric case load in state mental hospitals may, in the future, be relieved.[23, 26]

Prevention of disorders. More important than even the pressing problems of care and housing for our mentally ill is the prevention of emotional illness by the practice of sound mental health principles. The nurse must be alert to situations that may be precipitating an emotional crisis in the aged person. Sudden retirement from occupation, emancipation from responsibility for children, loss of husband or wife, and the increasing shortage of personal recreational activities are all factors that contribute to psychosis. The nurse has the confidence of the family almost more than any other worker, and her suggestions regarding the need for psychiatric consultation or mental health assistance may be heeded. Sometimes the nurse working in the public health agency is fortunate in having a mental health consultant in her agency with whom she may discuss the meaning of the behavior of her patients.

Most psychologic problems in the aged result from unresolved problems of earlier life. Physical illness, as well as social and emotional upsets, are often determining factors that produce personality disorder in the individual who has failed during his earlier life to develop a satisfactory integration of personality. It seems almost surprising that older people maintain as sound mental health as they do. Obstacles in the way of happiness for the person growing old are innumerable. Economic insecurity, loss of friends, failure of accomplishment during the active period of life, and loneliness are but a few. Loss of husband or wife, one of the most traumatizing experiences in living, often comes to the person 65 years of age or older. With physical restrictions appearing and time for achievement seemingly short, it is more difficult for the older person to resolve satisfactorily the conflicts that up to this time he may have dealt with more or less adequately. For with age there comes a time when a long series of physical, mental, economic, and social conquests must give way to gradual retirement from such activity and from concrete achievement.

Good adjustment starts at birth and continues until death. It is in infancy and early childhood that the foundations that will help to ensure emotional security in age must be built. Heredity is beyond personal control, but it is possible in childhood to develop such emotional stability as will contribute to sound mental health in the years to come. These may sustain the individual through an active and happy maturity and into the time beyond, when the next best must sometimes be substituted for the best. Resources with which the person is endowed at birth should be fully developed if good mental health is to be ensured in age. A study of early child development is, however, beyond the scope of this chapter.

Psychosis less often affects the person who has a working philosophy that gives him at least partial harmony with his environment. It less often befalls the person who has a faith that carries him through each day without undue peering into an uncertain future. The nurse cannot instill in each one she meets a sustaining faith and philosophy that will make life always seem worthwhile; but by her understanding, her interest, and her encouragement she can often help the aged person seeking peace of mind to guard against uncertainty and fear.

Maintaining interests is conducive to good mental health. Participation in learning, such as attendance at adult education classes, is of value in maintaining interest in life. Mental illness appears to be less of a threat to persons who continue a lifelong participation in mentally creative and intellectually stimulating pursuits than to persons whose recreation, as well as lifework, has comprised largely physical activity or manual skills, which old age may prevent them from continuing. Encouraging the older person to take an interest in people around him, in popular events of the day, and in his own personal appearance stimulates him and helps to ensure good mental health. Every effort must be made to preserve the feeling of personal worth so that the old person can recognize and accept the limitations of age without undue stress. Maintenance of personal dignity and purposeful activity are two important factors in mental health for the aged. In the home, younger members of the family must remember that the older person is happier when he is doing something. Permitting patients at home to do some of the cooking, some of the cleaning, and some of the simple household repairs and showing appreciation of their efforts adds immeasurably to their sense of usefulness and well-being and to their feeling of being essential to others.

Early treatment of chronic physical illness may contribute to prevention of mental illness. The constant wear from pain, irritation, discomfort, and frustration and the fear of becoming helpless or of dissipating financial assets for care make it much more difficult for a person to face other emotional problems satisfactorily.

Development of personality disorders. To help the older person who is suffering from either beginning or established mental illness, the nurse must have some understanding of normal personality and its changes with age. She must know when changes of personality are consistent with normal physical change and when they represent the first signs of mental illness. She must be able to interpret these changes to family members and others with whom the older person may be so that, if it is indicated, medical care will be sought, and so that she can assist the persons around the patient to adjust to him. She must help families to accept reality in facing both normal and pathologic changes in aging members so that family and community relationships are preserved. The school, the church, and the community center sometimes offer opportunities for teaching wholesome social attitudes toward older people.

Normal old age is marked by some inflexibility, some introspection, and a tendency to engage in long reflection, which are sometimes interpreted erroneously as sullenness or stubbornness. The older person may live a good deal in the past and recall early accomplishments with vividness. He may have an increased interest in himself and his organic functions as the struggle for survival goes on against mounting odds.

Mental illness in the aged is difficult to classify. Perhaps the most common diseases are senile psychosis, arteriosclerotic psychosis, and toxic and confusion states, though other forms of mental illness such as schizophrenia that have appeared in earlier life may reappear in old age. Involutional melancholia also appears, though its beginnings may usually be traced to early life, and it is not a disease confined to old age.

It is often impossible to say whether functional disease or organic disease is the main cause of the patient's symptoms. For instance, a patient may have shown a typical picture of arteriosclerotic psychosis, yet upon his death, little obvious brain pathology will be revealed at autopsy. Autopsy of another patient may reveal marked arteriosclerotic brain damage, yet he may have shown no signs of psychosis. There is usually a strong emotional or functional component in organic psychosis, and, in turn, an organic component is present in almost all psychoses in this age group.

Mental illness in age is often marked by slow onset of suspiciousness, weakening of the initiative, and concentrated attention on the fear of growing old and on bodily function. Impaired response and sometimes misinterpretation of the environment, poor appetite, and lack of interest in social functions and in personal appearance may be manifested. Sometimes an unbalanced interest in sex and impairment of judgment in other aspects of daily living are evident.

Mental illness may be preceded by organic disease, malnutrition, and conviction on the part of the patient that he is neither needed nor wanted. Depression is commonly seen in mental illness in age. This may be due in part to the inability to accept growing dependence and often accompanies psychosis without excessive organic deterioration. When organic deterioration is present, agitation is often present also. Psychotherapy to relieve anxiety often produces striking improvement, even when the picture looks far advanced.

Individual need for nursing care. Nursing for each patient must fit his particular needs and consider his individual problems. Since many patients are unable to give personal response to the care given them, satisfaction for the nurse's efforts must come from within herself. Qualities that will be present in many of her patients and which the nurse should anticipate and attempt to combat are forgetfulness, fear, insecurity and uncertainty, difficulty in expressing themselves and irrelevance in conversation, loneliness, reluctance to relinquish any established patterns of behavior, and a predisposition to accidents.

The seriousness of the illness may be determined partly by whether the acute psychosis has been brought on by a severe emotional crisis such as the loss of spouse or children, or whether it represents the climax of a lifetime of difficulty in adjustment. It will depend also upon how much organic deterioration has taken place. Nursing that applies generally to all psychoses in age will be considered and followed by descriptions of a few of the more common clinical entities and their particular care.

Certain characteristics that are not readily apparent under normal conditions may become pronounced in mental illness. A preoccupation with self is one of them. Most aged patients need to have attention drawn from themselves. They need to be engaged in group activities even though in many instances their participation in these activities may be trying for persons about them. The patient with senile psychosis may be worried and fearful. He needs constant kindly assurance of his worth within the group. With his fretful worry about details, he expresses a lifetime of insecurity and frustration that must be dealt with by encouragement.

Many elderly people are inclined to be careless of personal appearance, and, when they are mentally ill, this becomes marked. While feeling rejected and overly concerned with the impression they make upon others, they are careless of personal details that would make them more acceptable to their fellow human beings. They must be encouraged to clean their teeth, to brush their hair, and to be neat and appropriate in dress. A beauty parlor is of inestimable help to female patients. Having suitable locker space in the hospital and facilities in the home where the patient can take care of his clothing is extremely important.

The hoarding and hiding propensities, which are characteristic of age, present nursing problems. As infirmity advances, these seem to be natural protective mechanisms; perhaps it is a subconscious effort toward self-preservation, in anticipation of the time when it will be less easy to get about and to acquire the things essential to living. The patient with senile or arteriosclerotic psychosis may collect an amazing quantity of materials such as old rags, papers, crusts of bread, dishes, clothing, and the like. The older person living alone may collect stoves, wire, old furniture, and other articles to the point that they become accident and fire hazards. The principles of care of the patient should be the same whether he is in the home or in the hospital. Avoid making the older person unhappy by needless curtailment of hoarding. There must, however, be a limit because some of the materials hoarded are dangerous from a standpoint of pest and accident control.

Confusion and hurry must be avoided. The older person who is mentally ill may have hearing loss and may misinterpret sentences spoken to him. If the patient does have a hearing loss, use of a hearing aid may be recommended by psychiatrists. Conversation with the patient should be simple and unhurried. The patient should be protected from rush and excitement. Walks, meals, and other group activities should be prepared for in as quiet an atmosphere as possible. The nurse should repeat explanations yet avoid making them lengthy since this may lead to misunderstandings. Many other people have the fear, more apparent in mental illness, that younger relatives would be better off without them, and this sensitivity may cause them to misinterpret conversation.

Surroundings are important. Changes should be avoided since the confused and often frightened older patient may misinterpret shadows on the wall, strange sounds, and unfamiliar faces. If he is permitted to be up and about, he should have a place at the table that belongs solely to him. He should have his own bed, table, and chair and provision for his own things arranged to his liking, no matter how small that space may be. Furniture should not be rearranged, and the patient should be kept in the same room. His entire environment should be changed only when absolutely necessary.

Older patients often gossip, talk at length of the past, and indulge in repetition of sometimes meaningless conversation. This tendency may lead to trouble with the neighbors, with relatives, and with immediate family members. In the hospital, gossip is common when patients are allowed to congregate in groups and sit for hours with little to do. Persons who care for aged mentally ill patients must be tolerant. To attempt conspicuously to stop the gossiping or chatter is unwise since the psychotic patient may not accept logical explanation. It is better to say nothing, but to keep patients busy with sewing, listening to music, gardening, walking, improving their appearance, and such activities. Occupational or diversional therapy is a useful preventive for unproductive conversation.

Nutrition may be impaired since most patients with mental illness have poor eating habits. Many have lived for years on little besides tea or coffee and toast or rolls. Even when living in the homes of relatives, they have convinced their families that, because they are old and are doing little active labor, tea and toast is about all the food they need. Mental illness will often respond favorably to a diet that is high in vitamins, minerals, and proteins. Frequent nourishing fluids should be served, and the heavier meal should be planned for the middle of the day, with a light meal in the evening. Effort should be made to consider the food likes and dislikes of each patient. One with involutional melancholia, for instance, may have been a temperamental eater for years and have numerous notions of what does and does not agree with him. Accidents in eating should be avoided by cutting food into small pieces and being certain that all bones are removed.

Patients who are mentally ill are likely to be either incontinent of feces or to have constipation and to develop impactions. The patient who is agitated and the severely depressed person may ignore the stimulus to go to the bathroom. The nurse must take responsibility for checking her patient who is unreliable in personal habits and for teaching responsible members in the home, if the patient is being cared for by his family. Regular mild laxatives are usually preferred to frequent enemas, which may be disturbing to the patient, and exercise is helpful in ensuring regular bowel movements. The patient may need to be reminded to go to the bathroom at regular intervals, and fluids at supper may sometimes be restricted, since it is dangerous for the patient to get up at night as he may forget where he is, may fall, or may otherwise injure himself.

Effort should be made to combat infections and toxicity that may intensify mental symptoms, and the nurse should be on the alert for signs of chronic ills such as cardiac failure, urinary difficulty, gastrointestinal disease, or cerebral thrombosis. Eye disease may be present to add to the patient's confusion. It is important that the nurse be keen in her observation of his behavior.

Sleep and rest are essential. Aged patients sleep lightly, and mental illness increases this tendency; therefore great care must be taken to quiet these patients for sleep and not to disturb them during sleeping hours. The routine of an afternoon nap should be encouraged. The practice of having supper around five o'clock in the evening and having patients retire around seven o'clock is deplorable for any patient, but particularly so for those whose patterns of going to sleep at a later hour are firmly established. Forced to bed at this early hour, some patients thrash about and become so restless and agitated that sleep at even the normal hour is impossible, and sedation must be resorted to. In elderly patients, barbiturates may have cumulative effects and result in untoward reactions such as night-walking and confusion. If a sedative must be given, many physicians prefer that paraldehyde be used, despite its unpleasant taste and odor. Nursing measures that will induce sleep and rest without the use of sedative drugs should be employed. Among the most effective measures are complete body massages, warm bath at 37° C. (98.6° F.) for approximately an hour, followed by rubs with a lotion to prevent drying of the skin, warm drinks, and warm but light bedcovers. The patient who wishes to read himself to sleep should be permitted to do so.

Special effort must be made to protect the patient from injury and exposure. He may pay no attention to clothing and may become chilled. He may be uncertain in his movements and so preoccupied with his delusions or particular obsessions that he is utterly oblivious to normal accident hazards such as misplaced furniture and fluids spilled on the floor. Stairs, loose rugs, waxed floors, and bathtubs are particularly dangerous. Beds should be low to lessen danger of injury if the patient gets up at night. Impairment of judgment often results in accidents. For example, a person who is still living at home but is suffering from arteriosclerotic psychosis may drive the car, cross busy streets, climb ladders, and engage in similar activities that are not suited to his abilities. In the hospital many aged patients with mental illness are fearful and obsessed with their lack of worth. They may attempt suicide if given the opportunity.

The patient must be encouraged to be out of bed each day. He should have periods of rest alternated with change of activity and change of position. He is often easier to get out of bed if some attractive occupation can be presented, such as an hour in the garden, a drive, the theater, or church. Some elderly patients are depressed and fearful and prefer to remain in their beds and in their rooms. Remaining in bed may cause dangerous complications such as emboli or coronary occlusion and is definitely deleterious to physical well-being in age.

Some patients may have such irreversible brain damage that chances for recovery are truly hopeless. The nurse caring for the mentally ill in the hospital must remember not to force socially approved standards on a patient when for obvious reasons he is never going to return as an active member to society. For example, if such a patient has peculiar habits of dress, they should be tolerated if they are not harmful and if the patient is happier, no matter how bizarre the attire may appear to others. Despite their poor prognosis, however, many elderly patients with mental illness respond remarkably to skilled and thoughtful nursing care.

Disease conditions. In old age the brain becomes smaller, the dura mater is thickened, and senile plaques may appear. These changes do not appear to be related in any way to mental limitations that may develop. Generalized arteriosclerosis affecting the brain as well as other parts of the body, however, does alter mental function in varying degrees.

Senile dementia, or simple senile psychosis, and arteriosclerosis with dementia are the most common mental illnesses of old age. In a report released in 1957 by the National Committee Against Mental Illness it was found that 27 percent of all new patients admitted to public institutions for mental illness were suffering from one of these two conditions. It was found, also, that patients with senile psychosis comprised 13 percent of the resident population of all mental hospitals.[4]

In *senile dementia* there seems to be little if any correlation between the amount of mental deterioration and degeneration of brain cells. The condition is more common in women than in men. Onset usually is slow with a history of gradually increasing memory loss particularly for recent events, suspiciousness, night restlessness and insomnia, a tendency to live more and more in the past, stubbornness, weakening of the initiative, impairment of judgment, irritability, and change of mood with depression and feeling of uselessness. Carelessness and poor judgment in dress and grooming may occur and incontinence may develop. The prognosis is not good, although shock therapy sometimes brings about improvement. This treatment is not considered contraindicated as long as cerebral arteriosclerosis is not present. In this group are many patients whose condition is slowly progressing, who are beyond psychotherapeutic aid, and who profit little from confinement in institutions. The problem of their care and safety may be unsolved in many communities; therefore, they are finally placed in institutions for the mentally ill. Occasionally patients with senile dementia have pronounced improvement, even when little or no treatment is given.

Arteriosclerosis with dementia is more common in men than in women and occasionally occurs when the patient is in his fifties. There appears to be little relationship between the amount of arteriosclerosis and the degree of dementia; autopsies often reveal severe damage when no symptoms have occurred, and vice versa. The signs and symptoms of arteriosclerosis with dementia are similar to those of senile dementia except that they are often preceded or accompanied by usually short periods of confusion, aphasia, loss of consciousness, or loss of awareness of surroundings. The prognosis in this condition is poor, although some patients improve with improvement in their general health. The ataractic drugs are now used widely in treatment of this mental disorder.

Delirium reactions are fairly common in the elderly. Delirium is marked by sudden onset, though careful study of the patient's history may reveal that there were early signs that went unnoticed. These reactions may be due to organic cause and may follow abnormalities in nutrition, metabolism, electrolyte balance, or state of hydration. They may accompany infections or toxicity from other physical illness. They may be caused by drugs or alcohol; phenobarbital, bromides, and the very large variety of tranquilizers are but a few of many drugs that may cause sudden and severe symptoms.

Delirium reactions may follow an operation and may seem to be caused entirely by the operation, but in reality the surgery merely precipitated them. Control and treatment consist of finding and eliminating the causative factor. The nurse can be of assistance in anticipating these reactions by observing her patient closely before surgery and reporting accurately anything significant in his reactions or behavior. This condition may follow an operation on a patient who fears the operation desperately, but who says very little about his fears. The patient may have been reluctant to ask for a full explanation of the procedure, yet may have some completely erroneous ideas about it. He may have had a friend or relative who died following a similar operation, and so on. The patient who hesitates to tell his fears to the surgeon may sometimes mention them to the nurse, whose responsibility it then becomes to notify the doctor promptly.

Delirium reactions develop so suddenly that they are often mistaken for drug reactions. They may be aggravated in the aged by renal inefficiency and other physiologic limitations. The patient may be suspicious and delusional and may have auditory and visual hallucinations. He is likely to misinterpret his entire environment and may attempt escape even through an open window. Many patients recover within the relatively short time of a few days to a few weeks. Some authorities feel that because of the number of aged in the general hospital, there should be special provision in the general hospital for the safe care of these patients. Their illness seldom demands that they be sent to a hospital for the mentally ill; yet they require skilled treatment and nursing care.

The patient must not be restrained. If he has had a recent operation, some provision must be taken to prevent his tampering with the wound until healing has taken place. Paraldehyde is often used for this purpose. Physical measures such as warm drinks, warm baths, and massage are helpful. It is important to maintain food and fluid intake, and infusions of 500 ml. of 10 percent glucose are sometimes ordered. The patient must not be left alone, though he is often suspicious of the nurse or attendant in the room, and observations frequently must be done from outside the room. The patient must be approached carefully and kindly, and every procedure must be explained to him regardless of how apprehensive and uncooperative he may be. If possible, the same nurses should care for the patient since he is often distrustful of new faces.

Involutional psychotic reaction, commonly thought to be a disease of women at the menopause, is in reality a disease of both sexes. It appears in women most often between 45 and 60 years of age and in men after 55 years of age. The disease is usually characterized by an agitated depression, often a preoccupation with personal unworthiness, with sins of omission or commission in regard to sex, and often with suicidal tendencies. Involutional psychotic reaction in age is common in persons who have unresolved conflicts of early life, particularly problems relating to sex. The disease is most common in introverts who have struggled for perfection throughout a carefully planned and guided life and who cannot face the fact that the struggle for complete perfection must finally be lost.

The patient with involutional psychotic reactions should usually be kept in the hospital since he needs protection from injury to himself and also because he may in a carefully guarded environment develop some interests that will aid him when he leaves the hospital. Recovery is seldom complete or permanent unless the original conflicts can be resolved to some extent at least. Continued psychotherapy over a period of time is essential if permanent benefit is to be achieved.

Patients with involutional psychotic reaction are sometimes extremely clever in planning for their own destruction. The nurse must watch them very closely and at the same time must not permit her constant observation to cause further agitation or depression. The patient's meals are a nursing problem, and if the patient consistently does not eat, this omission must be reported to the doctor since tube feeding must often be resorted to in order to maintain the patient's strength.

At the present time involutional psychotic reaction is one of the mental illnesses of age that is most amenable to treatment. Electric shock therapy has been used with excellent results in these patients. One series reported indicates that 85 percent recovery can be anticipated, provided that continued psychotherapy is available and is accepted by the patient. Many patients show remarkable improvement after six to eight or ten shock treatments.

Electric shock therapy. Electric shock therapy is treatment by means of brief electrical stimulation of the central nervous system to the degree that convulsions are produced; this is followed by a period of sleep. The actual mechanism of the therapeutic effect of electric shock therapy is not well understood. Electric shock treatment must be accompanied by psychotherapy if lasting therapeutic benefit is to be obtained.

Electric shock therapy needs interpretation to the family and careful explanation to the patient. The treatment is neither shocking nor painful, though it is not entirely free of dangers, and the family of the patient should be acquainted with this fact. Many people fear intensely any procedure that has anything to do with the brain. They are under the impression that the patient suffers pain, that actual brain damage may occur, or that he may become paralyzed, and so forth. The nurse must know what the physician has told the patient in order that she may answer questions intelligently.

Great care must be taken that a complete physical examination has been done and that any signs of cardiac failure and of renal or vascular disease has been noted and investigated. However, experienced physicians do sometimes carry out electric shock treatment in certain patients when there are some signs of physical disease. Electric shock treatment is considered safer than Metrazol or insulin therapy and can be given to patients up to 70 years of age.

Treatments usually are given in the morning, and the patient may receive several treatments in a week. Sedatives must not be given before the treatment since sedative drugs may increase the amount of shock that is required to produce convulsions and may also tend to delay normal breathing at the end of the convulsion. The patient receives nothing by mouth for three hours prior to the treatment. He should void immediately prior to the treatment, and all hairpins, dentures, and bridges should be removed. Treatment should never be referred to as *electric* shock in the presence of the patient, since this word may produce fear of electrocution and arouse serious apprehension.

Treatment may be given either on a narrow, firm table, using one or more pillows under the thoracic spine to produce hyperextension, or else in the patient's bed, placing him head to foot in the bed and raising the knee Gatch to give the needed hyperextension. Electrodes are placed on the sides of the patient's temples, using either the special preparation for electrocardiograms or K-Y Jelly with salt. One physician usually holds the chin well forward and inserts the mouth gag as convulsions begin, and another physician watches the dials of the machine. A 90- to 125-volt current is turned on for an interval of 1 to 1.5 seconds. The nurse stands ready to hold the patient when convulsions begin. Oxygen is kept in the room and ready for immediate use. If the patient fails to start breathing at the end of the convulsion, artificial respiration is given at once and oxygen and respiratory stimulants are administered.

It is important that the equipment be removed from the room before the patient awakens, that he be left well covered, and that he is attended by the nurse or trained worker until he awakens fully. The patient usually awakens within one-half to one hour and may complain of dizziness and appear somewhat confused. After an hour or two he may be permitted to be up and about and should be given food. Because of the confusion often manifested in elderly patients, the treatments are seldom given more than two to three times each week. The patient may complain of muscle soreness following the treatment. Gentle massage with a mild lotion is helpful, and sometimes warm soaks in a tub of tepid water are useful if permitted by the physician.

It would seem that the fragile bones of the elderly would be prone to fracture with the intense muscular exertion during the convulsion, but this does not seem to be the case. Curare in the form of Intocostrin or other muscle relaxants may be given intramuscularly or intravenously to produce relaxation of skeletal muscles before shock therapy is given. If curare is used, it is necessary to have the physiologic antidote, neostigmine, on hand ready for immediate administration, since depression of the muscles of respiration can occur.

HOUSING THE MENTALLY ILL

It is a regrettable truth that there is little provision for care of persons of failing mental powers. This is largely because of the conditions under which we live, housing shortages, and lack of public interest. Some aged persons are placed in hospitals for the mentally ill, not because their condition may in any way warrant it, but because there seems nowhere else to keep them. Many older people cannot benefit from the psychotherapy that is available in our crowded mental hospitals, where it is almost impossible to provide even the minimum of physical care. In fact, the activity, the noise, and the constant change in placement and location in the hospital tend to increase their symptoms.

There is a slowly increasing interest in a plan whereby certain mentally ill people may be kept in carefully selected private homes in which care is supervised. The state pays for this care if private funds are not available. At present, many states are using such a plan though its possibilities have not yet been fully developed.

The outstanding world example of this humane plan for care is at Gheel (Belgium), where provision is made for mentally ill persons to be cared for in private homes. So many patients from the surrounding areas have been accepted that almost one third of the persons in the town are mentally ill. Life in the town and the community is geared to their presence, and their appearance on the main streets is not cause for comment. This plan seems to hold much promise for the future. It must be remembered that many mentally ill persons may not be different from normal individuals except for some fixed delusions or obsession. Many can be kept at productive activity if they live with persons who know and appreciate their delusions. Sometimes their delusions disappear in a sympathetic and kindly environment.

CARE OF THE SEVERELY DETERIORATED PATIENT

Medical and other scientific investigations, based on our present knowledge of the physical and emotional changes of age, have not determined whether senile dementia is preventable. There are examples of truly remarkable retention of mental faculties to a great age when heredity, physical state, and environmental factors are favorable. It is well known that many persons who are termed senile can be assisted greatly by improvement in diet, medical care, and pattern of living. Recent experiments in geriatric wards in several state mental hospitals throughout the country attest to the possibility of great improvement in the mental condition of many geriatric patients.[26] On the other hand, some individuals deteriorate eventually despite good nutrition, apparently good physical health, economic security, a loving spouse and attentive children, home living, mental challenges, and social participation with others. Intensive individual psychotherapy and skilled psychiatric nursing may help some of these patients, but for the present, at least, there are far too many patients for such services to be available generally.

Senile patients are housed and cared for in a variety of facilities. Many are in state mental hospitals and in federally supported housing such as veterans' hospitals and related federal domiciles. The 1954 survey of proprietary nursing homes conducted by the United States Public Health Service showed approximately 325,000 patients, 90 percent of whom were 65 years of age or older and whose median age was 80 years. In 20 percent of these patients, senility was a primary diagnosis, and in a large number of others it was a secondary diagnosis. Nonprofit nursing homes and homes for the aged also house many people who are very old and suffer from senility. No one really knows how many mentally deteriorated aged are cared for in their homes or in the homes of relatives or friends, but a survey of the case load of any visiting nursing agency indicates that the number is large. With an anticipated further increase in life expectancy, it can be assumed that the number of senile patients will increase in the near future. This is true despite some most encouraging results in improving the mental state of some elderly patients whose condition might have seemed hopeless even a few years ago.

Care of the senile patient consists of kindly and continuous nursing care. Much of this care is similar to what has been discussed in other chapters. Because it is more consistently needed for senile patients, it is summarized here. Professional nursing should and must assume more initiative for care of this sizeable segment of the total patient population if it is to fulfil its responsibility to all in the nation who are ill. This does not mean that all care of senile patients should be given by professional nurses. To so plan would not be feasible, practical, or necessary. There are many ways in which the professional nurse may contribute to better care of the senile patient. A few of them are:

1. By taking an active interest as a citizen and as a professional person in developments in legislation and community action that affect facilities for senile patients such as nursing homes, state hospitals, and home care programs.
2. By more and better teaching of relatives of patients, which may be done by hospital nurses when a patient is admitted to the general hospital, in the patient's home by the public health nurse, and by encouraging lay participation in home nursing courses like those offered by the American National Red Cross
3. By more actual participation in nursing care in the locations where senile patients are cared for and by more organized and effective teaching of nonprofessional personnel in these institutions

Approach to the patient. The patient who is senile should be treated with the same consideration for his feelings or for basic emotional needs as any patient of any age. This is an absolute rule of good care, and, if it were followed not only in actual doing, but also in the *way in which things are said and done,* it would result in improved care. This may sound impractical, for the physical needs of senile patients are so many, their living quarters are often crowded and ill-equipped, and they are obviously unaware of their surroundings much of the time. This consideration, however, is the right of every person living in a civilized society. It is well known that almost every senile patient, no matter how deteriorated he may be most of the time, has occasional and sometimes only fleeting periods of contact with reality. It is during these moments that he senses keenly where he is, that he is separated from loved ones, and that responses of those around him are varied. We do not know how much of what is heard or experienced during these periods of orientation affects the happiness, contentment, and peace of mind of the patient when contact with reality is again lost. We do know that the patient's response to kindliness, gentleness, and consideration is very real. This is so even with patients in whom one might first suppose no actual responses were possible.

Although nursing aides and other nonprofessional persons should not survey the personal records of patients too closely, it is useful for them to know what the patient did when he was 40 years of age. A good exercise is to have nursing personnel practice treating the patient exactly as if he were again that age in regard to informing him, asking him instead of telling him, and the like. It is interesting to note how quickly there is change in a patient when he is addressed as mister and his surname is used, rather than to be called by his first name or some other perhaps inappropriate term. The reason is that we are a status-conscious society, and most status is accorded persons in their middle years. It is a much more general practice to give the middle-aged patient an explanation of a treatment or a procedure than it is to similarly inform the very old and apparently senile patient.

The patient who is senile is entitled to the same regard for his privacy as any other patient, and it has been said that older people have a greater need for privacy than younger ones. Privacy may seem difficult to provide in a large ward where many patients must live together. But within any physical setting, some privacy can be provided if even a small effort is made. The patient who needs assistance in bathing should be protected from undue exposure by a small towel or other means if he is cared for by more than one person. The patient should have screens to give privacy when he uses a commode.

Genuine respect for the right of each patient, even when he is senile, to be different is one of the hardest things for both professional and nonprofessional personnel to cultivate. Perhaps this is because it is so much easier for the staff if everyone does the same thing at the same time and likes things done the same way. Yet, appreciation of the differences of individuals and of the right to these differences is essential to good care of the senile patient. For example, the patient has a right to reject participation in a certain group activity. The staff should provide for group activities and encourage participation in them, but they should not coerce. The patient who stoutly refuses to participate one day will often participate of his own accord on another occasion if left to his own devices.

Observation. The senile patient needs extremely close observation for several reasons. He usually has several chronic ailments, but, unlike the elderly person who is fully oriented, he will not complain about them or mention early symptoms of exacerbations of chronic illness. Often he has low resistance to new diseases, such as staphylococcic infection, and these may progress to a dangerous stage unless early signs are noticed by the nursing staff. Careful observation is necessary to anticipate and prevent accidents. Usually the patient is (or should be) out of bed in a chair or dressed and moving about where his exposure to accidents from falls is evident. The senile patient will seldom report when he is cold or chilled, and it is the responsibility of persons caring for him to notice whether a sweater is needed, whether there are drafts, or whether heating is faulty. The nurse or person caring for the patient must learn to think for the patient and anticipate his needs, yet not make this apparent. The problem is greater than for the irrational adult patient who is younger since usually the younger person, if disoriented by physical illness, is ill enough to remain in bed, and his environment can be studied and controlled more easily.

Nutrition and feeding. The mental condition of many patients improves remarkably with the regular intake of sufficient amounts of the right kinds of food. The senile patient needs the same essential foods each day as anyone else and probably appreciates attractively served food, even though he may sometimes mix foods in a bizarre way when left to his own devices. If the patient is in an institution, it is likely that food is not as well seasoned or as well prepared as when it is individually prepared in the home; thus it becomes doubly important that the nursing staff make a special effort to see that enough is eaten.

Foods should be arranged so that the patient may feed himself if possible. There is reason to believe that even the senile patient who has had a cerebrovascular accident gets real satisfaction from feeding himself although he may have to accomplish this in an awkward fashion with his left hand. If the patient is so confused that he tends to put all foods together, he can be served one dish at a time.

Some patients do eventually have to be fed. Whenever possible, it is best to raise the patient to a sitting position. It must be borne in mind that the gag reflex is much less sensitive than in the normal young person, and aspiration of food or fluid into the lungs occurs easily. The patient must never be hurried in efforts to chew or to swallow.

Urinary incontinence. Urinary incontinence is common and is a serious nursing problem in care of the senile patient. The study of proprietary nursing homes showed that fully one third of the patients were incontinent.[25] Urinary incontinence in senile patients has long been considered a nursing problem primarily, and only recently has there been serious medical effort to determine the causes and to suggest solutions. One physician[5] suggests that the following are the main causes of incontinence in the aged: (1) anatomic changes such as relaxation of sphincters, (2) increased reflex mechanisms of the bladder, (3) lessening of desire to void because of decreased awareness following cerebral clouding, and (4) a cerebral lesion that interferes with neurologic mechanisms between the bladder and the central nervous system.

Urinary incontinence may improve when bladder infection is treated. Usually, mild antiseptics such as methylene blue are used. It may decrease when alertness is improved by giving small doses of stimulating drugs such as ephedrine or Metrazol or by giving small doses of thyroid, under the direct supervision of a physician. Fluids should never be restricted since concentration of urine may cause irritation of the bladder and urethra and increase frequency of voiding.

Fluids are often moderately restricted during evening hours, but most very old people must void several times each night regardless of the amount of fluids withheld in the late afternoon or evening. Offering the patient a bedpan at regular intervals during the night, even if one must awaken the patient to do this, may help to prevent incontinence.

Getting the patient out of bed and into a sitting position is often surprisingly effective in controlling urinary incontinence.[5] Patients who have had cerebrovascular accidents and are incontinent have shown marked improvement when gotten out of bed and into a chair one to two weeks after the accident. Patients with fractures of the femur that were treated by pinning and who are out of bed within a week are less likely to develop incontinence than those who remain in bed for long periods of time. It is likely that these measures improve general circulation, increase the vital capacity of the lungs and hence the oxygen intake, generally improve the patient's physiology, and thus lessen the cerebral clouding that might otherwise occur. Excellent results in control of incontinence have been reported with patients who have been bedfast and incontinent for a long period of time—even years—and who have been gotten out of bed regularly. The use of commode chairs and commode wheelchairs permits patients to be out of bed even when urination is uncontrolled. It has been reported that the intradermal injection of procaine hydrochloride over the bladder stimulates a peripheral alarm system and helps to establish a regular pattern of voiding in some patients whose incontinence is of neurologic origin.[5]

When urinary incontinence persists despite medical treatment and the best of nursing measures, it presents very real problems. Care of the skin and subsequent prevention of pressure sores are paramount. The patient who is incontinent should have a tub bath at least daily. The water should not be too warm, and time in the tub should not exceed five to ten minutes lest the patient suffer exhaustion. Baths are best given by a team of two people since this provides better assistance and security for the patient and lessens danger of injury to personnel in lifting. Some institutions such as the Home for the Aged and Infirm Hebrews in New York City have equipped bathrooms with a tub that can be approached from three sides and that has a fixed seat at the sloped end (Figure 37). Thus the patient can be raised from the tub with ease by two people and can sit comfortably while being dried. The old-style tub with curved rim provides a firm, rough surface that can be grasped easily. If the patient is in his own home, tub baths may not always be given safely, and frequent local sponging must be substituted.

There are several commercial companies that distribute incontinence pads that can either be worn by the patient who is up or be placed directly on the bed under the patient; usually they consist primarily of a moisture-impervious material lined with disposable cotton or Cellucotton. These become costly when they are changed as often as desirable. Another form of "diaper" is now prepared commercially and consists of a rubber sheet covered with a muslin drawsheet that fastens to the bed. An open pantlike piece of material is then placed on the bed, lined with several thicknesses of muslin material, and secured to the patient as a diaper by means of tapes. Additional pieces of muslin can be placed

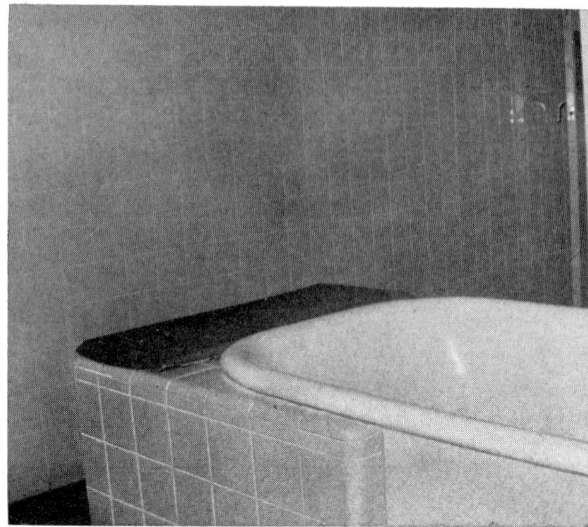

Figure 37. Note the seat at the sloped end of the tub on which the patient may sit while being dried. A space around both sides and the end of the tub helps to ensure safe, efficient care. (From Gubersky, Blanche D.: In Cowdry, E. V. [editor]: Care of the geriatric patient, St. Louis, 1958, The C. V. Mosby Co.)

between the thighs of the bed patient. Many large nursing homes now use commercial diaper services while others treat all diaper materials with Diaparene Chloride, which prevents the urine from breaking down into ammonia and thereby decreases skin irritation and unpleasant odors. Diaparene powder may also be sprinkled on sheets to delay the decomposition of urine.

Urinary incontinence in women is very difficult to deal with, and often absorbent pads must be used. So-called female urinals of rubber have been used, but they are likely to be uncomfortable, to irritate the skin if they fit tightly enough to prevent leakage of urine, and to retain odors. Uncontrolled urinary incontinence should not be a reason to keep the woman patient in bed. Pants made of waterproof material and lined with absorbent material may be used; thus the patient is permitted to be up and about and to attend group activities, such as eating in the dining room. Protective pads are sold by several commercial companies or can be made at home (Chapter 10, Care in the Patient's Own Home).

Very satisfactory drainage can be devised for men who are incontinent of urine. Since it may interfere with circulation, the penile clamp should not be used for senile patients who cannot be relied upon to report symptoms. The best device for external drainage is made with an ordinary condom, a glass connector, a piece of rubber tubing, and a receiving bottle or rubber bag. It is prepared as follows. Tie the closed end of the condom firmly over one end of the glass connector, using linen thread or fine tie material, and make an opening in the condom to drain the urine. Invert the equipment and attach the glass connector to the tubing and this to the bottle or bag. Cleanse and thoroughly dry and powder the penis before putting the condom on; leave about one-half inch between the urinary meatus and the opening made by the glass connector. The upper end of the condom may be anchored to the skin with adhesive after tincture of benzoin has been applied. A very soft rubber band with several notches that permit it to fit snugly but not tightly is now available from commercial companies. Manufactured equipment to substitute for the condom and glass connector can also be obtained, but at the present they are somewhat thicker and less flexible than the condom and are less satisfactory. The condom should be removed, and the penis should be washed and examined for skin irritation at least once daily. This device is comfortable, and most patients do not attempt to remove it.

The male patient who has trouble with dribbling may be cared for by using a condom or even a rubber glove loosely but carefully anchored and changed frequently. Occasionally, reminding the patient to remain for a few moments at the conclusion of voiding before rearranging his clothing will help to prevent dribbling.

Indwelling catheters occasionally are used for women who are incontinent, since the female urethra is short, and there is less danger of infection than in the male patient. Men frequently develop urethritis and epididymitis when an indwelling catheter is used for even a few days.

Bowel elimination. Since the senile patient cannot be relied upon to report bowel elimination accurately, a commode is more satisfactory than the toilet, which may be flushed at any time. Stools should be examined. It must be remembered that variation in normal elimination exists. It may be perfectly normal for one patient to have a bowel movement only every three or four days, whereas another one must have a movement daily. If the stool is soft and formed, it can be assumed that bowel elimination is satisfactory. If the stool is hard and dry, it usually means that the patient is constipated and may be dehydrated, regardless of how often he has a movement.

The relatively new drug bisacodyl is now being used widely for patients confined to bed and who must have some stimulation for regular bowel evacuation. Often the common trade name of Dulcolax is used. This drug may be given by mouth or in a suppository. It acts by reflexly stimulating the bowel musculature upon contact and its regular use does not appear to increase tolerance to it. In care of the severely deteriorated and incontinent patient it is most often used as a suppository placed high in the rectum with a gloved finger. Protective material is then used until the patient's bowels move. This procedure has been found helpful in enabling patients to be up and around more if they are ambulatory and can mingle with others, in preventing repeated small bowel evacuations, and in reducing impactions.

A real problem in care of the senile patients is impactions. These seem to occur sometimes regardless of the care taken and the diet eaten. Any patient who is incontinent of small amounts of liquid stool at repeated intervals should be suspected of having an impaction, and manual inspection with a gloved finger should be made. Policies of institutions vary as to who is permitted to break up impactions manually; serious lacerations and trauma have followed attempts by untrained persons. It is sometimes best for the nurse or the untrained person to remove the impaction gradually by breaking only a part at a time and follow each attempt by giving a small amount of enema solution, rather than attempt to break up a large impaction completely at one time. Treatment of an impaction can be an exhausting experience for all concerned, and the nurse or her assistant must watch the patient for signs of fatigue such as diaphoresis, skin color changes, or change in pulse. If these occur, the procedure should be delayed, and medical advice should be sought. If possible, the patient should be in bed during this procedure rather than sitting on a toilet or commode, since this permits him to rest more easily.

REFERENCES AND RELATED BIBLIOGRAPHY

1. Bluestone, E. M.: Hospitalization. In Cowdry, E. V. (editor): The care of the geriatric patient, ed. 2, St. Louis, 1963, The C. V. Mosby Co.
2. Bojar, Samuel: The psychotherapeutic function of the general hospital nurse, Nurs. Outlook **6**:151-153, 1958.
3. Bureau of the Census: Statistical Abstract of the United States, 1965, ed. 86, Washington, D. C., 1965, U. S. Department of Commerce.
4. Busse, Ewald W.: Mental disorder of the aging. In Johnson, Wingate M. (editor): The older patient, New York, 1960, Paul B. Hoeber, Inc., Medical Book Department of Harper & Row, Publishers.
5. Eckstrom, Sten: Urinary incontinence in old persons, Geriatrics **10**:83-85, 1955.
6. Friedman, Jacob H., and Bressler, David M.: A geriatric mental hygiene clinic in a general hospital; first two years of operation, J. Am. Geriatrics Soc. **12**:71-78, 1964.
7. Gitelson, Maxwell: The emotional problems of elderly people, Geriatrics **3**:135-150, 1948.
8. Goldfarb, Alvin I.: Responsibilities to our aged, Amer. J. Nurs. **64**:78-82, 1964.
9. Haas, Adolph: Management of the geriatric psychiatric patient in a mental hospital, J. Am. Geriatrics Soc. **11**:259-265, 1963.
10. Hamilton, James Alexander: Psychiatric aspects. In Cowdry, E. V. (editor): The care of the geriatric patient, ed. 2, St. Louis, 1963, The C. V. Mosby Co.
11. Havighurst, Robert J., and Albrecht, Ruth: Older people, New York, 1953, Longmans, Green & Co., Inc.
12. Hulicka, Irene M.: Fostering self-respect in aged patients, Amer. J. Nurs. **64**:84-89, 1964.
13. Hulicka, Irene M.: Psychologic problems of geriatric patients, J. Am. Geriatrics Soc. **9**:797-803, 1961.
14. Lemkau, Paul V.: Follow-up services for psychiatric patients, Nurs. Outlook **6**:149-150, 1958.
15. Litin, Edward M.: Mental reaction to trauma and hospitalization in the aged, J.A.M.A. **162**:1522-1524, 1956.
16. MacCallum, D. V.: Proprietary and nonprofit homes for the aged. In Cowdry, E. V. (editor): The care of the geriatric patient, ed. 2, St. Louis, 1963, The C. V. Mosby Co.
17. Macleod, Kenneth I. E.: Well oldster health conferences, Nurs. Outlook **6**:206-208, 1958.
18. Marchesini, Erika H.: The widening horizon in psychiatric nursing, Amer. J. Nurs. **59**:978-981, 1959.
19. Mereness, Dorothy, and Karnosh, Louis J.: Essentials of psychiatric nursing, ed. 6, St. Louis, 1962, The C. V. Mosby Co.
20. Overholser, Winfred, and Fong, Theodore C. C.: Mental disease. In Stieglitz, Edward J. (editor): Geriatric medicine, ed. 3, Philadelphia, 1954, J. B. Lippincott Co.
21. Riccitelli, M. L.: Modern concepts in the management of anxiety and depression in the aged and infirm, J. Am. Geriatrics Soc. **12**:652-657, 1964.
22. Riccitelli, M. L., and Rosen, James M.: Integration of the general hospital and the nursing home in the total care of the aged and the infirm, J. Am. Geriatrics Soc. **9**:611-614, 1961.
23. Simpson, William S., and Moulun, Roberto D.: Opening nursing home doors to psychotic patients, Nurs. Outlook **7**:367-368, 1959.

24. Smigel, Joseph O., and Russell, Anna: The do's and don'ts of therapy for decubitus lesions with emphasis on use of the electric lamp, J. Am. Geriatrics Soc. **10**:975-982, 1962.
25. Solon, Jerry, and others: Nursing homes, their patients and their care, Public Health Monograph No. 46, Washington, D. C., 1957, U. S. Government Printing Office.
26. Tibbitts, Clark: Social change, aging and public health nursing, Nurs. Outlook **6**:144-147, 1958.

Chapter 18

Nursing in orthopedic disabilities

Orthopedic disabilities are exceedingly common in old age. Since earliest recorded times, orthopedic ills have occurred to plague the lives of persons who lived to become old. In Egyptian hieroglyphics of 1500 B.C., a thin, stooped individual leaning on a staff was used to signify old age. The use of a variety of crutches to support old and orthopedically handicapped persons has been recorded through the centuries.

From the standpoint of nursing at least, the most important orthopedic conditions are hypertrophic arthritis due to degenerative joint changes, osteoporosis following bone atrophy, extra-articular pathology of obscure origin including fibrositis and bursitis, and fractures caused by trauma and disease. Diseases of unknown or uncertain origin such as Paget's disease and osteomalacia are also considered diseases of age. Multiple myeloma and metastatic malignant bone lesions occur, and their care is considered with that of fractures. Orthopedic diseases that usually occur in younger life such as rheumatoid arthritis may persist into old age. It is not too unusual for this form of arthritis to make its first appearance when a person is over 50 years of age, and many people with rheumatoid arthritis are now living to be old. Recent estimates indicate that at least 97 percent of the persons over 65 years of age have some form of rheumatic disease causing varied amounts of discomfort and disability.

DEGENERATIVE ARTHRITIS

Degenerative arthritis is really a misnomer in that it implies an inflammation of the joints. In reality the pathologic state of the joints is due to a degenerative process of unknown cause. It is often aggravated by excessive use of the joints and by trauma from direct injury or from poor functional use of the body including the joints. Synonyms are osteoarthritis and hypertrophic and senescent arthritis.

Some authorities believe that most people over 35 years of age have degenerative changes in the joints. The disease is more common in women than in men.

In degenerative arthritis there is a gradual thinning and deterioration of the articular cartilages, bringing the working surfaces into closer approximation. This may produce pain upon use of the joint. The nurse will be aided in distinguishing this condition from atrophic arthritis if she recalls that the cartilage has no established blood channels; therefore an inflammatory reaction cannot occur in the main structures involved. This is in contrast to rheumatoid arthritis in which pathology is initially in the vascular synovial membrane. In degenerative arthritis, excess bone deposit may form on the articular margins of the joint, producing the "lipping" commonly seen on radiographs of the hip, the knees, and the spine.

Signs and symptoms. Degenerative arthritis usually comes on slowly. The first symptoms may be pain, often following excessive use of weight-bearing joints, and stiffness after prolonged rest. Pain may be caused either by close approximation of atrophied cartilages, by reaction on surrounding tissues, or by pull or pressure on nerves when bone alignment is altered. A severe occipital headache sometimes accompanies degenerative arthritic changes in the cervical vertebrae.

Symptoms of pain may be out of proportion to the apparent changes in the joint. Some people may have severe pain and disability with apparently little joint change, whereas other persons may complain of few symptoms and yet have very marked changes in the joints. Associated conditions in surrounding tissues, such as bursitis and fibrositis, may contribute to pain.

Pathology produces pain, discomfort, and the "old-age stiffness" that is so often most apparent to the patient upon awakening and during cold, damp weather. Usually there are no constitutional symptoms unless there is additional disease.

Degenerative arthritis is seen frequently in the person of stocky pyknic build who is moderately obese. This has led to speculation as to an endocrine factor as the cause of the disease. Many patients with degenerative arthritis also have marked arteriosclerosis, but no direct connection between the two conditions has been demonstrated.. The most constant and obvious outward sign besides the general stiffness and limitation of motion is the presence of Heberden's nodes or a proliferative deposit around the distal phalanxes of the fingers. This is an extremely common finding in women patients that causes distress primarily because of cosmetic disfiguration of the hands.

Degenerative disease of the hips is a most disabling form of the disease. In advanced stages, as frequently seen in very elderly women, it is commonly referred to as malum coxae senilis. Pain on motion or weight bearing may become severe and is often referred to the groin, the distal anterior surface of the thigh, or medial surface of the knee. Patients rarely complain of pain in the hip joint. Loss of abduction, extension, and internal rotation of the hip joint are common and are associated with rigidity of the opposing muscle groups.

Treatment and management. There is no cure for degenerative arthritis. Better control of obesity in early and middle life and more attention to good body mechanics during the hard-working years of life would probably help to make old age more comfortable for some people. The elderly person with painful joints needs reassurance since often he fears becoming completely crippled.

With attention to a few modifications in living as prescribed by his physician, the patient will probably be able to live with his arthritis quite well and suffer only moderate or slight discomfort.

Occasionally, marked changes in plan of living have to be made. The work of the patient may have to be decreased and in some cases may have to be altered entirely. The dentist with arthritis of the hip and upper spine may have to decrease the number of hours of active work. The typist with arthritis of the shoulder joints may have to change her means of livelihood.

Accidents must be guarded against by the person with degenerative arthritis. Several factors predispose to falling or injury. Muscle rigidity and reduced range of motion especially at the hip joints, thinning cartilage of the knee joints, and loss of strength especially of the quadriceps muscle all contribute to instability and faulty weight bearing. With these limitations the patient may easily lose balance when walking on uneven surfaces, going up or down curbs or steps, or hurrying across streets. The added loss of neuromuscular coordination further reduces his ability to regain balance or adapt quickly to change of pace on uneven walking surfaces. Malposition of a weight-bearing joint may cause sudden sharp pain or injury to the knee structures. It is often helpful for an old person with degenerative arthritis and associated faulty posture and gait to use a cane. In addition to widening the base of support for improved balance, the person obtains added proprioceptive stimuli via his hand. He is better able to judge body position and has a ready support in case of need.[9] Most orthopedists and physiatrists believe that an exercise routine is essential for all older people in order to maintain good general health and muscle strength and to help keep them limber, as well as to restore function in the event of disease. Authorities are agreed that many regular exercise programs are too strenuous for the aged person and that his general physical condition must be carefully appraised before exercise is prescribed.

Rest is of the greatest importance in the treatment of degenerative arthritis. Painful joints must be relieved of their burden at frequent intervals during the day. It is seldom necessary, however, and in most instances definitely harmful, for the aged person with degenerative arthritis to remain in bed. He may need assistance from the physical therapist or the nurse in learning how to get about if marked limitation of motion in certain joints is present. For example, he may have to be taught how to get from bed to chair or to a standing position without losing his balance and possibly suffering injury.

Trauma from poor posture and body mechanics cannot be undone, but further damage may be decreased by close attention to posture. If changes have occurred because of alteration of alignment of the vertebrae and subsequent pain, a firm bed is often helpful. If the pain is in the upper spine, rest without a pillow may be ordered. This may cause more pain at first, and the nurse must urge the patient to continue to follow his doctor's instructions. Pain in the neck caused by faulty alignment of arthritic joints will often disappear in a reasonable time with this treatment.

The patient with degenerative arthritis should give special attention to his shoes. Shoes should have a straight last, low rubber heels if the posterior heel cords are not contracted, and should be carefully fitted. A tendency to bunion formation is increased when arthritic changes are taking place. Alterations in joints of the foot may make the type and size of shoe usually worn by the person uncomfortable. The patient must know that, though changes have developed, comfortable and satisfactory shoes that accommodate individual foot changes can be obtained by careful selection.

Drugs are of limited use in the treatment of degenerative arthritis. Most physicians feel that habit-forming drugs should never be prescribed. The patient should not rely upon codeine or even aspirin to tide him over periods of pain that might be better handled by controlling weight or by increasing rest periods. Aspirin, however, is often ordered to combat symptoms. Phenobarbital may be ordered occasionally for sleeplessness and apprehension.

In the absence of scientific data about the relationship of diet to degenerative arthritis, special diets are not usually ordered by the doctor. The patient too frequently suffers dietary deficiency, particularly in protein and vitamin B. This may be the result of edentia, loss of energy and incentive to prepare meals, financial difficulties, and other reasons. He may need some assistance in planning adequate meals and considerable encouragement to eat them. Following food fads is likely to increase further the discrepancy between body requirements and food eaten.

Obesity aggravates degenerative arthritis since weight puts an added burden on joints, particularly on weight-bearing points, and not only increases pain, but may also further the degenerative process. Obesity should be corrected in most patients with degenerative arthritis. In the hospital and in the home, the nurse can explain the need for weight reduction and help the patient to plan a satisfactory diet as directed by the doctor. It is helpful when the diet does not differ too radically from his established dietary patterns.

Generally speaking, surgery occupies a small place in the treatment of degenerative arthritis. Occasionally a joint is surgically fused because of pain. Bony or cartilaginous bodies (joint mice) that have broken off from the joint surface may be removed. Osteophytes or spurs may require surgical removal to alleviate pain if they form on the heel or other locations subject to pressure or friction.

When extensive destruction of the head of the femur has occurred, an arthroplasty of the hip or insertion of a prosthetic cup or head may be done in selected cases. The increased joint motion and relief of pain often results in improved function and general health. Physical therapy procedures offer comfort to many patients with degenerative arthritis. Heat is often helpful, but general procedures that raise body temperature must be used with caution when there is cardiovascular disease. Also, when peripheral vascular disease is present, local application of heat should be given cautiously to avoid increasing the demand of the tissues for oxygen beyond the capacity of the vessels to supply it. The paraffin bath is an effective means of supplying heat to local areas when needed. The details of this procedure are discussed in Chapter 12, Special Treatments. Massage is useful in the treatment of degenerative arthritis, but should be employed with moderation in the older person. Degenerative arthritis often affects the lumbar and cervical spines. Mild traction on the neck may help to relieve pain in cervical involvement. Apparatus for this can be set up in the patient's own home.

EXTRA-ARTICULAR DISEASES

Fibrositis. Fibrositis is an orthopedic affliction that seems common in the elderly. There is difference of opinion as to the etiology and significance of fibrositis, but excessive muscular activity combined with poor digestion and toxemia and aggravated by chilling seem to be generally considered predisposing factors. Fibrositis is a condition that has not been accorded much space in medical literature in this country until recently. It is a most important disease among the aged from a standpoint of physical discomfort. Fibrositis is classified by some physicians as a nonarthritic rheumatic disease similar in some ways to tenosynovitis and bursitis. Many times it may occur in conjunction with these allied conditions.

Steinbrocker defines fibrositis as a nonsuppurative, low-grade inflammatory disease of fibrous supporting tissue anywhere in the body. It exists in the acute form in young persons and is usually aggravated by strenuous exercise. In the elderly, a chronic form of the disease is much more common.

The cause of fibrositis is obscure. The feeling of fatigue and malaise so common in fibrositis has caused speculation as to the possibility of a virus origin. Elderly persons suffering from fibrositis are often found to be harboring low-grade infections of some nature, to be living on inadequate diets, and to have poor posture and body mechanics that result in persistent strain on and increased work of certain muscle groups. Impaired circulation with inability of the circulatory system to provide sufficient nutrition to fascial structures and to remove waste products effectively has been given as another possible cause of the disease. Prevention would then indicate guarding against excessive use of individual muscles or muscle groups, teaching the need for moving about at intervals so that different muscle groups will be brought into use, and teaching effective ways to accomplish particular daily work with a minimum of strain on muscle groups.

Chronic fibrositis may come on suddenly, as for example the stiff neck that may remain with little relief for many months. Or it may come on so gradually that the patient cannot recall its beginning. Fibrositic nodules can be felt by the experienced doctor, nurse, or physical therapist in many patients. These nodules are small masses of connective tissue lying within the fascia or embedded within the muscle. Fibrositic nodules may occasionally have to be surgically removed, though in many instances they disappear with vigorous massage. Such massage should of course, be given only as specifically prescribed. Some physicians question the belief that fibrositic nodules are significant in fibrositis, pointing out that nodules may occur in young people in the absence of pain.

The person who is troubled with fibrositis would do well to remain indoors in wet weather and avoid chilling whenever possible. Automobile rides are excellent for many aged persons who are chronically ill, but drafts on the neck, shoulders, and other parts of the body must be avoided.

Physical therapy in the form of heat, massage, and stretching are invaluable in relieving the symptoms of fibrositis. The infrared lamp is often used. Following a treatment, it is extremely important that the patient be protected from chilling. The patient who is using a small lamp for heat in his home needs to be reminded of this.

Bursitis. Bursitis is a condition in which there is irritation of the bursa with accumulation of fluid and calcium salts. The disease is not confined to the aged, but is most common in persons over 40 years of age. The most frequent cause is thought to be trauma, but in a few cases rather severe bursitis can appear in the absence of any evidence or history of trauma. In this country bursitis of the shoulder is by far the most common.

Bursitis can be a most distressing chronic ailment that is often slow to respond to treatment. Pressure or stretch on the bursa causes pain and marked limitation of motion of the affected joints. Physical therapy is by far the most effective form of treatment, although roentgen treatment is sometimes helpful also.

Usually the patient is not hospitalized. The nurse most often meets him in the clinic or in his home. One of her most important responsibilities is to encourage the patient to continue to follow his doctor's orders and to perform exercises as specifically directed by the physical therapist. Constant pain is demoralizing. Patients with bursitis become discouraged and are likely to turn to patent remedies and to persons not qualified to care for them adequately. They may fail to carry out instructions as given and fail to keep clinic or physical therapy appointments. The inevitable result of disuse will be contracture of the muscles that control the joint—the so-called "frozen" shoulder.

FRACTURES

Fractures with accompanying injuries and complications frequently snuff out the life of the aged person, but perhaps not before a distressing period of time has intervened between injury and death. The outlook for the aged patient with a fracture has improved markedly in recent years, however. Modern surgical methods, careful consideration of the aging physiology, and expert nursing care have contributed to this improvement.

Fractures result from accidents, from bony metastasis of malignant lesions elsewhere in the body, and from conditions of the aged bones themselves, such as osteoporosis. Mineral starvation seems to take place, although blood calcium and phosphorus levels are normal. This may be the result of poor nutrition with high intake of carbohydrate, endocrine changes, or achlorhydria with the resultant poor use of the small amount of essential food taken.

The treatment and nursing care of fractures in the older patient present specific problems. The slow rate of bone repair and the extreme danger of serious complications from immobilization are ever present. Though the general condition of the patient determines choice of treatment, the older person is no longer considered a hopeless surgical risk. The physician selects treatment that will permit the patient to move about as soon as possible. For example, nailing the hip in fracture of the neck of the femur has largely supplanted immobilization in a cast. Russell traction is widely used since it permits moderate freedom of movement. When cardiac or other disease makes it necessary that the patient's head be elevated, it is possible to raise the head of the bed a few degrees and still maintain moderately effective traction. Russell traction is used quite effectively for many patients whose general condition does not permit surgery. In some instances when the patient is extremely old and there is no displacement of fragments, a suspension sling is the treatment of choice for fracture of the neck of the femur.

Fracture of the neck of the femur is extremely common in old age, and by far the larger number of cases are among women. The older person has usually known a friend or relative who suffered a fracture of the hip and from which he failed to recover; thus the diagnosis is linked in the mind of the patient with suffering, permanent helplessness, and eventual death. He needs quiet reassurance that he will again be able to move about independently. The best way to give him this reassurance is to start activities in preparation for independence from the first day of injury or hospitalization. The doctor may need to assure the patient that activity is safe and necessary, especially if the patient or a close friend or relative had a fractured hip treated with prolonged rest and immobilization.

Before the fracture is surgically nailed, the patient may be placed in either straight traction (Buck's extension) or Russell traction to relieve muscle spasm and prevent or reduce displacement of the fragments. If there is no displacement or spasm, only minimal immobilization may be required. This can be achieved by placing a folded blanket under the extremity from buttocks to below the knee, a pad above the heel, a support for the foot such as a padded box, a bolster, or a pillow, and a soft roll under the greater trochanter of the femur to hold the extremity in neutral rotation. If neutral rotation cannot be achieved easily, it should not be forced. The patient may have, as many adults do, an outward rotation contracture. Patients with hip fractures, if not in Russell traction, may be turned safely onto the affected side. The bed serves as a splint for the extremity. However, the patient will need to be assured of this. Turning him slowly and gently without force or discomfort will usually establish his confidence. The person should be turned in this manner not only for back care and linen change, but also for placing the bedpan. A flat (fracture) pan should be used if available. In any case, pillows should be placed above the pan to support the upper trunk and head, and below the pan to support the thighs. The patient should be rolled back onto the pan, taking care to support the fractured extremity during turning and when the position on the pan is assumed. To remove the pan, the patient should be turned again onto the fractured hip.

When Buck's extension is used prior to reduction of the fracture, care must be taken to maintain the traction at all times. The weights should hang free of the bed and should not be removed without the permission of the doctor. Friction of the heel on the bed can be prevented by placing a pad about two inches thick the full length of the extremity from gluteal fold to the ankle joint. A trochanter roll should be placed to prevent extreme outward rotation at the hip. The same procedure for placing the bedpan as already described may be used safely when Buck's extension has been applied. Some physicians will permit

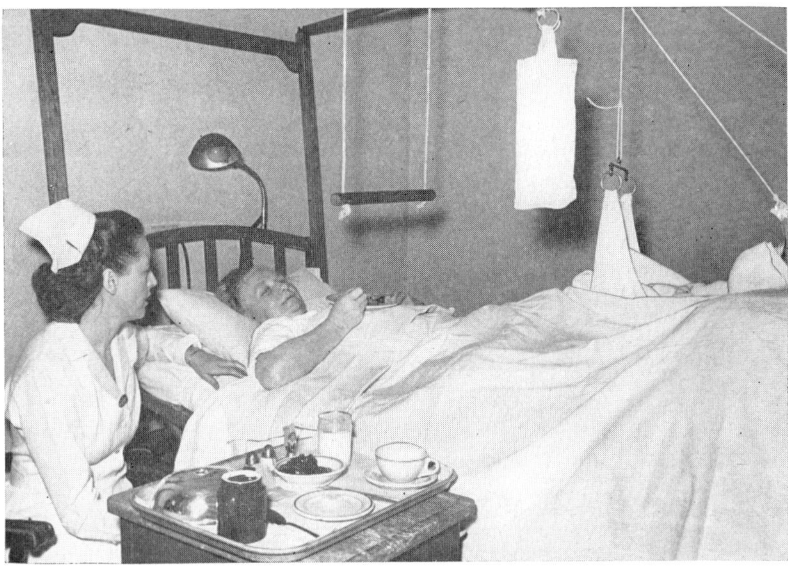

Figure 38. This patient requires only a small amount of assistance with her meals and enjoys the independence that feeding herself gives. (Courtesy American Journal of Nursing; photograph by Julius Huisgen.)

patients in traction to have the head of the bed elevated slightly for meals and to facilitate use of the bedpan.

Russell traction may be used before the hip is surgically nailed. If this is so, the nurse can teach the patient how to hold onto the trapeze and lift himself enough to take weight off the base of the spine for a few moments or for placement of the bedpan. Elevating the head of the bed slightly will make it easier for him to reach and use the trapeze. The patient who has been told that he has a hip fracture may be afraid to move for fear of causing pain or increasing the damage. The nurse should remain with him until he is confident in reaching for the trapeze and understands which type of activity and motion is safe. Free movement and use of all uninvolved extremities should be encouraged to maintain muscle tone, strength, and circulation. Even while in traction the patient can be taught exercises that will prepare him for using a walker or crutches.

The body may be turned only slightly in either direction for care of the back. Therefore, the nurse should give particular attention to frequent massage and the maintenance of a dry, smooth, clean bed to prevent pressure sores from developing. The patient can be instructed and encouraged to raise his body slightly from the bed every hour or oftener. Although only slight change of weight distribution may occur, even short duration of relief from pressure will permit circulation of blood to the tissues and reduce the likelihood of occurrence of pressure sores. Movement of the noninvolved extremities for useful activities or for exercise to maintain muscle tone and circulation should be encouraged. Many elderly persons, especially those of advanced years, tend to remain very still in bed. This may be due to preexisting muscle rigidity that is

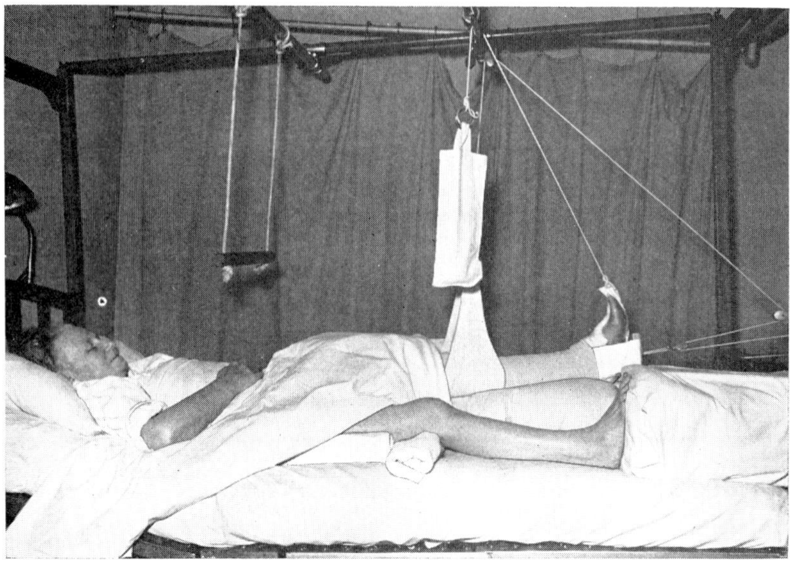

Figure 39. This patient is in Russell traction. Note the trapeze that enables her to change her position, the device to prevent foot drop on the affected side, and the good alignment of the unaffected extremity. (Courtesy American Journal of Nursing; photograph by Julius Huisgen.)

normal for the individual or to fear of pain or displacement of the fracture. Old persons can rarely be expected to assume full responsibility for activity, exercise, or the maintenance of changes of position.

Although patients may be in traction for only a few days prior to surgical fixation of a hip fracture, nursing responsibilities related to the application of traction and care of the patient in traction as described in orthopedic nursing texts should be meticulously observed. Nurses caring for an elderly person in a cast should review recent nursing texts on orthopedic nursing.[7] Although rarely used today, occasionally a patient may be placed in a hip spica cast, a well-leg splint, or other cast for treatment of a fractured hip.

The patient must be prepared for fairly early mobilization following fracture of the neck of the femur. He may be both frightened and encouraged by the news that he will in a day or two begin to exercise his affected extremity, to sit in a chair, stand in a walker, use crutches, and prepare to go home. Each step must be explained carefully, and adequate competent nursing supervision is necessary in order that the patient does not stumble, lose his balance, or injure himself when each new activity is attempted. The patient may be confined to a chair for eight to twelve weeks and then progress to a walker and then to crutches and a cane in three to six months following the accident. But for many whose physical and mental condition permits, the progression to ambulation in a walker or crutches with bearing weight on the affected extremity may begin within a few weeks.

Early mobilization is often considered essential from the standpoint of prevention of cardiovascular, urinary, and other complications. It must be borne in mind, however, that the elderly person has decreased elasticity of muscles and connective tissue. Too vigorous activity may cause spasm and retard progress. Sometimes moving about in bed may be better for the patient than getting into a chair or on crutches too early.

The extent of the patient's activity should be discussed with the physician. If permission for sitting up for meals and using the commode at the bedside for elimination can be obtained it has been found that older persons eat better and maintain regular habits of elimination more successfully. This is true not only for the mentally alert and responsible person, but even more so for those who are confused. Assisting an alert, physically able person from the bed to a chair or commode and back presents few problems, especially if the bed is chair

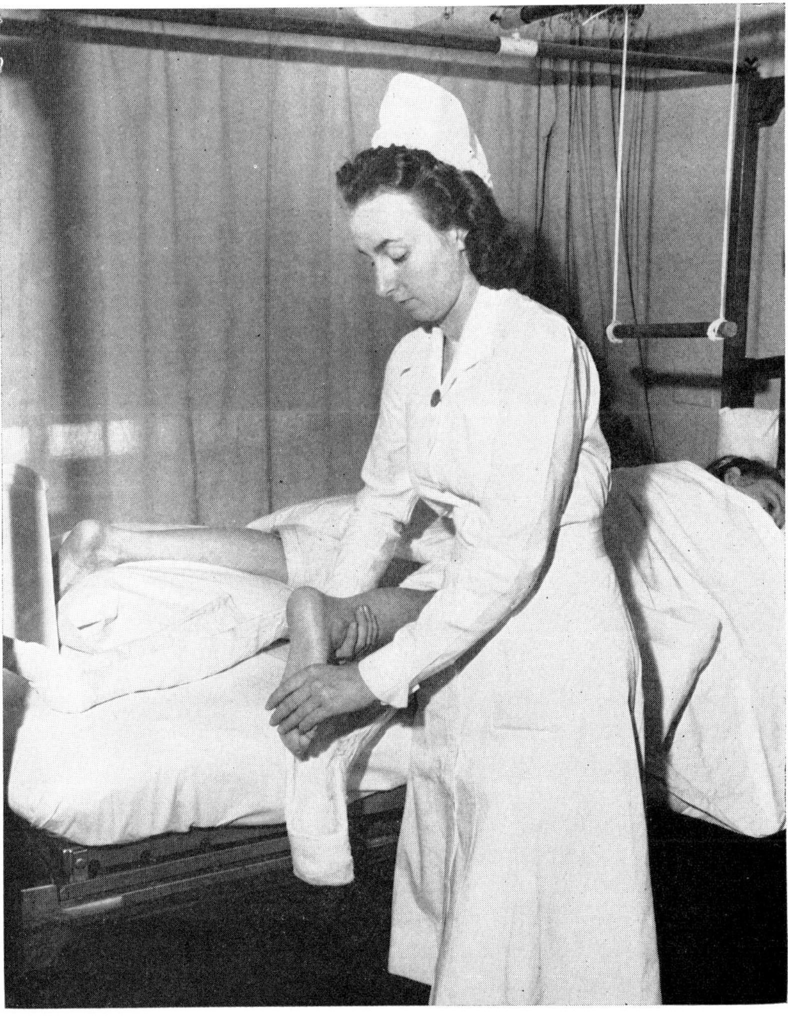

Figure 40. Casts may be bivalved to permit removal of the limb for passive exercise and movement through range of joint motion.

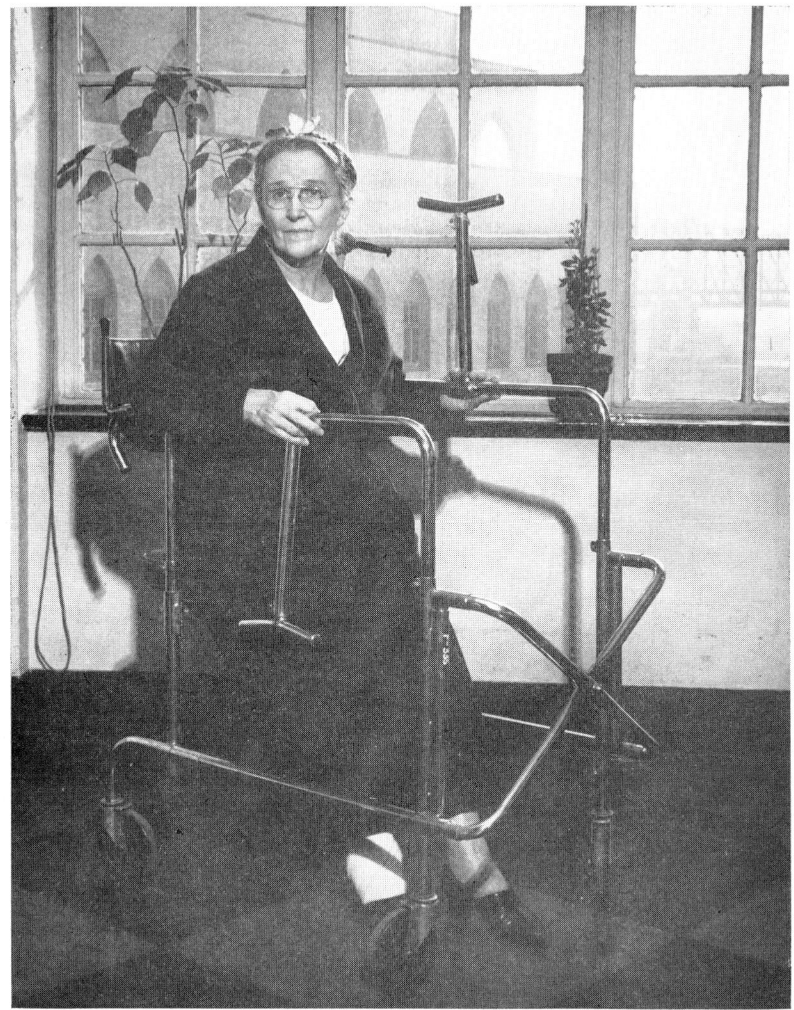

Figure 41. This patient, recovering from a fracture of the femur, uses a walker before progressing to crutches. Note her security; she is using the drop seat for a rest period.

height. Whenever possible the bed should be lowered to standard bed or chair height, whether in the hospital, nursing home, or the patient's own home. Until weight bearing is permitted, it is helpful to have the patient wear a shoe only on the uninvolved or weight-bearing extremity. A warm sock, felt slipper, or boot on the affected side will help to remind the patient that he is not to place weight on this foot. The less alert or somewhat confused person will need to be reminded each time he stands that he is not to bear weight on the affected side. If a person cannot be prevented from weight bearing he should be lifted or assisted to transfer to the chair using a sliding board or other device rather than be left in bed.

When helping a person with a fractured hip to move to the side of the bed and come to a sitting position, it is well to direct him to turn onto his affected hip, flex his hips and knees to a right angle, extend his heels over the side of the bed, and push himself sidewise to a sitting position. The chair or commode to which he will transfer should be placed at his unaffected side to enable him to pivot on the weight-bearing extremity and so reduce the tendency to use the affected one. Before he returns to bed the chair should be moved so that the bed is in the same relation to the chair.

When getting patients out of bed, it is extremely important to see that they are adequately clothed. Most elderly persons are extremely modest and will resist any activity that threatens bodily exposure even to a well-known and well-liked nurse or attendant. Consideration of this fact is just as important when turning the patient in bed, assisting with bed exercises, bath, or other activities even when they are carried out behind closed doors or drawn curtains.

In addition to verifying specific written orders from the physician for activities, the nurse should record on the nursing care plan any particular choices of method or physical limitations of individual patients such as a stiff shoulder that are cause for special changes in helping him with any activity. This assures transfer of essential information from one nurse to another and consistency in care of the patient.

Regardless of the method of fixation of fractures or the rate of mobilization out of bed, the nurse must remember that the patient in bed must move about frequently. The rule should be to turn him or help him to turn every few hours. Some effective method of checking this should be adopted, such as listing on the treatment card. Many hospitals have special assignments for nurses during the afternoon, evening, and night hours that consist of turning or helping patients turn at hourly intervals. This is a most important function that should never be delegated solely to practical nurses or orderlies until they have demonstrated their skill and reliability. The prime responsibility rests with the nurse, even though the patient can be taught the need for frequent moving and can take some responsibility for his activity. The extremely old patient is likely to doze the day away more or less, and his personal reports on how much he has moved may be inaccurate. Deep breathing and coughing at regular intervals should be taught, but must be checked upon also.

The doctor decides when and for how long the patient is to be out of bed. It then becomes the responsibility of the nurse to be certain that he is up regularly and for the desired length of time. It is often much easier to let the patient lie in bed, to bring him a bedpan, and to otherwise wait on him than to see that he is suitably clothed and appropriately assisted in getting up and about. Sometimes he may not want to get up, may wish to be up too long, may prefer to wander about during the night, or may rebel against assistance offered. The patient often needs tactful handling, and the thoughtful nurse will assume personal responsibility for supervising his needs and will not delegate it to unskilled or untrained workers.

Skin care is extremely important in the care of patients with fractures. The delicate skin of the elderly breaks down easily, and healing is slow and often impossible. Prevention is the best cure. Change of position is again essential, and frequent light massage over bony prominences should be listed as a regular nursing function. The patient is often awkward in handling the bedpan; he adjusts to this unpleasant necessity with difficulty; and he is sensitive to the least sign of impatience on the part of the nurse or the attendant. He may lie in a soiled bed rather than let anyone know that an accident has occurred. Any incontinence or accident with the bedpan must be cared for immediately, the skin should be sponged and dried gently, and the bed linen should be changed. Soft, fresh linen should be used. Occasionally a Foley or indwelling catheter may be used for the extremely old woman patient who is troubled with incontinence and whose skin threatens to break down as a result of being constantly wet.

Pressure on any area must be prevented. Though frequent change of position is the most important factor in alleviation of pressure, support to take pressure off bony prominences should be used. Use of cotton "doughnuts" is usually unfortunate. They become wadded and hard and are difficult to keep in place when the patient moves, and the adhesive often needed to keep them in place is irritating to the skin. Good results may often be obtained from placing a piece of rubber sponge under the ankle, heel, sacrum, elbow, or other bony prominence. A water or air mattress is also a valuable adjunct to care of the patient with a fracture; the air mattress is probably preferable since the motion in the water mattress is disturbing to some patients.

Untreated sheepskin with the wool still in place is excellent in prevention of pressure areas. The wool adds buoyancy, and it is believed that the lanolin in the wool is also protective. It is well to cut two pieces of the sheepskin of sufficient size to be used alternately. When soiling has occurred, the sheepskin can be washed in a mild soap and should be worked a little before drying is complete. Sheepskin is particularly useful for the very thin person with dry skin. A synthetic product that has resilience similar to that of sheepskin is now available.

Attention to nutrition is important. The aged person often eats slowly and should not be made to feel that his slowness is interfering with hospital or household routine. Often, in the position his fracture forces him to assume, he finds that it is just too much bother to try to eat. He should be encouraged to feed himself, even when he cannot sit up for meals. Assistance should be given when necessary. Fluid intake and urinary output should be noted carefully by the nurse. Adequate nutrition, fluid intake, activities, and use of the commode should prevent fecal impactions from occurring. Occasionally, when the patient is very inactive, the surgeon requests that the patient receive an oil retention enema weekly.

Contractures develop more quickly in older people than in the young. Joint stiffness and muscular weakness appear with alarming speed and persist to hamper the progress and rehabilitation of the patient after the fracture has healed. Bed posture is important. Pillows must be arranged behind the back so that forward bending of the cervical spine is not increased and the chest is held forward, which enables the vital capacity to remain as normal as possible. Care must be taken that external rotation of the hip does not occur, that hyperextension of the knees is not permitted, and that contracture at the shoulder joint is not allowed to develop. Limitation of abduction and extension of the shoulder can occur quite easily in the older person who remains in bed day after day with the head of the bed elevated. Contracture at the hip is a common difficulty presented when the patient begins to walk. This must be prevented. The patient who cannot be turned over on the abdomen should lie for a period of time each day with the bed flat and without a pillow under his head. The nurse nowadays is well aware of the danger of contracture of the knees when large, soft pillows are used beneath the knee and of other potential deformities, though she may have to explain the disadvantages to the patient. The drop-foot position may become fixed and still occurs with dismaying frequency in many hospitals and homes. Elaborate equipment is not necessary, but a firm foot support should be provided against which the patient may push when in the dorsirecumbent position. A cardboard box covered with a sheet serves the purpose very nicely. A foot support supplies the added advantage of keeping covers from pressing against the patient's feet. Cradles are less satisfactory if they tend to limit freedom of movement, and many aged patients complain that chilling from drafts accompanies their use. The nurse must remember that no position, no matter how correct, should be maintained for an extended period. The position must be changed frequently if contractures are to be prevented.

All joints should be put through complete range of motion at least twice daily if there is no joint pathology. This is preferably done actively and can in part be accomplished when the bath is being given. The nurse must herself have adequate knowledge of the normal range of joint motion as illustrated in basic nursing texts. Regular exercises to help in maintaining muscle tone are taught and must be supervised by the nurse. Checking from time to time to be certain that regular prescribed exercises of noninvolved parts of the body are being performed is an essential nursing responsibility. If a physical therapist is teaching and supervising therapeutic exercises and ambulation, the nurse should keep her informed about the patient's general condition. She should discuss the nursing follow-up of the therapeutic exercises as well as the physical nursing measures being carried out for general conditioning of the body. These measures are discussed in Chapter 11, Rehabilitation. If there is a department of physical medicine in the hospital, the nurse may obtain assistance from the physical therapist in checking the effectiveness of exercises as demonstrated by the patient.

Many elderly patients leave the hospital before the fracture has healed completely. The nurse has a responsibility to teach the patient and his family members about care at home. For example, the doctor usually wishes the patient who has a hip fracture to use a bedboard under his mattress and to follow a regular exercise regimen in preparation for weight bearing. The public health nurse prepared in orthopedic nursing can often be very helpful in giving practical suggestions in the home about keeping safe balance and using the limb effectively when the patient goes through the somewhat fearful stages from crutches to cane and in turn to independent walking.

Keeping occupied is tremendously important to the progress and well-being of the aged orthopedic patient. For women, knitting and crocheting are popular since they do not tax the eyesight of experienced workers, and patients derive pleasure from seeing something attractive that they have created. Other examples of useful and satisfying activities are making Christmas cards and dressing dolls.

These may be sold, used in the home, or given away to compensate for minor obligations that are worrying the patient. Making anything that can be sold or used gives them a feeling of security and accomplishment. Needed things that can be done about the ward also yield genuine satisfaction.

The alert nurse will devise occupations that help to preserve joint motion. For example, she may arrange a mirror and help her patient to a position in which she herself can curl and arrange her hair. This activity gives shoulder exercise and yields the psychologic benefit of improving appearance. The use of an electric sewing machine, the patient activating the control with the foot on the affected side, is good exercise for the ankle joint.

In caring for the aged person with an orthopedic disability, the nurse must have constantly in mind not only his present comfort, but also his future comfort. She must think of helping him in every way to return as a self-sufficient, self-respecting member of society. From the first day of his illness, this must be borne in mind, and functional activities that will minimize any feeling of helplessness and dependence must be devised. In the home, the nurse can make many helpful suggestions as to how household facilities may be adapted to individual limitations. The public health nurse should visit the home before the patient leaves the hospital so that plans can be made with his family to avoid feelings of helplessness and frustration when he first returns home. He may, for instance, need assistance in learning to climb stairs, in getting in and out of the bathtub, and in sitting comfortably in his favorite chair. For persons who do not have suitable homes to which they can go, there is need for more and better nursing homes to provide convalescent and long-term chronic care.

REFERENCES AND RELATED BIBLIOGRAPHY

1. Beck, E. D.: General principles of fracture management in the aged, Surg. Gynec. & Obst. **106**:343-346, 1958.
2. Committee of the American Rheumatism Association: Primer on the rheumatic diseases, New York, 1964, The Arthritis Foundation.
3. Hollander, Joseph Lee, and others: Arthritis and allied conditions, ed. 6, Philadelphia, 1960, Lea & Febiger.
4. Larsen, Loren J., Schoettstaedt, Edwin R., and Abbott, LeRoy C.: Diseases of the bones. In Stieglitz, Edward J. (editor): Geriatric medicine, ed. 3, Philadelphia, 1954, J. B. Lippincott Co.
5. Larson, Carroll B.: The wearing-out of joints, J. Am. Geriatrics Soc. **11**:558-566, 1962.
6. Larson, Carroll B., and Gould, Marjorie L.: Fractures of the hip and nursing care of the patient with a fractured hip, Amer. J. Nurs. **58**:1558-1563, 1958.
7. Larson, Carroll B., and Gould, Marjorie L.: Calderwood's orthopedic nursing, ed. 6, St. Louis, 1965, The C. V. Mosby Co.
8. Mayo, Richard A., and Hughes, Joanne M.: Intramedullary nailing of long bone fractures and nursing care after intramedullary nailing, Amer. J. Nurs. **59**:236-240, 1959.
9. Peszczynski, Mieczyslaw: Why old people fall, Amer. J. Nurs. **65**:86-88, 1965.
10. Robin, Gordon C., Bar-Maor, A., and Weinberg, H.: Morbidity and mortality rates for internal fixation of femoral neck fractures, J. Am. Geriatrics Soc. **11**:560-569, 1963.
11. Rudd, J. L.: A better method for cervical traction in the aged orthopedic patient, J. Am. Geriatrics Soc. **11**:283-286, 1963.
12. Sister Mary Francis: Nursing the patient with internal hip fixation, Amer. J. Nurs. **64**: 111-112, 1964.
13. Solomon, Walter M.: Diseases of the joints. In Stieglitz, Edward J. (editor): Geriatric medicine, ed. 3, Philadelphia, 1954, J. B. Lippincott Co.

Chapter 19

Nursing in disease of the gastrointestinal system

In older persons, the entire gastrointestinal tract undergoes atrophic changes that may interfere with the efficiency of its function. On the whole, though, it has been shown that if an older person eats the right foods in the right combination, the gastrointestinal tract can carry on its functions quite effectively. A few disease conditions such as hiatus hernia, diverticulosis of the large bowel, inguinal and femoral hernias, and prolapse of the rectum may be caused in part by the loss of tone of supportive structures as age advances. Treatment for these conditions usually is conservative, with surgical intervention undertaken only when symptoms become pronounced.

Mesenteric vascular occlusion occurs fairly often in the aged person who has extensive arteriosclerosis, and in this condition the blood supply to a portion of the bowel is cut off and necrosis follows quickly. Disease of the gallbladder with cholelithiasis and its complications occur frequently, and the incidence of cancer throughout the gastrointestinal tract is higher. The treatment for these conditions is usually operative, and the problems encountered in extensive surgery of the elderly are discussed in Chapter 13, Anesthesia and Operative Care.

General hygiene that should help to maintain the gastrointestinal system functioning at maximum efficiency into old age is discussed in Chapter 6. Included in that chapter also are a few of the common problems that trouble elderly people, such as care of dentures, general appetite, and constipation. In this chapter only a few disease conditions occurring frequently will be discussed briefly and their nursing care described.

DISEASE OF THE MOUTH

Older people are likely to have poor mouth hygiene, due in part to lack of necessary and regular cleaning of the mouth and teeth, to irritation from broken or decayed teeth, to achlorhydria and gastritis, to atrophic changes in mouth structures, and to other causes; nutritional deficiency is fairly common and may cause symptoms. Some older people seem either to become used to an unclean and uncomfortable mouth or to lose their sensitivity to minor irritations in the mouth. The result may be that lesions develop and are ignored by the patient for months, during which extensive growth of malignant cells may then have occurred. The older person is inclined to think that any unusual sore in the mouth is a canker sore and that it will clear up within a few days. Often he is unable to tell when he first noticed the lesion, as each succeeding day he hoped it would disappear. It is true that many irritating lesions of the oral cavity are the result of causes other than cancer. It is important in all health teaching, however, to emphasize that lesions in the mouth or on the lip that do not disappear completely within a few days (at the most two weeks) should be referred to a physician for investigation as to their cause. Regular visits to dentists by older patients would result in detection of many oral lesions that are left to develop into advanced malignancies.

Many malignant lesions of the lips and mouth appear where there has been persistent irritation or trauma. Carcinoma of the lip is most likely to occur on the lower lip of pipe smokers where the warm stem of the pipe rests; irritation from a broken or jagged tooth may cause malignancy on the inside of the lip. Malignancies occur anywhere within the mouth and are often present on the gum surface where a dental prosthesis has caused irritation or pressure, on the inner surface of the cheek particularly if this has been traumatized at intervals by the patient's bite, on the tongue particularly the part that may rest next to a jagged tooth, and on the floor of the mouth. Lesions on the posterior pharynx, about the base of the tongue, and on the floor of the mouth are often highly malignant and metastasize at an early stage. Sometimes the first sign of such a lesion is a swelling of the neck seen on the outside.

Pain is not an early characteristic of malignancies of the mouth. The lesions are often slightly raised ulcers with a definitely raised edge and may be sore upon pressure or disturbance and may bleed easily. The nurse must never take the responsibility of determining whether a lesion may be cancer, but must refer all patients with any persistent lesion to a physician.

Leukoplakia is a condition of the mouth that occurs most often in older patients. Elevated flat white patches appear on the mucous membrane, may be scattered or diffuse, and vary a great deal in size. Since leukoplakia is considered a precancerous lesion, surgical excision is the treatment of choice if the areas are not too large. If they are quite extensive, surgery may not be possible, and radiation must be resorted to. The lesions of leukoplakia may be extremely painful, and their successful treatment is exceedingly difficult.

Treatment of malignant lesions of the lip and mouth depends upon the extent of the lesion, the age and condition of the patient, and the nature of the lesion. Tremendous variation in the necessary treatment exists. Small lesions, for example, may be successfully treated by radiation therapy alone; others in which control of metastasis is attempted may include a removal of the affected area, as well as dissection of the lymph nodes of the neck. Operative treatment usually is either preceded or followed by radiation therapy.

General nursing for oral surgery

Because the nursing care for patients having extensive surgical treatment for conditions such as cancer of the mouth and throat are discussed fully in texts on medical and surgical nursing,[19] only a few aspects that have to be watched particularly carefully when caring for the aged patient are included here.

Preoperative care. It is imperative that the patient develop confidence in the nursing staff before surgery is done. Many questions arise and these must be answered and often repeated for the patient. It is best if he has the same nurse or group of nurses caring for him before the operation and when he returns from the recovery unit to his own room. He must be assured that he will not be left alone for some time following surgery. He should be told that speech may be difficult, painful, or impossible for a few days after surgery and that he will have to write or otherwise indicate his needs. The nurse must get to know the patient and give instructions accordingly. For example, some patients may benefit a great deal from learning names of equipment, even designating a few signs indicating needs, such as the desire to be moved, while others may become upset at discussion of the situation where speech for them may be impossible. If the patient is deaf, has a tremor that makes writing difficult, or has other physical problems, this should be considered in preparing him preoperatively for the circumstances he will likely encounter postoperatively.

Mouth hygiene is important before surgery is done, and in many hospitals a dental hygienist is called upon when such attention is necessary. Local preparation usually consists of mouth irrigations with saline solution every two hours for a period of two days preoperatively. If mouth infection is evident, sodium perborate, compound sodium borate solution (Dobell's solution), or potassium permanganate solution 1:10,000 may be ordered as frequent irrigations, and antibiotics may be given. The nurse should be certain that irrigations are given thoroughly since many older patients may perform an irrigation quite superficially unless they are carefully instructed.

Elderly patients are particularly susceptible to infection, and the postoperative mortality from this complication following major surgery is substantially above that of younger patients. Care must be taken to wash the hands thoroughly before any treatment and to use only equipment that has been sterilized in order that infection may not be introduced into the mouth.

If a lesion in the mouth is so advanced that there is pain, bleeding, and drainage, nutrition may be impaired and may need attention before surgery is performed. If extensive surgery is contemplated, such as a radical neck dissection, the most careful attention is paid to nutritional status and to blood protein level and blood volume, as well as to the more routine determinations such as hemoglobin. Liquid foods may be given preoperatively (and postoperatively) by means of a nasogastric tube that bypasses a lesion in the mouth. In some instances a gastrostomy is done preoperatively to assure the introduction of food into the stomach.

Postoperative care. Immediately after surgery the patient usually is placed well on his side with face turned downward so that drainage from the throat and mouth is facilitated. The nurse should check with the doctor if no specific instructions for position have been written. Pneumonia caused by the aspiration of mucus or foreign material is one of the most common and most disastrous complications of extensive mouth and neck surgery, and inadequate pulmonary ventilation is a frequent problem in the operative and postoperative treatment of the elderly. If the same position must be assumed for several hours, the nurse should attempt to support body parts to avoid strain and discomfort. Moving limbs that can be disturbed through range-of-joint motion and shifting body weight and position, if only very slightly, at frequent intervals helps a great deal to allay discomforts such as backache that many older patients report are worse than the operation.

Many older patients have a cough, which may be due to a chronic chest disease, to the prolonged use of tobacco, or to an acquired habit of coughing. When surgery of the mouth has been done, severe coughing may cause pain and seriously disturb healing tissues. It is sometimes necessary to give codeine sulfate for a cough, and, when this is done, it is imperative that the patient be turned at frequent intervals and assisted in coughing *occasionally* in order that congestion of the lungs does not develop. The patient must be urged to take deep breaths and to cough at hourly intervals. Pain and apprehension may be alleviated if the nurse places one hand at the back at the patient's neck and the other firmly on the dressings as he coughs.

DISEASE OF THE ESOPHAGUS, STOMACH, INTESTINE, AND RELATED ORGANS

General nursing care

One of the major problems in the diagnosis and treatment of elderly patients with disease of the gastrointestinal system is that symptoms frequently are atypical and misleading. Pain may not be pronounced even when disease is far advanced, while other symptoms may be absent entirely. One study, for example, showed that more than half of a group of elderly patients having malignant lesions of the lower bowel had no signs or symptoms. Yet most of these lesions could be seen when a sigmoidoscopy was done. The nurse should encourage all elderly people to have physical examinations at regular intervals and to follow the physician's suggestions for special tests, roentgen studies, or examinations such as gastroscopy or sigmoidoscopy.

Special examinations to detect disease of the gastrointestinal tract include barium swallow and examination under a fluoroscope, esophagoscopy, gastroscopy, gastric analysis, gastrointestinal series of roentgenograms, barium enemas, and cholecystograms; also sigmoidoscopy, proctoscopy, and anoscopy. Essentially the preparation and nursing care needed is the same as described in medical and surgical nursing texts for all patients. A few aspects need special emphasis, however. Tests and the preparation for them must be explained to the patient, and often this explanation must be repeated. The ambulatory patient may be bewildered by the haste and activity in a clinic and may not remember instructions given. It is best to have instructions written for the patient, and then the nurse should sit down with the patient in a quiet room and go over the instructions with him. He may not, for example, realize that "nothing by mouth" before a test means he should not take water. He may not have equipment or sufficient knowledge to give himself enemas, and it may be necessary to have a public health nurse give him assistance. Often a relative or a friend accompanying the patient needs to know the preparation that is necessary.

Food must be withheld for most of the tests and examinations of the gastrointestinal system. This presents a problem in caring for the elderly patient. Older people do not tolerate going without food for long intervals. They may develop tremor, weakness, and faintness, all of which predisposes them to anxiety and to accidents. Repeated enemas are tiring to the elderly patient and they remove electrolytes and fluids. Most physicians now believe that enemas should not be repeated more than once, and preparations such as "Fleet's enema" are prescribed widely, since they are easy for the patient to use and usually produce good results with a minimum of fatigue and exhaustion. Bisacodyl (Dulcolax) suppositories have been found quite effective also.

If the patient is ambulatory it is best for another person to accompany him to the clinic, laboratory, x-ray department, or other location where the procedure is to be done. In the outpatient clinic or in the hospital, the nurse should do all she can to expedite the carrying out of the procedure as scheduled, and she should encourage the patient to take some food as soon as is permissible. In the clinic the patient should rest a little while before walking, and the hospitalized patient should remain in bed until after he has had food. The nurse should observe the elderly patient very carefully while procedures are being done and for a time thereafter. If the patient appears weak, or becomes dizzy or faint he should lie down at once.

Positions that must be assumed for some tests and examinations are uncomfortable at best. The dorsirecumbent position with hyperextension of the neck that is required for esophagoscopy is almost intolerable for some elderly patients with limitation of motion from arthritis of the spine. The nurse should note any limitation of free movement and question the patient if joint stiffness is suspected. She should explain the necessary position to the patient and have everything in readiness so that anxious and uncomfortable waiting is avoided. Sometimes small pillows used to support such contours as the lumbar curve can be used to add to the comfort of the patient. If the patient has real difficulty in assuming a position such as the knee-chest position for a proctoscopic examination, the doctor should be consulted since this examination can be done with the patient in a more comfortable position (Sims position). Sometimes it is helpful if the nurse reminds the patient to mention his limitations to the x-ray technician, who may be proceeding with a busy schedule and may not think of the patient's possible difficulty in free movement.

Some positions for examination such as the knee-chest position alter circulation to the extent that the elderly patient may become dizzy and faint. He should never be left unattended on the examining table during or after the examination and should be assisted most carefully from the table to a chair where he should rest for a few minutes before moving about.

Throughout the gastrointestinal tract the mucous membrane may be thinner in the elderly patient. This makes it easier for trauma and even perforation to be sustained when instruments must be passed for diagnostic purposes. Perforation is most likely to occur when stricture or other anomaly such as the presence of a tumor are found. Trauma is less likely to occur when the patient is relaxed and unafraid. Complete explanation of what will be experienced and constant thoughtful attention during the procedure help to allay apprehension and enable the patient to relax more fully. Care must be taken also that medication ordered for their sedative and relaxing effect are given as prescribed, so that the patient may receive their full benefit. Symptoms of perforation of the esophagus, stomach, or bowel are pain that may come on suddenly and be severe, and shock. The treatment for this rare complication is operation as soon as is possible.

The care of the elderly patient who must have an extensive operation performed is discussed in Chapter 13. If the patient must have a permanent gastrostomy, jejunostomy, ileostomy or colostomy, the care he needs will not differ materially from that of younger patients with these conditions, as discussed fully in current medical and surgical nursing texts.[19] The elderly patient, however, who has any of these operations may be expected to progress more slowly toward self-care than the younger patient. His general response and overall recovery from major surgery is slower than the younger person and he may be discouraged easily. He needs a great deal of kindly, thoughtful attention and encouragement as he progresses in each small step of his care, such as preparing his own meals to be taken by gastrostomy tube, administering his fluid meals, or caring for a jejunostomy.

Long-term health care and supervision of the elderly patient who has an operative procedure like a gastrostomy may lead to particular difficulties. This is because he may live alone or with another person who may also be old and unable to assume responsibility for his care. The nurse in the hospital should attempt to learn all she can about the patient and the human, as well as the economic, resources he has available to him when he leaves the hospital. She can suggest to the patient or to his doctor that the patient needs contact with the medical social worker to help him plan for the time when he leaves the hospital. If she is to assume responsibility for assistance with nursing care and general health supervision in the home, the public health nurse in the community should visit the patient in the hospital before he leaves.

Disease conditions

Hiatus hernia (diaphragmatic hernia). There are several types of hiatal hernias, but the most common is the *sliding hiatus hernia,* which occurs at the normal hiatus where the esophagus passes through the diaphragm (see Figure 42). Normally, there is a small amount of motion or moving up and down, but the hernia develops when muscle weakness and increased abdominal pressure cause the tissue around the hiatus to become incompetent. It is suspected that the primary cause may be a congenital weakness of the muscles surrounding the hiatus. This condition, in which a portion of the caria of the stomach becomes displaced upward through the diaphragm hiatus, is now known to be one of the most common pathologic conditions of the gastrointestinal tract. Most cases occur after the age of 50, although it is suspected that many people have the condition in a mild degree but have no symptoms in their early years. The patient may recall that for years he has had a tendency to have heartburn or

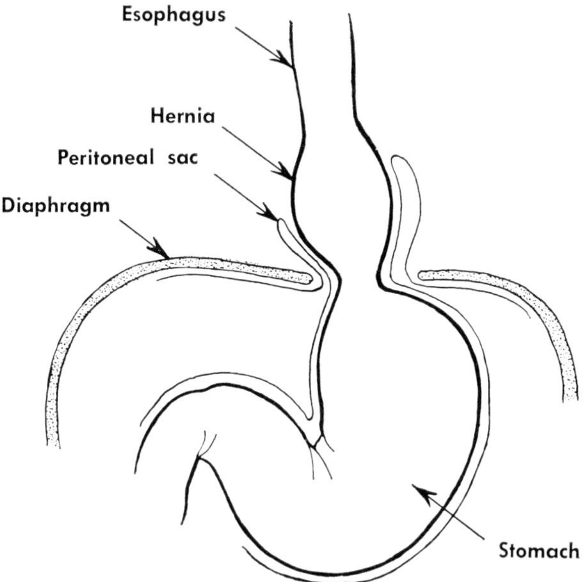

Figure 42. Schematic drawing to show displacement of a portion of the cardia of the stomach through the normal hiatus into the thoracic cavity in a sliding hiatus hernia.

even to regurgitate small amounts of food, particularly when bending sharply forward after meals. He may have heartburn and general discomfort after eating large meals or taking large amounts of fluids. Other symptoms resemble those of peptic ulcer or of some cardiac disease; occasionally, there is pain particularly on the left and sometimes radiating down the left arm as in anginal disease. Often the patient complains of a feeling of pressure over the left side of the diaphragm. If acid secretions from the stomach have seriously affected the mucous membrane lining of the esophagus, severe esophagitis with stricture, hemorrhage, or even perforation may occur.

The treatment for hiatus hernia depends upon the severity of the symptoms and the age and condition of the patient. Many patients respond very well to conservative treatment, which may include weight reduction, avoidance of increase in abdominal tension, and changes in eating patterns. The patient may be advised by his physician to avoid tight constrictive clothing about the trunk, which may increase abdominal tension, and to take a mild laxative to prevent straining at defecation if constipation is a problem. Usually the patient is advised to eat slowly, take fluids mainly between meals, avoid large meals, and remain in an upright position for two hours after eating. A rocking chair with footstool is ideal for the elderly person who tends to enjoy a brief nap after meals but who should not lie flat after eating if he has this ailment. Heartburn that awakens the patient during sleeping hours is sometimes the first noticeable sign of a hiatus hernia. If this occurs, the patient is advised to use several extra pillows when sleeping and to avoid large or late evening meals. If the patient has heartburn and discomfort, he may be placed on a peptic ulcer regimen by his physician, with frequent small meals containing milk and antacid drugs between meals. If symptoms persist despite careful adherance to conservative measures, an operation usually is performed in which the hernial opening is repaired.

Gastric atrophy, peptic ulcer, and cancer of the stomach. Gastric atrophy occurs occasionally and causes symptoms of general indigestion and discomfort. Often it is associated with achlorhydria and pernicious anemia. Upon gastroscopic examination the surface of the stomach wall appears hardened and flattened, so that function is impaired.

Peptic ulcer, or gastric ulcer, contrary to popular opinion, is not solely a disease of the young. It is estimated that one fourth to one half of all cases of this condition occur in those over 50 years of age.[4] Diagnosis and treatment are similar to those for younger age groups, except that operative intervention may be undertaken more often, because this condition may be difficult to distinguish from cancer of the stomach, which occurs most often in the older age group.

Carcinoma of the stomach is essentially a disease of later life, with 90 percent of all cases occurring in those over 50 years of age.[4] Carcinoma of the stomach has the extremely high mortality rate of between 93 and 95 percent within five years. This is because the extensive blood supply of the stomach often permits metastasis to occur before symptoms are noted. Early diagnosis and surgical removal of the affected portion of the stomach gives the only hope of cure. X-ray therapy is of limited value in treatment of malignant lesions of the stomach.

When partial or complete resection of the stomach is impossible, a gastroenterostomy or jejunostomy may be performed, depending upon the location of the lesion and the symptoms it is producing. If a total gastrectomy has been done, the jejunum is brought up and anastomosed with the esophagus. If the cardiac end of the stomach and the lower esophagus are both affected and the lesion is inoperable, a jejunostomy may be done.

Carcinoma of the esophagus. Carcinoma of the esophagus is rare before the age of 50 years. The incidence of this disease, which causes 2 percent of all deaths from cancer, is highest in the seventh and eighth decades of life. It occurs more frequently in men than women in the ratio of five to one. By far the most common symptom is difficulty in swallowing. This may come on gradually and not be noticed by the patient for a time. When hoarseness, pain, and marked weight loss occur, metastasis has usually developed and the prospects for the patient are poor. The treatment is esophagectomy with wide excision of the affected portion of the esophagus. If possible, a portion of the stomach is brought up to meet the remaining esophagus. If this is not feasible a gastrostomy may be done, through which the patient can receive food. Because of the extensive surgery necessary and the frequency of metastases, the mortality from the complications of surgery and from the original condition are fairly high.

A gastrostomy is a new opening into the stomach. It is used for a patient with inoperable malignancy of the esophagus in order that food may be introduced into the stomach. There are several methods of performing a gastrostomy. The stomach may be sutured to a small incision in the abdominal wall, and an opening is then made into the stomach through which a catheter is passed and sutured. A flap of stomach can be used to form a tube which is then brought out to the abdominal wall. The advantage of this method is that the opening will

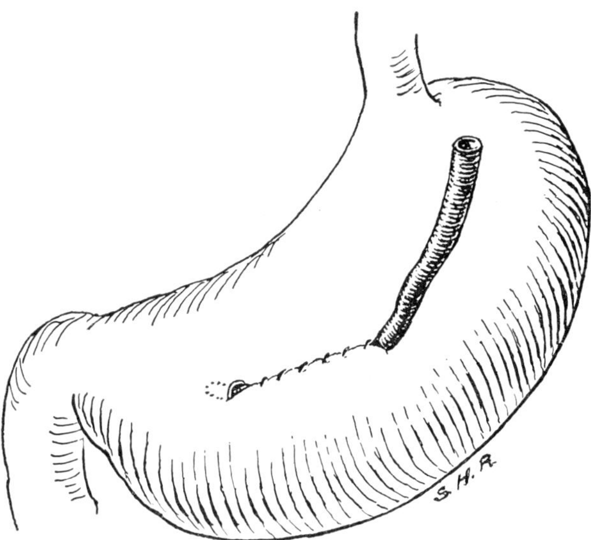

Figure 43. The Witzel procedure for gastrostomy. Note that the catheter lies in a tunnel made from the outer stomach wall.

not close if the catheter is removed between feedings. In another method, the Witzel procedure, the catheter is placed in the stomach from which it lies for a short distance in a tunnel made from the outer stomach wall before it opens through a stab wound in the abdominal wall. The advantage of these two methods is that gastric contents are less likely to be extruded to the outer surface where they produce a disagreeable odor and may cause irritation of the skin. Other methods are described in current nursing texts.[19]

The nurse needs knowledge of the anatomy and physiology of the stomach if she is to give skillful care to the patient following surgery. She needs to know what has been done at the time of operation and how it will affect normal processes. She will recall that the normal adult stomach holds from 1,000 to 1,500 ml. and that it empties in from fifteen minutes to four and one-half hours, depending upon the kind of food taken. Water, for example, remains in an otherwise empty stomach for only about ten minutes, whereas fatty fried foods may remain four and a half hours or even longer. These normal processes are altered by disease, and there are wide individual variations. Normally the stomach relaxes in anticipation of food when the wave of muscle action in the esophagus that is to carry the food to the stomach starts. Consequently, when swallowing does not precede the entrance of food into the stomach, relaxation may not occur, and a feeling of fullness and nausea may follow, particularly if feedings are given rapidly.

In brief, it should be recalled that the saliva contains ptyalin, which begins the digestion of starches, and the stomach secretes three products: mucin, hydrochloric acid, and gastric ferment. Hydrochloric acid soften protein foods in preparation for action upon them by gastric and intestinal digestive juices, inhibits bacterial growth, and stimulates the flow of pancreatic enzymes. The person who does not have the benefit of hydrochloric acid in the stomach is more likely to have bacterial growth in the stomach and upper intestine, which may contribute to formation of flatus and to diarrhea. The patient who has a jejunostomy may have diarrhea, which may be improved by eating sterile foods and by boiling equipment before use. Gastric ferment contains pepsin, which starts the breakdown of protein substances to simpler forms; rennin, which splits milk to curd and whey; and lipase, which is a weak fat-splitting enzyme. It is apparent that the patient who cannot swallow saliva or who has a gastrectomy suffers from definite handicaps in digestion. Some relatively normal people, however, have no gastric secretions and get along fairly well, though they fare best when simple and easily digested foods are eaten.

The surgeon decides the time at which food should be taken after a gastrostomy has been done. This may be the day of operation, or it may be a few days later, depending upon whether the stomach was opened at the time of surgery or whether it was attached to the abdominal wall and adhesions were permitted to form prior to making the opening into the stomach. Usually only 50 ml. of water are given at first. Feedings are gradually increased until the patient is taking six to eight daily, and the average amount of each feeding is about 400 ml. of food and 50 to 100 ml. of water, which is taken after the food. The amount varies with each individual and with the extent of the malignant lesion.

If the tube is left in the gastrostomy opening to prevent closure of the opening or for any other reason, it is important that the tube be clamped securely to prevent leakage of gastric contents. A rubber band is easily adjustable and effective for this purpose. The catheter should rest within a gauze dressing and not against the skin of the abdomen. If excoriation of the skin around the opening occurs, aluminum paste, codliver oil, or castor oil and zinc oxide ointment are often applied. Brewer's yeast has also been found to be helpful in protecting the skin from the injurious effects of gastric secretions. The powder or the cake can be used. A thin paste is made and spread fairly thickly on the skin around the opening. It is also helpful to place a dressing across the wound that will help draw the edges slightly closer. Sometimes, however, this may encourage closing of the new aperture. The gastrostomy opening is usually made through the rectus muscle, which should develop a sphincterlike action that will help to prevent the leakage of gastric contents.

Careful attention must be given to the mouth when a patient is fed through a gastrostomy tube. Before the gastrostomy is performed, he is often dehydrated and is likely to develop parotitis or other mouth infection. Saliva may be decreased during this time, but after surgery, when he is receiving adequate food, the saliva may increase. Many patients can swallow saliva even when they cannot swallow enough food to avoid starvation; in others the obstruction is complete. The constant accumulation of saliva is most annoying to a person who cannot swallow it, and inconspicuous provision for expectoration must be made. A soft towel that can be put under the face during sleep will lessen the patient's apprehension over the possibility of soiling the linen.

The nurse may be called upon to plan complete and acceptable meals for the patient and to help the family to do so when the patient returns home. Feeding the patient is not difficult. It does, however, demand imagination on the part of the nurse since she must be able to place herself in the position of the patient and anticipate what he would like to have. She must consider the cost of food and the time it takes family members to prepare foods. With the low cost and the large variety of strained and tasty baby foods now available, it seems unnecessary to give the patient large quantities of foods that may increase caloric intake but cause gastric distress and diarrhea, such as oil, cream, and other foods that human beings do not normally ingest in large quantities.

In most instances, foods should be as similar to those normally eaten as possible. The patient should be fed and not be given a treatment. He should sit up as he does for meals and not lie on his side as he might for a treatment. The tray should resemble a usual meal tray. It is psychologically harmful, many times, to assemble the requirement of food for the entire day and then divide the mixture into so many "feedings" for the day. The patient should see a glass of orange juice on his tray at breakfast. Often he can be taught to give his own feedings, and being able to do so before he leaves the hospital adds to his happiness and self-sufficiency when he returns to his family.

Meals should be given at regular times. The amount given may be altered to fit normal meals more closely. For example, a larger amount may be given at noon if the patient has been used to dinner at that time. Foods should be warmed to body temperature, but not overheated. Hot and cold foods are normally held in the mouth until they almost reach body temperature, and in addition food that is too hot or too cold for the sensitive tissues in the mouth will be almost automatically removed. Attractive small pitchers in which separate foods are placed on the tray add to the patient's appetite and increase the acceptability of tube feedings. Air should be removed from the tube before food is given, and food should flow slowly by gravity through the tube, though sometimes gentle pressure with the Asepto syringe is necessary.

No effort should be spared to give the patient what he likes and thinks he needs. Feedings for the elderly patient must take into consideration the food habits of a lifetime. With the assistance of a food blender (if it can be afforded) or similar equipment, it is possible to give the patient many foods. Often foods that are "easily digested" are not so much simple foods as those that the patient likes and thinks agree with him. If he has been used to having oatmeal for breakfast, then gruel should be substituted for some other cereal requirement that may be in the sample menu. Many physicians and nurses believe that the elderly patient should be allowed tea and coffee through a gastrostomy tube if he has been accustomed to their use and believes that they aid his digestion. One elderly man was having difficulty with nausea following his meals. He was very fond of tea and believed that if he could have it with his feedings his digestion would improve. Tea was given and the nausea improved. The effect may have been purely psychological, but, if so, it was equally important. The patient who has habitually taken a glass of sherry before dinner for the larger part of his life may benefit from being given this before his dinner meal.

Certain facts should be considered in preparing tube feedings for elderly people. Diarrhea occurs fairly often in persons who live on liquid foods. Diarrhea may be partially controlled by boiling fresh milk, by using canned milk instead of fresh milk, and by giving pectin. Plain pectin can be obtained in popular jelling products on the market such as Certo. A diet high in fat often is not well tolerated by the elderly person. It may cause nausea and loss of appetite and may contribute to diarrhea. It should also be remembered that the ingestion of fat slows both the motility of the stomach and the production of digestive secretions.[2] A diet high in carbohydrate may also contribute to diarrhea. Often if carbohydrate must be increased to raise total calories, pectin must be added to the diet to prevent diarrhea.

The day's requirements of food may be put together and divided into equal "feedings." This is necessary for short intervals in the hospital when the patient is being prepared for surgery and when detailed planning for him is impossible. Some elderly persons living alone and preparing their own food do not wish to be bothered with adapting their feedings to normal meals. They would rather mix a quantity of food once during the day and be done with it. Some families do not have the money or the time to use the equipment necessary in planning and preparing individual meals.

The following low-cost diet has been prepared for the patient with cancer who must be given tube feedings with as little time, effort, and equipment as possible. The protein content of this diet may seem high. It must be remembered that the patient has usually lost a great deal of body tissue. Estimated protein needs are based primarily on optimum weight and not on actual weight. One gram of protein per kilogram of body weight per day is the estimated need for maintenance of body tissue. The patient needs large amounts of additional protein if he is to rebuild lost tissue. The diet is also high in calcium, and it will be recalled that the older person requires larger amounts of calcium than the young adult since absorption and utilization of calcium seem to be less effective with age. Caloric value of this diet could be increased by the addition of cream if the patient could tolerate the extra fat. Protein might be reduced as the patient regained lost weight by reducing the number of eggs and the amount of milk. Dark corn syrup is cheaper than light, but light might be used if diarrhea is present. If no good refrigerator is available, the yeast would be put into a single feeding, since otherwise it might start fermentation of the mixture.

New York State Department of Health
*Suggested Low-Cost Gastrostomy Tube Feeding Formula**

This formula is designed for use in the home where there is no special equipment available and could be prepared with an ordinary eggbeater and sieve. It is not a palatable dish and is for tube feeding only.

The suggested formula is as follows:

1 can (3½ oz.) strained liver (baby food)
2½ cans (14 oz. cans) evaporated milk
4 eggs, beaten

*Reprinted with permission of the New York State Department of Health, Nutrition Bureau.

5 oz. canned or fresh orange juice
*2 oz. applesauce or 1 oz. Certo
1 teaspoon salt
1 cup dark corn syrup
4 oz. strained peas
†2 tablespoons dried brewer's yeast
4 drops fish liver oil concentrate (given in one feeding)

The volume totals 2 quarts, 4 ounces, including a cup of hot water for dissolving the corn syrup and ½ cup warm water in which the yeast is soaked.

It is suggested that the formula be divided into six feedings and refrigerated, to be warmed slightly before each feeding. About 100 ml. of water should be given after each feeding for fluids and to wash the tube.

Food Values of Formula

Calories	2,820
Protein	127 Gm.
Fat	109 Gm.
Calcium	3,067 Gm.
Iron	24.8 mg.
Vitamin A	11,840 I.U.
Thiamine	4.351 mg.
Riboflavin	7.682 mg.
Niacin	17.25 mg.
Ascorbic acid	83 mg.

Equipment

Tray
French catheter, size 16 or 18
Asepto syringe

Cleaning the equipment: Wash the catheter and Asepto syringe well with warm water and soap. Rinse well. Return to tray and cover with a towel after each feeding. Boil the catheter and Asepto syringe once daily.

With this excellent diet as a basis, possible modifications for a two-day period are given as illustrations of how modifications can be made so that the patient's meals resemble those of a normal person. These diets yield roughly between 80 and 90 grams of protein and approximately 2,700 calories. The normal basic caloric requirements are about 25 calories per kilogram of body weight; light to moderate activity increases this requirement by 50 to 75 percent. The patient whose normal weight is 60 kilograms would need 1,500 calories as his basic requirement and 750 to 1,025 additional calories for his activity, which thus makes his total caloric needs about 2,600 per day.

In the following diet, ¼ can of evaporated milk and ½ cup of water can be substituted throughout for the whole milk. It cannot be overemphasized that diet must be modified to suit the individual. In the following menus, effort has

*This ingredient is added to prevent diarrhea and must be adjusted to the individual.
†If considerable distention or diarrhea develops, substitute with equal amount of wheat or corn germ.

been made to place the richer foods during the earlier hours of the day, since most elderly people sleep better if a light evening meal is taken.

First day

Breakfast	½ glass orange juice 1 egg, 1 cup milk, 1 T. dried brewer's yeast 1 cup coffee, 2 T. corn syrup
10:00	eggnog (1 cup milk, 2 eggs, 2 T. corn syrup)
Dinner	1 can liver baby food, ¼ cup tomato juice, ½ cup water, 4 drops cod-liver oil concentrate, ½ tsp. salt 1 cup milk, 2 T. corn syrup
3:00	1 cup skim milk, 1 T. dried brewer's yeast, 2 T. corn syrup
Supper	cream soup (½ cup strained peas, 1 cup milk, ½ tsp. salt) 1 cup tea, lemon, 2 T. corn syrup
8:00	banana milk shake (one ripe banana, 1 cup skim milk, 1 small scoop ice cream)
10:00	1 cup skim milk, 2 T. corn syrup

Second day

Breakfast	½ glass orange juice 1 egg, 1 cup milk, 1 T. wheat germ 1 cup coffee, 2 T. corn syrup
10:00	eggnog (1 cup milk, 2 eggs, 2 T. corn syrup)
Dinner	1 can beef baby food, ½ cup broth, 4 drops cod-liver oil concentrate, ½ tsp. salt 1 cup milk, 2 T. corn syrup
3:00	1 cup skim milk, 1 T. brewer's yeast, 2 T. molasses
Supper	cream soup (½ cup strained beans baby food, 1 cup milk, ½ tsp. salt) 1 cup tea, lemon, 2 T. corn syrup
8:00	apple milk shake (½ cup strained applesauce, 1 cup skim milk, 1 T. pectin, 1 small scoop ice cream)
10:00	1 cup skim milk, 2 T. corn syrup

Some patients enjoy the aroma of food; a pleasing aroma of food is important in stimulating gastric secretions that aid digestion, and, if saliva can be swallowed, it also helps digestion. Some patients with a gastrostomy who cannot swallow saliva are annoyed by salivation and would rather not smell food in preparation. Saliva may be collected and introduced into the stomach through the gastrostomy tube, but this is not often psychologically acceptable to the patient.

Disease of the biliary tract and the pancreas. Cholelithiasis and its complications are common in the elderly. One study showed that of 200 elderly patients who had complaints of severe abdominal pain, 55 had the pain from this cause.[16] Cholecystitis and its complications are often treated conservatively in the elderly patient, with operation delayed until acute inflammation has subsided. Cirrhosis or other liver failure may lead to liver coma, which is treated by giving fluids, combating electrolyte imbalance, and attempting to eliminate intestinal organisms that produce ammonia that in turn must be disposed of by the liver.

Carcinoma of the biliary tract is relatively rare, but carcinoma of the pancreas is fairly common in elderly persons. Slowly progressing, painless jaundice is often the first sign of the disease. The lesion may progress until obstruction of the duct entering the duodenum interferes with the flow of both bile and pancreatic juice. Part of the pancreas can be removed surgically, but involvement is usually in the head of the pancreas, which is so closely related to large blood vessels and other structures that surgery is difficult, and metastasis to surrounding tissues occurs easily. It is possible, in some instances, to perform operations that reestablish the flow of bile into the intestinal tract and thus relieve the obstructive jaundice and improve digestion. This is called pancreaticoduodenectomy or Whipple's operation. It must be remembered that malignancies in older persons progress less rapidly than in young persons, and patients may have a relatively long period of relief from purely temporary or palliative procedures.

Diverticulosis and diverticulitis. Diverticulosis is a condition in which tiny areas of weakness develop in the muscle wall of the large bowel. Usually these are at points where blood vessels pass through the muscle. The lower or sigmoid portion of the bowel is most often affected. It is believed that as many as one person in every five over the age of 40 may have diverticulosis.[4] Diverticulitis occurs when bowel contents become trapped in the diverticuli where they may decompose, cause pressure, and set up inflammation and infection. Approximately two thirds of those who have symptoms of diverticulitis are over the age of 60. Symptoms of diverticulitis include pain and persistent soreness in the lower abdomen, particularly on the left side over the sigmoid, alteration of bowel function including alternating diarrhea and constipation, and passage of mucus and sometimes blood in the stools. Nausea may occur and if inflammation and infection are severe, the patient may feel generally ill and the temperature may be elevated. Some elderly patients may develop complications, such as severe hemorrhage or even perforation with no previous history of abdominal discomfort. Complications of this condition include hemorrhage and severe infection with perforation of the bowel and subsequent peritonitis. Occasionally, strictures and obstruction occur with large scar tissue masses resembling tumors being found at operation.

Treatment for diverticulitis usually is conservative. A bland, low-residue diet is recommended. If the patient has no signs of increased intraocular tension, the antispasmodic drugs such as the belladonna preparations are often prescribed, as well as small doses of barbiturates or the ataractic drugs. If signs of acute infection occur, the patient may be given one of the sulfonamide drugs. Often the doctor orders one of the mild bulk laxatives containing agar agar or psyllium seed to keep the stools soft and ensure regular elimination. If severe complications occur, such as perforation, or if the symptoms are severe and do not respond to conservative treatment, operative treatment may be resorted to. If only a portion of the large bowel is affected, this may be resected and an

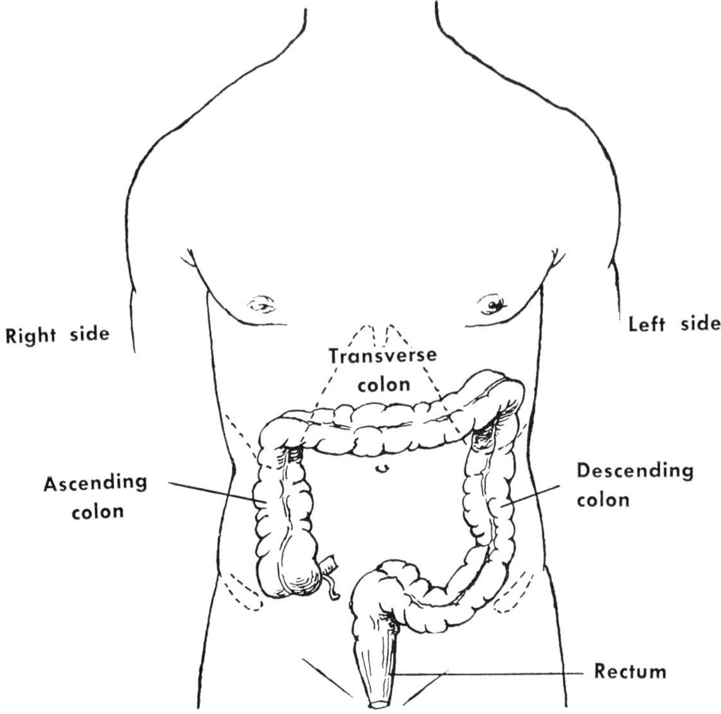

Figure 44. Normal position of the large bowel.

end-to-end anastomosis done. If a large part or all of the large bowel is affected, a colostomy may sometimes be necessary.

Carcinoma of the large bowel and rectum. Carcinoma of the large bowel is common in the elderly. Some cancer detection clinics are performing proctoscopy examinations routinely on all men patients over 35 years of age, since the disease occurs more often in men than in women. Malignant lesions occur anywhere throughout the large intestine, though they appear most often in the sigmoid colon and rectum.

Cancer of the colon can often be cured if it is discovered and treated surgically in its early stages. Routine physical examinations for all elderly people would help in early discovery of this disease. Older people are inclined to blame alteration of bowel habits on old age, lack of exercise, change of diet due to edentia, and innumerable other factors. They may have hemorrhoids that they think are responsible for new signs and symptoms. The hemorrhoids may have been present for years, and thus the patient is likely to delay seeking medical attention.

No specific signs or symptoms of cancer of the bowel are uniformly present. There may be changes in bowel function including distention, constipation, which may alternate with diarrhea, and change in the shape of the stool caused by partial obstruction of the lumen of the intestine. Loss of weight and appetite may follow. If the lesion is high in the bowel, tarry stools may be passed; if it is low, bright blood may be evident. Sometimes, rather sudden and complete intestinal obstruction may be the first sign of malignancy; occasionally, the lesion may perforate into the abdominal cavity, and peritonitis may be the first evidence that anything is wrong. Pain is not an early sign of malignancy of the colon. Metastasis to the liver is frequent, and jaundice may be the first sign of illness.

The emotional reaction of the patient to necessary surgery may be severe, particularly if a permanent colostomy is to be done. The surgeon prepares the patient for the possibility of a colostomy, and the nurse must know what explanation he has given the patient. Few patients refuse necessary surgery if effort has been made to develop their confidence in the hospital and its staff, and time has been taken to give a thorough and complete explanation of the procedures as they are done. It may seem to the nurse that the information that is given to the patient is incomplete at times. She must remember that the surgeon often does not really know exactly what has to be done until he operates. The lesion may be inoperable; on the other hand, it may be less extensive than is anticipated, and a colostomy may not be necessary. Without giving misinformation to the patient, it is possible to emphasize positive features and avoid discussion of circumstances that may not occur. The nurse must be extremely careful in what she tells the patient. The elderly patient may misunderstand and be made apprehensive by misinterpretation of statements. Time must be taken to carry out any explanation, once started, to a conclusion satisfying to the patient.

Surgical procedures for excision of a malignant lesion in the bowel may vary with the location and extent of the lesion. Surgical removal of a malignant lesion of the colon may be accomplished by a resection and anastomosis of the large bowel. Often, however, the patient must have a colostomy or permanent new opening for the removal of intestinal waste products. A colostomy may be performed in the cecum, the transverse colon, or the descending colon. A loop of bowel may be brought to the exterior through a stab wound and the lumen of the bowel is not opened for forty-eight to seventy-two hours. This allows closure to occur about the opening so that contamination from the contents of the bowel will not infect the abdominal cavity. When this is done, there are two loops to the colostomy—a proximal loop that continues upward to the duodenum and stomach and a distal loop that continues onward to the rectum.

An abdominoperineal resection may be done if the malignant lesion is in the rectum or lower part of the large bowel. In this operation the lower segment of the bowel, the rectum, and surrounding structures are removed, leaving a single colostomy opening, or stoma. This stoma will be open and will begin to drain fecal material immediately upon the patient's return from the operating room.

The nurse has an important responsibility in assisting the patient to adjust to his new situation and in teaching how he may care for himself so that his independence may be continued. In order to help the patient effectively, the nurse must know the position of the large bowel, as well as its function. She must remember that the large bowel ascends on the right side of the abdomen, crosses, and descends to become the sigmoid colon on the left side. If she remembers, it will help her to avoid confusion in determining which direction in the double loop colostomy is toward the small intestine and which is toward the rectum.

Many patients believe that a colostomy is a rare and terrible operation. They fear that they will no longer be able to mingle with their fellows, eat normally, or do any of the things that make life worth living. It can be explained that a colostomy is not really a tremendous variation from normal; diet will probably require very little change. Many people who have had colostomies live very normal lives for years.

The patient should be told early that he will be able to care for himself and that the problems he first encounters in the hospital will not continue. If this is not done, his emotional reaction to the sudden appearance of fecal drainage through the abdomen may be severe. He may be disturbed by the odor and may become convinced that difficulties with drainage and with dressings will persist for the rest of his life. The patient should be told that the bowel will develop regularity in evacuation, just as it does in normal excretion of feces, and that many persons need little if any protection since evacuation through the stoma occurs at a definite time each day. In some instances the abdominal musculature may take over some of the action of the rectal sphincter.

The elderly patient must not be hurried in learning to care for himself. Too much haste may result in apprehension and discouragement. Often, talking with another patient who has had a similar operation and has made a good adjustment is most helpful in early adjustment to the colostomy. The patient must be assured from the beginning that each step of care of his stoma will be carefully explained to him and that he will be cared for until he is able to care for himself and has learned to do it. He may have hearing and visual limitations that hamper his progress. He may have joint stiffness and general fatigue that make irrigations and any other procedures exhausting.

Drainage from the stoma may at first be loose and unpredictable. This is more likely to occur when an operation has been done high on the bowel, such as a cecostomy, since reabsorption of fluid in the large bowel has not yet occurred. Gauze dressings should be fluffed and arranged circularly around the openings so that the tendency of fluid to run under the dressings onto the bed or the rest of the abdomen is minimized. The patient must be told that many individual variations exist; if he finds that certain foods cause diarrhea or otherwise disagree with him, he should avoid them. If diarrhea is troublesome, boiled milk may be taken instead of whole fresh milk. Many patients find that little if any alteration of diet is needed, and the trend is toward allowing a solid diet as soon as a day or two after surgery in order to prevent liquid stools.

Skin around the stoma must be kept clean by changing the dressings as soon as they are soiled until regularity of evacuation has been established. Soap and water are most satisfactory for preserving the health of the skin, though zinc oxide and castor-oil ointment and aluminum paste are useful in protecting the skin if signs of irritation appear.

Most patients have better results in control of bowel function if the colon is

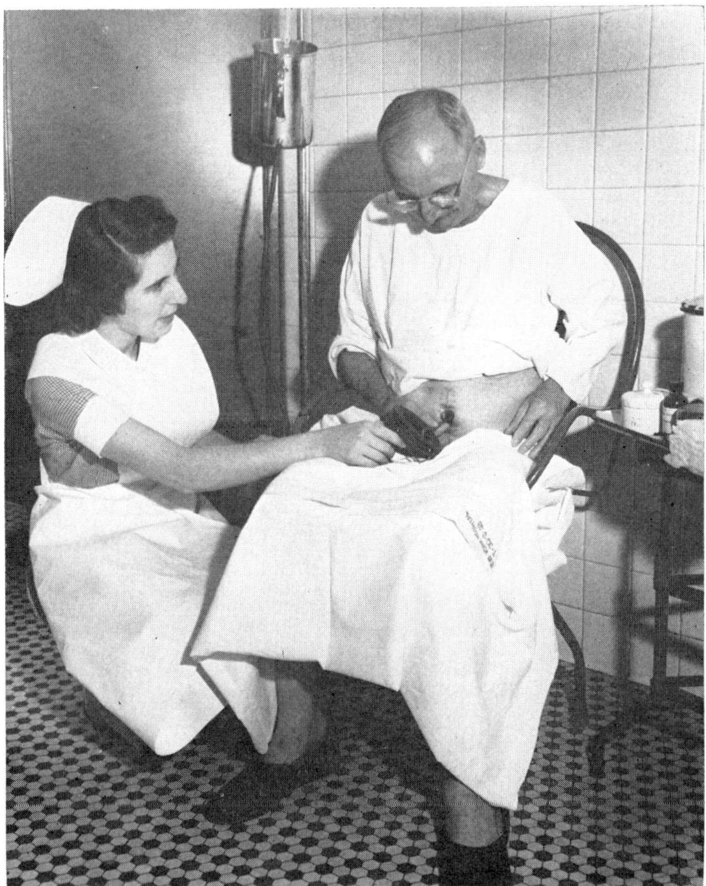

Figure 45. The patient with a colostomy learns to care for himself through careful teaching and encouragement at each new step of the procedure.

irrigated at regular intervals, though some find that irrigation is not necessary. Usually irrigations are given in the hospital, and adjustments are made as they seem necessary for the individual patient. Irrigations must be done at exactly the same hour each day in order to establish bowel regularity. The time required for a satisfactory irrigation varies from a very short time to several hours. The elderly patient must be watched closely since lengthy irrigations can be exhausting. When the patient is able, he begins to irrigate his colon in the bathroom, using the equipment that he will use when he returns home. Irrigations should be given in the hospital at a time that will be convenient for the patient in his home or rooming house and that will permit him to carry on normal activities, such as work if he is still employed.

Even though he has learned to care for himself in the hospital, the average patient with a colostomy is apprehensive at the thought of being completely on his own. The public health nurse can be called upon to visit him in his home and help him in necessary adjustments to his home situation.

Irrigating equipment made of thin plastic material is now available; the small dome that fits over the stoma is made of hard, transparent plastic material. This equipment is easier to keep clean and free of odors and easier to handle than equipment made of rubber. An inexpensive irrigation set can be devised as follows.[13] Cut off the bottom of a plastic cup that is about four inches in diameter, leaving a depth of approximately two inches; attach to this a tube of plastic waterproof material, securing it with two rubber bands. Using a sharp, round instrument such as an icepick, make a small opening in the side of the cup about halfway up through which a catheter may be inserted. A belt can be improvised by making a slit in a wide band of elastic to fit over the cup and securing it behind the patient with a safety pin. This obviates his need to use one hand to hold the dome in place for long intervals.

Whether the patient must wear a colostomy bag at all times depends upon him, his general condition, and the location of the colostomy. He should know that many patients manage with no bag and only a small dressing. Disposable plastic bags are now available at low cost. An elderly patient who is retired from work and remains at home all day sometimes has less incentive to control the colostomy than the person who goes out to work. Regulation, however, is recommended for psychologic reasons, regardless of the living pattern of the patient.

Patients and their families would be spared a great deal of worry, apprehension, and needless expense if the nurse in the hospital would inquire about the patient's home situation and suggest suitable dressings and equipment before he goes home. Many family members buy expensive gauze, not realizing that Cellucotton pads are adequate and available. The nurse should know the resources of her community. For example, the local chapter of the American Cancer Society will often supply unsterile dressings without charge. Referral to the public health nurse should be made before the patient leaves the hospital so that she may visit the home if necessary to be certain that the patient and his family can manage their situation.

REFERENCES AND RELATED BIBLIOGRAPHY

1. Beeson, Paul B., and McDermott, Walsh (editors): Cecil-Loeb textbook of medicine, ed. 11, Philadelphia, 1963, W. B. Saunders Co.
2. Best, Charles Herbert, and Taylor, Norma Burke: Physiological basis of medical practice, Baltimore, 1961, The Williams & Wilkins Co.
3. Boros, Edwin: Hiatus hernia, Am. J. Gastroenterol. **34**:438-441, 1962.
4. Cayer, David: Disorders of the gastrointestinal tract and digestive organs. In Johnson, Wingate M. (editor): The older patient, New York, 1960, Paul B. Hoeber, Inc., Medical Book Department of Harper & Row, Publishers.
5. Dagradi, Angelo E., and Stempien, Stephen J.: Symptomatic esophageal hiatus sliding hernia, Am. J. Digest. Dis. **7**:613-633, 1962.
6. Davis, Loyal (editor): Christopher's textbook of surgery, ed. 8, Philadelphia, 1965, W. B. Saunders Co.
7. Eyerly, James B., and Breuhaus, Herbert C.: Diseases of the esophagus, the stomach and the small intestine. In Stieglitz, Edward J. (editor): Geriatric Medicine, ed. 3, Philadelphia, 1954, J. B. Lippincott Co.
8. Fansler, Walter A.: Special problems in the proctoscopic examination of the geriatric patient, J. Am. Geriatrics Soc. **10**:567-570, 1962.

9. Greene, George W., Jr.: Diagnosis of oral lesions, J. Am. Geriatrics Soc. **11**:131-139, 1963.
10. Ingles, Thelma, and Campbell, Emily: The patient with a colostomy, Amer. J. Nurs. **58**:1544-1546, 1958.
11. Klug, Thomas J., Magruder, Lucinda, and others: Gastric resection; and nursing care, Amer. J. Nurs. **61**:73-77, 1961.
12. Kurihara, Marie: The patient with an intestinal prosthesis, Amer. J. Nurs. **60**:852-853, 1960.
13. Lindner, Janet: Inexpensive colostomy irrigation equipment, Amer. J. Nurs. **58**:844, 1958.
14. McHardy, Gordon, and others: Geriatric gastrointestinal therapy, including observation of the effect of dicyclomine, J. Am. Geriatrics Soc. **11**:199-210, 1963.
15. Nutrition Bureau, New York State Department of Health (mimeographed material).
16. Ponka, Joseph L., Welborn, J. Keith, and Brush, Brock E.: Acute abdominal pain in aged patients: an analysis of 200 cases, J. Am. Geriatrics Soc. **11**:993-1007, 1963.
17. Puestow, Karver: Geriatrics, gerontology and gastro-enterology, J. Am. Geriatrics Soc. **9**:101-109, 1961.
18. Robinson, Hamilton B. G.: Oral disease of the aging patient, J. Am. Geriatrics Soc. **11**:120-130, 1963.
19. Shafer, Kathleen Newton, and others: Medical-surgical nursing, ed. 3, St. Louis, 1964, The C. V. Mosby Co.
20. Stahl, William M.: Major abdominal surgery in the aged patient, Am. J. Geriatrics Soc. **11**:770-779, 1963.
21. Warren, Richard: Surgery, Philadelphia, 1963, W. B. Saunders Co.
22. Wirtz, C. Wilmer: The aging intestinal tract; esophagus, stomach and small bowel, J. Am. Geriatrics Soc. **9**:933-939, 1961.
23. Wolfman, Earl F., Jr., Flotte, C. Thomas, and Hallburg, Jeanne C.: Carcinoma of the colon and rectum and the patient with surgery of the colon, Amer. J. Nurs. **61**:60-66, 1961.
24. Zuidema, George D., and Klein, Marilyn Kitching: A new esophagus, Amer. J. Nurs. **61**:69-72, 1961.

Chapter 20

Nursing in diseases of the ear, nose, and throat

THE EAR

Older people can be affected by the same diseases of the ear that affect younger persons. Otitis media occurs much less often than in children, but can be severe in a debilitated elderly patient. Meniere's syndrome is seen in the aged; treatment and care for this condition is similar to that for a patient of any age.

Deafness is by far the most common condition that affects the aged. Many older people accept hearing loss as a part of growing old that must be endured, but skilled medical care can do much for the older person with a hearing loss. Even if hearing cannot be fully restored, other means are available to assist the old person in preserving contact with other persons and with the world about him.

Two kinds of deafness have been described. Perception deafness is due to failure of nerve endings in the inner ear to register sound. Neurologic disease such as meningitis can cause this type of deafness, though nerve degeneration is the most common cause in older people and may be part of the normal process of aging. Some of it may be prevented when more is known about the degenerative changes of age.

Conduction deafness is caused by some disturbance or interference with transmission of sound impulses before they reach the center of hearing in the cochlea. These impulses can be transmitted through both air and bone. At present, conduction deafness is more responsive to treatment and control than perception deafness. Prompt attention to infection in the middle ear, the nose, the sinuses, the throat, and the eustachian tubes is helpful in the prevention of disease and its early diagnosis.

Perception deafness has been considered to be difficulty in the inner ear, and conduction deafness has referred to disease in the middle ear. Deafness may be due to a combination of perception and conduction impairment. Otosclerosis is an example of ear disease that primarily causes conduction defect (from bony interference with conduction) and that secondarily may cause perception defect (from pressure on the end organ in the cochlea). The term progressive deafness is now usually used.

It is estimated that between 15,000,000 and 20,000,000 persons in the United States have defective hearing, and of these between 5,000,000 and 8,000,000 have serious hearing loss. There are 800,000 persons who wear hearing aids, and it is thought that probably many more need to use them. This number will probably increase considerably in the future. It is believed that many persons who suffered hearing damage during World War II will need assistance in hearing by the time they reach old age. Limitations in hearing are common in the aged. By the time they have reached 80 years of age, far more people have defective hearing than have normal hearing. Some persons, however, retain excellent hearing capacity until they are 90 years of age or older.

Causes of hearing loss. Much hearing loss in age is from three main causes. The person who has hearing limitations needs to be referred to a skilled otologist, who can discover the cause of his trouble, prescribe treatment, and outline assistance. Catarrhal deafness follows acute infections in childhood, and in adult life follows recurrent acute or chronic otitis media. Injury to the eardrum and pathology of the eustachian tube may also further aggravate the condition and contribute to an increasing hearing loss. Damage from repeated and continued infection may not be noticed until age advances and nerve changes appear to make the presence of hearing limitation apparent.

A second cause of hearing loss among older people is otosclerosis, though the disease is really one of youth and middle life. A predisposition to develop otosclerosis is inherited, and it occurs more commonly in women and is aggravated by puberty, pregnancy, and the menopause. There is absorption of the bony capsule about the labyrinth, which is replaced by spongy bone. Hearing loss for low tones is noted first, and the condition is often accompanied by tinnitus, rumbling, and other raucous and disturbing sounds. Operative procedures have proved helpful in carefully selected cases, but many people with otosclerosis progress to total deafness in old age.

Eighth nerve deafness, senile deafness, and *degenerative nerve deafness* are names used to designate a type of deafness common in age. The pathology is in the nerve cells of the organ of Corti in the cochlea. Neurologic degeneration occurs and is similar to that which appears in the optic nerve in age. There is early loss of high register tones. Nerve deafness seems to be increased by the presence of other conditions, such as nutritional inadequacy, nephritis, diabetes, vascular disease, and chronic systemic infection.

Emotional factors in loss of hearing. For each individual the emotional implications of loss of hearing are tremendous. The inability to hear what is going on about him and to share in informal group conversation seems to set the person apart more than does even partial or total blindness. The person with a hearing difficulty is often irritable, insecure, and defensive. He may come to believe that persons around him are talking about him, and he becomes suspicious and avoids the association of others. These tendencies may be increased in age. The older person may already be insecure and often suffers from the feeling that the world about him has little need or desire for his active presence. He may suffer from fatigue, discouragement, and impatience, which make the frustration from hearing loss even more acute. The older person needs constant encouragement in his attempts to learn lipreading and to adjust to the use of a hearing aid if it has been prescribed.

Some people refuse to admit that they have serious hearing limitations. They may accept the necessity for dentures stoically, but refuse to accept the necessity for a hearing aid and are reluctant to admit that they engage in lipreading. Helping in the adjustment of the patient to the point that he will admit that he has hearing limitations and is willing to accept hearing assistance is a major step in the rehabilitation of the individual.

As the medical and nursing professions assume more and more responsibility for the patient from the time of illness or injury to complete rehabilitation, it becomes necessary that the nurse know what resources are available to the person who has a permanent hearing loss. She cannot be an expert in the selection and use of hearing aids or in teaching lipreading, but she should be able to direct her patient to suitable sources of information and assistance.

A serious and frustrating problem arises for the husband or wife or for any other person living intimately with an elderly person who becomes hard of hearing. He is saddened because sounds and experiences previously shared can now be shared only in part or with difficulty, and he, too, tends to become isolated in his social contacts.

Establishing communication. Preservation of emotional health is important. Success in this may be partially determined by the kind of person the patient was before he became hard of hearing. Many people with no hearing loss have severe emotional disturbances, and it should not be supposed that all personality difficulty encountered in a patient is the result of the hearing loss, although much of it often is. The person with hearing loss must be helped to feel that he is not separated from the persons around him. Group activities are important and should be participated in before the person has had much time to retreat and to develop antisocial tendencies. Occupational therapy that demands group participation is helpful while the patient is hospitalized for treatment of a hearing ailment. Social clubs where persons with hearing loss can mingle with others who also are hard of hearing makes them feel less isolated and less different from the world around them. Many theaters and churches have special seating arrangements for the hard of hearing where attachments for the use of earphones are provided. Silent group participation in activities, such as attending concerts, lectures, church, and the theater also help to foster the feeling of comradeship with others and yet does not make carrying on a conversation necessary. Interest fostered in others and activities participated in away from home help to prevent introspection and preoccupation with frustration and failure.

Lipreading often helps to retain communication with others. Unfortunately, many people believe that, with the use of hearing aids, lip reading is no longer necessary. It is beneficial to almost all who are hard of hearing. If for any reason a person is unable to use a hearing aid or receives no benefit from it, lipreading is essential. Some people learn lipreading very quickly, whereas others find it a rather difficult and tedious procedure. All persons can learn a good deal from regular instruction, and except for the individual who has marked visual or intellectual loss, the majority of persons can learn lipreading with persistence and practice. Individual instruction is helpful, but the social factors in group learning are important. A teacher with special preparation is necessary, and such a person is not always easy to find, particularly in the less populated parts of the country. Interest in the subject is growing. It may be possible in the future that arrangements can be made for teachers specialized in this kind of work to spend a few days or weeks of the year in areas where suitable arrangements for courses will have been made in advance. The nurse will be invaluable in directing persons with hearing difficulties to such courses when and if they are to be given.

The first electric hearing aid was produced in Vienna in 1900. Since then, many varieties have been produced and marketed. For example, in recent years a transistor or small electronic device has largely replaced the vacuum tube type, which was larger. One is now made that fits into the frame of glasses, with the receiver and battery incorporated in the part behind the ear. This hearing aid is expensive, but is sometimes chosen by a person who is particularly sensitive to the appearance of a hearing aid. Some persons use transparent devices that fit into the ear and connect by means of a tiny cord to a receiver hidden in the hair.

The nurse who is caring for an older person may be asked many questions regarding the individual merits of hearing aids. The question of whether he needs or should use an aid should be referred to his physician. Usually a hearing aid is recommended when hearing loss in the good ear reaches 25 percent of normal.

The nurse may be asked which type or make of hearing aid is the best. There is no *best* hearing aid for everyone. Each person must be fitted individually and must be taught how to use his own equipment. For this reason in large cities where agencies such as the American Hearing Society or the American Speech and Hearing Association have chapters, the patient is often referred to them by the physician. Some local chapters or Leagues for Hard of Hearing provide a consultation service in which individual problems are discussed, and a suitable hearing aid is chosen in accordance with the patient's particular needs. It may be that the person will have to try out several aids before he finds a suitable one. This discrimination is rarely permissible when he purchases his aid from a commercial company. In areas where this service is not available, the patient may be referred by his physician to one or more companies that market worthy and effective hearing aids. He may, however, shop around and finally purchase an aid that does not turn out satisfactorily for him, and he then may become discouraged and bitter. The Council on Physical Medicine of the American Medical Association maintains a list of hearing aids, their efficiency and the ethics of advertising in their sales. Whether or not a certain hearing aid is approved can be learned by contacting a hearing clinic or the Council. The trend in some parts of the country is for otologists to maintain a fitting and supply service for hearing aids in connection with their offices or with the otology clinic where the use of the hearing aid is taught. A follow-up service is continued until the patient is able to use his aid satisfactorily. A plastic mold of the ear canal, made from an impression obtained by using a pliable material, is a part of some hearing aids.

This is the only part of the equipment that can be washed. It should be removed and cleaned regularly; pipe cleaners are useful in cleansing the canal in the mold.

The elderly patient is likely to be concerned about the cost of hearing-aid equipment and its maintenance. At the present time (1966) hearing aids cost from $75 to $600. Many are now made with a tiny transistor and are quite inconspicuous and comfortable. The cost of maintenance depends upon how much the aid is used. For the older person this cost usually is less, particularly for those who are inclined to isolate themselves or are retired and may use the aid only when they go outdoors or when entertaining friends. The older person who is fighting introspection and loneliness needs to use his hearing aid more often than he feels he can afford. It must be remembered that hearing voices on the street, the noise of cars, the ticking of the clock, and the clatter of crockery all are part of our living and contribute to a normal outlook on life. In some cities the department of welfare confines its purchases of aids to the least expensive type available and to rebuilt ones. Thus the attention to individual need may be lost, and frustration in the use of the aid may result.

The patient may ask whether or not he will hear as well as he did in youth if he uses an aid. No device for hearing completely takes the place of normal hearing. This does not mean that hearing aids are not useful. They have contributed immeasurably to human happiness and enjoyment of living. The patient should be told from the beginning that, though an aid will help his hearing and will enable him to hear much that was otherwise impossible, it will not restore perfect hearing. Patience, practice, and persistence in the use of a hearing aid will eventually yield big dividends to the user. The aid should be used for a limited time at first, and the periods of use should be gradually increased. The user should also experiment with his hearing aid in groups, out on the street, and at home. He may, for example, find his particular aid invaluable when he is out on the street, but the use of earphones may give him better service when he wishes to listen to the radio because of the exclusion of external sounds, instead of amplification.

Each year hearing aids are made more effective and useful. The important limitation of hearing aids at the present time is that they are, after all, only mechanical devices that amplify sound. Unfortunately, the person who has progressive deafness does not usually lose both high and low tones equally or simultaneously. The modern hearing aid would be much more satisfactory if it were more adjustable to such a contingency. Many older people have loss of the high tones at first, and therefore an aid that picks up high tones will magnify the low ones to such a degree that adjustment to the hearing aid is sometimes difficult. Distant noises may be amplified enough to be most distressing; yet amplification may be barely sufficient to make close conversation satisfactory. Hearing aids do have the ability to register differences of pitch and volume. Tone qualities also vary and give the individual a certain amount of personal selection.

Much more has yet to be done in the education of the public to the acceptance of hearing aids. Glasses are accepted without comment, and even dentures are seldom a cause for secrecy. Hearing aid devices are linked in the public mind with pitiful decrepitude and are, therefore, stubbornly avoided until sometimes personality reactions to deafness have progressed to where an acceptance of the hearing aid is almost impossible.

Most hearing aids are easily controlled with a little practice. The tiny dial can be turned through the clothing. Women usually wear the dial (and often the battery) between the breasts in a special pocket built into a brassiere; men wear theirs in a vest pocket. Most elderly people need practice and repeated instruction in the care of their aid. They need to be reminded to turn off the battery at night and must know how to replace the batteries; they should know that using batteries that are almost worn out and low in efficiency is poor practice. Any person who uses a hearing aid should have extra batteries on hand.

THE NOSE AND SINUSES

Nasal conditions. Atrophic changes in the nose occur but are less troublesome than those occurring in many other parts of the body. Acute rhinitis is rare in older people, while a chronic mild rhinitis is common. This causes a dripping nose which, probably because of lessened sensation, appears to go unnoticed by the patient. Atrophic rhinitis is a chronic condition of the nose characterized by severe atrophy of the mucous membrane, crusting, and ozena (offensive discharge). Rhinitis sicca is excessive drying of the mucous membrane of the nose with the appearance of dry, thin, white crusts. Because of the excessive dryness of mucous membranes the elderly person may develop the habit of sniffing unconsciously at frequent intervals, and this habit may become most annoying to those about him. Increasing the humidity of air breathed and inhalation of aromatic drugs such as menthol are sometimes helpful. Glycerin and alcohol preparations may sometimes be used as sprays. Applications of glucose solution to the nasal mucosa seem in some instances to decrease the odor of discharges.

Dryness of the entire nasal and throat mucosa is often increased because of low household humidity, especially in winter when homes are heated artificially. This may predispose to nasal hemorrhage, to difficulty in speaking, and to a rasping voice that may frighten the older person, who may believe he is developing a serious illness such as cancer. Nasal hemorrhage occurs relatively frequently in older people. Medical advice should be sought if nosebleeds recur, since arterial hypertension is sometimes the cause.

Sinal conditions. Older people have less trouble with the sinuses than do younger persons. This is thought to be because atrophic changes permit better ventilation and better drainage. The mucous membrane of the sinuses atrophies and becomes drier and less vascular. The atrophic tissues seem to respond less readily to irritating influences. Infection acquired earlier in life may persist. An older person may continue to have drainage from a chronic sinus infection that he has harbored for years. A morning headache that disappears after a person has been up and about for an hour or two is indicative of sinusitis since the erect position and head movements facilitate sinus drainage. Occasionally sinusitis causes chronic infection of the throat, and even the eustachian tube may become involved. With age, the reflexes of the posterior pharynx become less sensitive, and there is danger of aspiration of infected material to the lungs. It is thought that bronchiectasis can be traced in some instances to chronic sinusitis. Chronic sinusitis may become worse in rare instances; it is thought that poor nutrition and lowered resistance to infection in age may be causes.

Treatment of sinusitis in age includes the use of bacteriostatic drugs, inhalation of medications such as benzoin or menthol, and effort to ensure a constant temperature of the air breathed. The elderly patient with severe sinusitis often has less difficulty if he can spend the winters in a warm, humid climate.

THE THROAT

Disease of the larynx. The larynx becomes firmer and smaller in age. The voice loses some of its fullness and is usually of higher pitch. Voice change may be the result in part of hearing loss, as well as of actual physical changes in the larynx.

There are many causes of hoarseness, but two are particularly important. Tuberculosis of the larynx may be the cause, though this occurs most often in younger people. A tumor should be suspected in anyone over 40 years of age who has persistent hoarseness of over two weeks' duration. It is important that the nurse bear this in mind, since early referral of people with hoarseness to a physician may result in complete cure if carcinoma of the larynx is present. The disease is much more common in men than in women and appears most often after 60 years of age. Carcinoma is often of the squamous cell type, and because of the lack of vascularity of the larynx and the fact that hoarseness is often produced early in the disease, the prognosis is more favorable than in malignancy in many other parts of the body.

The treatment for carcinoma of the larynx is surgical. Nursing care of the elderly patient includes thorough explanation of all procedures. He may not be able to hear well and may become agitated and apprehensive if he does not understand what to expect. Explanation will depend upon the surgery that is to be performed. The patient should be told that he may not be given food for a short time and that he may be fed through a tube passed through his nose into the stomach or intravenously. He should know that he may not be able to talk. This may be because of edema of the larynx or because a complete laryngectomy has been done. He should be provided with a pencil and pad or a Magic Slate on which he may write if he wishes to communicate with the nurse or with others. He should be told that he may have a tracheostomy opening and that it will be uncomfortable, but that he must make the effort to cough in spite of the discomfort, which will be of short duration.

Every patient who has either a partial or a total laryngectomy should be constantly attended for at least forty-eight hours and longer if there is much secretion and any danger of his being unable to eliminate the secretions that will form. After surgery the patient must be assured that he will have continuous supervision and not be left alone. He needs constant reassurance since he fears that he may choke or be unable to breathe. The patient is usually given a local anesthetic or a very short-acting general anesthesia so that he is awake when he returns to his room. He usually responds immediately to the nurse who by her

loss of voice and the use of a permanent tracheostomy tube is sometimes difficult. The patient's adjustment is usually similar to his response to other difficulties in his life. One difference is that the older person may be facing a large number of adjustments and handicaps, and this additional one may seem overwhelming. The patient is often cheered if it is pointed out to him that the vocal cords are not the only parts involved in effective speech. Speech of the person with a cleft palate demonstrates the fact that vocal cords by themselves do not produce a pleasing tone of voice. The patient still has his tongue, his lips, a firm roof to his mouth, and his nose and sinuses to give the necessary resonance to the new voice that he can develop successfully if he will make the effort to do so.

REFERENCES AND RELATED BIBLIOGRAPHY

1. Gardner, Warren H.: Rehabilitation after laryngectomy, Public Health Nurs. **43**:612-615, 1951.
2. Greene, James S.: Speech rehabilitation following laryngectomy, Amer. J. Nurs. **49**:153-154, 1949.
3. Heatley, Clyde A.: Diseases of the ear. In Stieglitz, Edward J. (editor): Geriatric medicine, ed. 3, Philadelphia, 1954, J. B. Lippincott Co.
4. Holinger, Paul H., Johnston, Kenneth C., and Mansueto, Mario D.: Cancer of the larynx; surgical treatment; Jimison, Carmin: Nursing the patient after laryngectomy, Amer. J. Nurs. **57**:738-741; 741-743, 1957.
5. Jackson, L., and Jackson, C. L. (editors): Diseases of the nose, throat, and ear, ed. 2, Philadelphia, 1959, W. B. Saunders Co.
6. Manhattan Eye, Ear, Nose, and Throat Hospital: Nursing in diseases of the eye, ear, nose and throat, ed. 10, Philadelphia, 1958, W. B. Saunders Co.
7. Markle, Donald M.: Hearing aids, Amer. J. Nurs. **57**:592-593, 1957.
8. Martin, Hayes, and Ehrlich, Harry E.: Nursing care following laryngectomy, Amer. J. Nurs. **49**:149-152, 1949.
9. National Institute of Neurological Diseases and Blindness, National Institutes of Health: Hearing loss, Washington, D. C., 1964, U. S. Government Printing office.
10. Plum, Fred, and Dunning, Marcelle F.: Technics for minimizing trauma to the tracheobronchial tree after tracheotomy, New England J. Med. **254**:193-200, 1956.
11. Riley, Edward C.: Preventing deafness from industrial noise, Amer. J. Nurs. **63**:80-84, 1963.
12. Ronnel, Eleanor C.: Hearing aids, Amer. J. Nurs. **63**:90-93, 1963.
13. Shafer, Kathleen Newton, and others: Medical-surgical nursing, ed. 3, St. Louis, 1964, The C. V. Mosby Co.
14. Shambaugh, George E., Jr.: Surgery of the ear, Philadelphia, 1959, W. B. Saunders Co.
15. Shepard, Mary Estelle: Nursing care of patients with eye, ear, nose and throat disorders, New York, 1958, The Macmillan Company.
16. Tatman, Laurence E., and Lehman, Roger H.: Tracheostomy care, Amer. J. Nurs. **64**: 96-98, 1964.

Chapter 21

Nursing in diseases of the chest

The older person who develops chest disease faces some distinct disadvantages in comparison to persons of lesser years. Certain physiologic and anatomic changes have occurred that hamper ability to ward off or withstand disease. The rib cage becomes more rigid and lacking in elasticity; costal cartilages may finally become ossified. The stooped posture of the upper thoracic spine, so often observed in the elderly, allows the ribs to fall downward and forward, thereby decreasing the chest capacity. Atrophy and fatigue of respiratory muscles may result in poor respiratory action, and poor tone of the abdominal musculature may interfere with the action of the diaphragm and hinder adequate respiration.

Changes in the lungs occur with age. The lungs become smaller in size and in weight. The bronchioles may lose elasticity, and pulmonary fibrosis may follow bronchitis, pneumonia, or any chronic irritation that has persisted for a period of time. The alveoli become larger and less elastic, and the walls become thinner. The vital capacity of the lungs decreases with age, and this means that more air remains within the lungs instead of participating in the exchange of gases normally occurring at each respiration. All of these changes lower the efficiency of the respiratory system and predispose to disease. Rhythmic activity is altered, which further impairs function and delays the elimination of accumulated secretions.

Many elderly people have arteriosclerotic changes in blood vessels that make circulation through the lungs less efficient. Impaired function of the blood vessels and the lungs places a burden upon the heart. The right ventricle may enlarge and this may lead to cardiac failure if extra strain is placed upon the heart by infection or other causes.

Chronic respiratory disease appears to be increasing among the aged. For example, it has been found that chronic respiratory disease among white men aged 65 to 74 years increased by 153 percent between 1950 and 1960.[14] Usually two or more chronic diseases occur together. There are really no pulmonary diseases that are those of old age specifically, although some disease conditions such as emphysema occur more often in the older age group. Nursing care for patients with specific diseases of the pulmonary system are described in medical and surgical nursing texts and will not be repeated here.[21] Only a few differences in care that are specific to the elderly for some of the more common diseases will be mentioned. Because several diseases, such as asthma, bronchitis, and emphysema, may occur together, the problems for the elderly patient and for those who care for him are compounded. Cancer of the lung occurs more often in middle age than in old age. Its treatment in the geriatric patient is the same as for younger patients, except that the operative risk is greater, as described in Chapter 13, Anesthesia and Operative Care.

PREVENTION OF DISEASE

It is difficult to measure accurately the damage caused by the constant inhaling of irritants. It is suspected, however, that total damage over a long period may be quite extensive. General hygiene for the respiratory system should exclude irritants taken into the lungs, such as excessive smoke; extremely dry fetid air as in some offices and industrial plants; chemical and industrial fumes as in some printing, dyeing, and cleaning establishments; and overheated air as in some bakeries. Experts in industrial health are working diligently to eliminate these harmful factors that may be damaging to the lungs of workers by improving everyday living and working conditions of employees of all ages.

Regular breathing exercises may help to protect the aged person from acute and chronic involvement of the respiratory system. Postural correction, adequate diet, weight reduction if necessary, and change in climate, particularly for the winter months, may also be of benefit. If the muscle tone of the abdomen is poor, an abdominal belt to support the viscera and assist the action of the diaphragm may be of help, and exercises to strengthen the weakened muscles may be prescribed.

The elderly person must avoid exposure to respiratory infection. For an older person the common cold may be a serious affair even when no other chronic disease exists. It is dangerous for the nurse, family members, or anyone else with a cold to be in contact at such a time with an older person. Protection from exposure to colds is difficult to carry out in the home where so often young children with colds are anxious to make a family visit to their grandparents.

Many older people have a chronic cough. In spite of the number of factors that contribute to the chronicity of chest conditions in the aged, specialists in geriatrics feel that it is unwise to assume that chronic cough and breathing difficulty are simply the accompaniments of age. Thorough investigation may reveal bronchiectasis, lung abscess, malignancy of the lung, or tuberculosis to be the cause of a cough. The nurse in the community has a duty in general health supervision of families to urge the older members who have chronic chest symptoms to visit a physician.

GENERAL NURSING

Cough. Coughing can be most exhausting to the patient. It is well to remember that the cardiac reserve is decreased with age, and rigid structures make coughing less effective. The patient should try to relax between periods of coughing and avoid ineffectual short coughs in which nothing is expelled and energy is dissipated. It is helpful sometimes for the nurse to assist the patient in coughing by applying manual compression to the lower thorax and abdomen. The nurse should explain what she is going to do and should place one hand firmly against the thoracic spine and the other against the anterior chest. The patient is then instructed to breath deeply and to cough as forcefully as possible. Any marked rise in pluse rate or pulse irregularity must be reported at once. Codeine sulfate and morphine sulfate may be used for severe coughing in which exhaustion is imminent. Ammonium chloride, syrup of ipecac, and potassium iodide are medications given to loosen the secretions and make expectoration less difficult. Hot sweet drinks and syrups may aid the patient in making the cough effectual. Hot fluids may help by causing vasodilation and also in producing general relaxation. Sweet substances cause the mucous membrane of both the mouth and respiratory passages to increase its output of secretions and thus help loosen the cough.

If the patient has severe cough associated with asthma or pulmonary emphysema, a positive pressure machine may be used. By means of this machine full inflation of the lungs can be obtained at 30 to 40 mm. Hg, and this is followed by negative pressure breathing. It has been found that the positive pressure machine is more effective than the most forceful and productive cough. These machines are now available in portable form for home use. The nurse must be certain that she herself understands the action of the machine and must caution the patient to never under any circumstances alter the pressure gauge without medical approval.

Steam may be ordered for the patient with a chronic cough, and aromatic medications such as tincture of benzoin or menthol may be added.

A number of safe and inexpensive steam humidifiers are now available for easy purchase. If the nurse is improvising in the home it is unwise to use a good teakettle that may be damaged by the benzoin. Use instead a large tin can with an opening into which a paper spout can be inserted; this makes a good and adequate container and may be heated on a small electric plate. When steam is being used, it is necessary to be certain that windows are closed and that the patient is well covered during and following the procedure. Many older people resist wearing a towel about the head to help concentrate the steam to be inhaled. A sheet can be used to improvise a canopy or tent, which is often more comfortable. The reason for the treatment should be explained, and the patient's position should be adjusted comfortably before inhalation of steam is started. Extra pillows may be needed to support bony prominences. Often the patient can continue the treatment best if an over-bed table on which he can rest his arms while leaning forward in an upright position is used. It is possible with the humidifiers now available to have one equipped with a long, flexible tube that is adjusted easily to any position the patient assumes comfortably. Some patients cannot tolerate steam close to the face, even when no covering over the head is used. It sometimes is necessary to use two or more humidifiers and to increase the moisture level of the air in the entire room. If the patient has bathroom privileges or can move about outside his room, the greatest care must be taken to avoid chilling after exposure to the warm moist air in a room where humidifiers are used.

Older people sometimes become careless about the details of hygiene in the disposal of sputum. This may be because of fatigue and discouragement, but more often it is because appropriate equipment is not available. The older person may have poor vision, and he may be unsteady in his movement so that it is imperative that a suitable sputum container into which he can expectorate with ease be provided. Paper tissues should be placed on both sides of the bed; they can be pinned to the bed and placed under the pillow. Paper bags for disposal of tissues should also be placed on both sides of the bed. Often the patient does not have the energy to turn to reach for necessary equipment.

Mouth hygiene is important for any patient with respiratory disease. Repeated expectoration of sputum and chronic cough are not conducive to a good appetite. An aromatic mouthwash should be used routinely before meals and the patient should be given an opportunity to wash his hands before he handles food.

Bronchoscopy. A bronchoscopy may be performed as a diagnostic procedure to obtain a specimen for examination, to break up adhesions, or to remove plugs of mucus in order to facilitate drainage from the lungs. The preparation is similar to that of the younger patient and is described in texts on medical and surgical nursing.[21] The utmost care must be taken that accidents do not occur during this procedure. The patient should be in his bed or in a wheelchair while the local anesthetic is applied to the pharynx; an extra pillow often is necessary when he is on the table to enable the patient to assume a position of hyperextension of the thoracic spine and to support him. If the procedure is done to facilitate drainage, the patient is not permitted to sit up immediately after it but is placed in the position prescribed for postural drainage. The patient must be prepared for the procedure and should know that he may not be able to speak for a few hours and that he should not swallow until the gag reflex returns. Equipment should be placed conveniently so that he can expectorate saliva as it accumulates. Before any fluids or food are taken by mouth the return of the gag reflex should be tested. This is done by gently touching the posterior pharynx with a tongue blade or applicator. Wide variations exist, but usually the reflex returns within about two hours after the procedure is completed.

Postural drainage. Postural drainage for the geriatric patient must be gently administered. Position for drainage must be individual for each patient, depending upon the part of the lung involved and his general condition. Elevation of the foot of the bed, which thus places the patient in shock position, often produces good results. The patient may also lie with his head to the foot of the bed and on his side, with the affected lung uppermost, and the knee Gatch of the bed raised. This position is satisfactory for draining the lower lobes of the lung if it is certain that the patient lies so that the upper chest is sufficiently lowered to facilitate drainage by gravity (Figure 47). One possible limitation to this method is that the patient may become tired and uncomfortable in a short time and may move until his chest is no longer being assisted by gravity in the drainage of the accumulated secretions in his chest.

Postural drainage may be poorly tolerated by many elderly patients when too great an alteration from a normal posture is demanded. The unusual position may cause dyspnea, palpitation, sweats, apprehension, and headache. The vas-

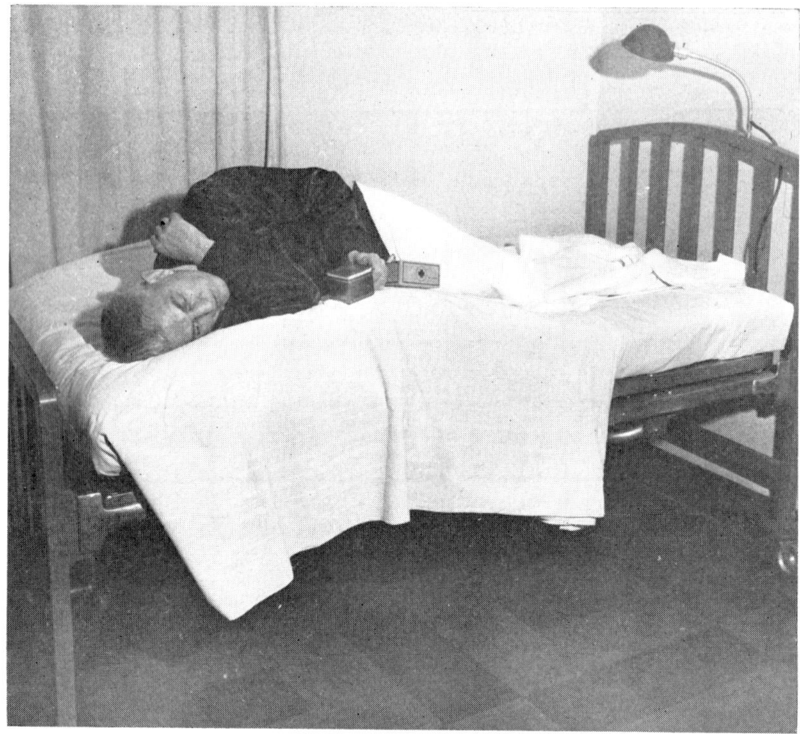

Figure 47. This method of postural drainage is effective and is well tolerated by the elderly patient.

cular system may not be able to accommodate to the sudden marked change in position. The nurse should report any unusual signs of distress to the physician immediately. Whatever the particular method desired by the doctor, the nurse can help to make the patient moderately comfortable by the arrangement of pillows. Unless it is specifically ordered, the older patient should not be placed for postural drainage on the abdomen, crosswise over the bed with the head resting on the floor, as is done for drainage in younger persons. Even with the addition of a stool on which a pillow can be placed and on which the patient's head and arms can rest, this position may be too strenuous for aged people.

Oxygen. Oxygen is prescribed for many elderly patients with pulmonary disease. Discretion in its use, however, is employed widely by physicians since it is known that too much oxygen may decrease the stimulus to respiration and thereby increase the accumulation of carbon dioxide in the lungs and in the blood. This may lead to a reduced use of oxygen and to respiratory acidosis.

Oxygen is sometimes prescribed to be used by the patient in his own home for emergency. When this is done, the nurse should be certain that the patient and members of his family know how to use the equipment correctly and also that they are aware of the safety precautions that must be taken. The danger of explosion or fire from lighted matches must be stressed.

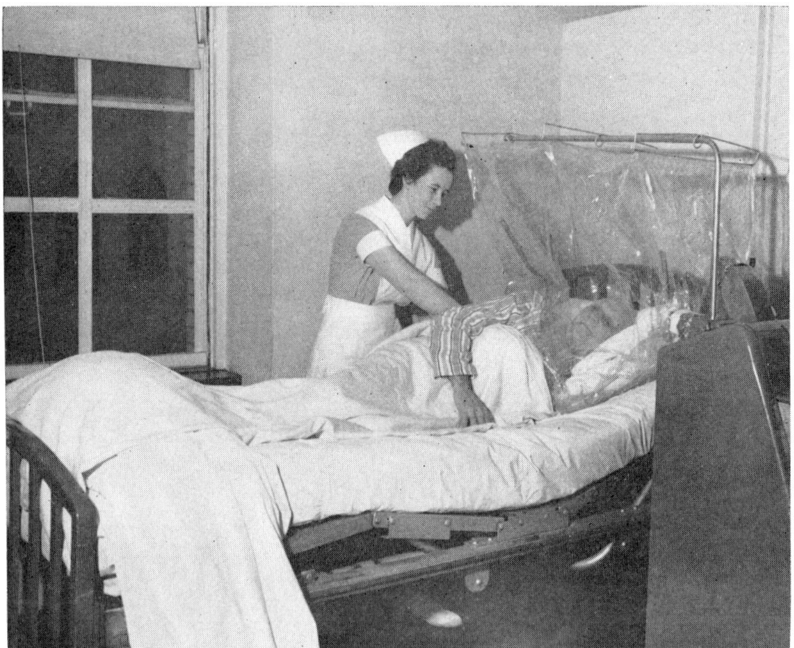

Figure 48. Nursing care can be given while the patient remains in the oxygen tent.

Oxygen may be prescribed in a mixture of helium; since helium has lower molecular weight than nitrogen, the patient can inhale the gas with less effort than is necessary when inhaling air. Oxygen may be given in a variety of ways, including mask, mask with intermittent and positive pressure, by nasal catheter, by catheter through a tracheostomy opening, and by tent.

The geriatric patient needs reassurance if oxygen is ordered. He often may have the mistaken belief that oxygen is a last resort and that his condition is therefore critical. When the oxygen tent is used, the patient should not be taken from the tent for any purpose until it is ordered by the physician. It is not difficult to tuck the tent canopy about the patient's neck and give him skin care and other attention without removing his supply of oxygen (Figure 48). Care must be taken, too, to see that the tank of oxygen is not allowed to become empty and thus interrupt the flow of oxygen to the patient.

Many elderly patients with chronic pulmonary diseases have drugs prescribed that must be inhaled through a nebulizer as liquid sprays, or as aerosols or dust sprays. Some elderly patients who have poor strength in their hand muscles have difficulty in using hand sprays. Treatment may be more effective if pressure can be obtained from a mechanical device such as the oxygen tank in the hospital or the clinic. In the patient's home, the small tank of oxygen that is now available may be ordered, or other mechanical means may be provided. The patient usually benefits most from the treatment if he inhales approximately half of the medication and then rests for five to ten minutes before completing inhalation of the drug.

DISEASE CONDITIONS

Asthma. Asthma is an adverse pulmonary reaction to some substance to which the individual is sensitive and which is termed an antigen. This reaction is characterized by edema of the bronchial mucosa, production of sputum, and spasm of the muscles of the bronchi that in turn obstructs the free flow of air upon attempted exhalation. This produces the wheezing sound upon exhalation which is so characteristic of the disease.

Asthma may have persisted since youth, or it may come on spontaneously in the later years of life. Usually, however, it is *intrinsic* in origin or caused by factors already within the body, such as bacteria that may have been harbored for years. *Extrinsic* factors, or those outside the body such as foods and pollens, are more common causes of asthma in young people. Occasionally, asthma may follow a change in climate and living conditions in which unfamiliar dust and pollens are encountered. In some cases it may follow retirement from work, which brings the person in contact for longer periods with some aggravating substance about the home.

The inability to exhale normally places increased pressure on the alveoli, which may become distended, and emphysema may develop. Bronchiectasis may complicate asthma as a result of constant pressure of air upon the weakened bronchial walls, and infection may then rapidly follow the accumulation of fluid in the dilated bronchioles. Asthma in the aged is often complicated by, or followed by, heart enlargement and signs of increased burden on the cardiac system. In the elderly person, cardiac function may be barely adequate to carry on the demands of the body under normal circumstances and it may be ill equipped to cope with the strains imposed by the severe bouts of coughing, the diminished supply of oxygen, and the secondary infection.

Treatment of asthma always includes search for the cause of sensitivity by careful questioning regarding the patient's environment and often by skin testing. Epinephrine, the drug which is so specific in relaxing the bronchioles, is as effective in the aged as in the younger patient, and usually the patient or some member of his family is instructed in how to give the drug hypodermically. Antihistamine drugs are of no value for this type of allergic disease. Other drugs that are useful and are used include ammonium chloride and potassium iodide by mouth to loosen secretions, bronchodilating drugs such as isoproterenol hydrochloride (Isuprel Hydrochloride), and liquefying agents such as normal saline solution or Alevaire, and aminophylline, a bronchial relaxant given by mouth, intravenously, or as rectal suppositories. Antibiotic drugs such as penicillin may be given intramuscularly and also by inhalation. Adrenocorticosteroids are prescribed occasionally for severe cases.

Bronchiectasis and lung abscess. Although bronchiectasis is really a disease of the young, it also occurs quite often in the elderly. It is thought to be primarily caused by a congenital weakness of the walls of the bronchioles that results in the breaking down of the alveoli and the bronchiolar walls. Aspiration of a foreign body, chronic bronchitis, and asthma may also lead to bronchiectasis. Secretions accumulate in the distended bronchioles and become infected with pyogenic organisms. Large amounts of sputum with a foul odor are often produced.

Lung abscess may be caused by unresolved pneumonia, the aspiration of foreign material, an area of atelectasis following anesthesia, malignancy, trauma to the lung, or tuberculosis. Signs of lung abscess are loss of appetite, weight, and strength. There may or may not be production of sputum; this depends upon whether or not the lesion opens into a bronchus through which sputum can drain.

Patients with bronchiectasis or lung abscess may have increased temperature and also a chronic cough. Differential diagnosis is usually made upon x-ray examination. Sometimes a radiopaque substance is used to visualize the extent of involvement in bronchiectasis.

Treatment of bronchiectasis and lung abscess may be surgical. Nursing care is then similar to that described for malignant lesions of the lung, or tuberculosis. Many older patients with bronchiectasis and lung abscess are not good candidates for surgery and must be treated conservatively. Sometimes involvement in both lungs makes surgery unsuitable. Supportive treatment often consists of attention to nutrition, postural drainage, and avoidance of additional infection that may make the condition more serious. The patient may be advised by his physician to winter in a warm climate if he can afford to and wishes to do this.

Emphysema. Emphysema, which is a common disease in old age, is caused by a decrease in the normal elasticity of lung tissue. Other factors such as changes in the size of the thoracic cavity and postural changes may also contribute to its development. Air is held in the distended and nonresilient bronchioles, exchange of air is reduced, and hypoxia follows. Dyspnea and cough are the most troublesome symptoms. The dyspnea differs from that seen in cardiac disease in that it is not relieved by assuming a sitting position. It appears that the incidence of emphysema is increasing, and there is evidence that it may be aggravated by smoking, the inhalation of toxic and noxious fumes during work hours, and the constant inhalation of the polluted air so often present in our large cities. There is no cure for the disease, which is slowly progressive. Fatigue increases gradually and is followed by lack of appetite and loss of weight and further fatigue until the patient becomes a total invalid.

There is no specific treatment for emphysema, although there is much research going on at present to seek better methods of prevention and treatment, and there are hopes that in the future the disease may be slowed in its progress or even reversed. Vigorous and prolonged coughing should be avoided because it may cause additional injury to the alveoli and because it contributes to fatigue and to discouragement. Because the patient is less likely to cough if he limits activity, he usually is advised by his doctor to avoid any exertion that causes dyspnea. The doctor may suggest that the patient lie most of the time in the position that favors drainage from the bronchi in the involved portions of the lungs, and occasionally percussion over the chest wall can be used to good effect. The patient or a family member may be instructed to assist with this.

Abdominal supports to elevate the diaphragm sometimes help the patient use the diaphragm more effectively in exhalation. The patient may assist himself manually in exhalation by placing his hands below the costal margin and pressing up and in during the last third of exhalation. Several other specific exercises have been described and recommended by some physicians,[27] and pamphlets describing exercises are available for patients, if permitted by their own physician.[6] Other medical authorities, however, believe that the benefit from exercises is quite limited.[3]

Oxygen, drugs such as aminophylline and ephedrine to control bronchospasm, and antibiotics such as penicillin may be used. Positive pressure breathing may also be ordered, and air and oxygen, or oxygen and helium may be given. This may be given continuously (upon inhalation and upon exhalation) or intermittently (upon either inhalation or exhalation) for varying periods of time.

The patient who has emphysema needs to avoid situations in which he is exposed to upper respiratory infection. Family gatherings must occasionally be missed, and recreation should be planned to avoid crowded indoor spaces and also to avoid undue exposure outdoors. The patient must also try to avoid emotional stress that may increase his respiratory needs. Depression is a problem encountered often in the care of the patient with emphysema.

Pneumonia. Pneumonia is still fairly common in older people, though the use of antibiotics has produced a striking reduction in the number of persons suffering from this disease. Among many factors contributing to pneumonia in old age are poor chest expansion, poor circulation, and decreased sensitivity of the pharyngeal reflexes that make the inhaling of foreign material more likely, particularly during sleep. Because pneumonia often follows a mild upper respiratory infection, the elderly person must be cautioned to avoid exposure to colds and to take particular care of himself if an upper respiratory infection does develop. Bronchopneumonia in the aged is more common than lobar pneumonia. Pain may not be severe, and other symptoms may either appear suddenly or come on gradually. Respirations are rapid and usually are out of proportion to temperature and pulse increases. The onset and progress of pneumonia in the older person is often much less dramatic than in the younger one. Slight cough, drowsiness, and apathy may be the only symptoms, and the patient may not appear as ill as he really is.

Many physicians believe that at the first signs of pneumonia the older person should be taken to a hospital, since it is difficult to transport him if the disease becomes severe and complications develop. If this is not possible, nursing care can be given in the home. Usually both penicillin and one of the broad-spectrum antibiotics such as Aureomycin are given.

The patient should be kept comfortable, with a minimum of sedation. Bed position may contribute greatly to the comfort of the patient. Often he is comfortable in a low Fowler's position with a pillow against the lower back. This brings the chest forward and permits better lung function than when the viscera are crowded against the diaphragm as so often happens when a Gatch break is used to secure a high Fowler's position. The patient may respond favorably to elevation of the head of the bed on shock blocks. When this is done, the abdominal viscera are crowded very little. Sometimes the patient is more comfortable sitting at intervals in a chair. If this is permitted, he must avoid exertion in getting in and out of bed since pneumonia places a severe strain upon the heart of the elderly patient.

Paralytic ileus is a complication of pneumonia in the elderly. The results of paralytic ileus in the geriatric patient may be serious, and effort should be made to prevent the condition from developing. This is one reason why an older person with pneumonia is now often permitted out of bed. The patient should be observed closely for symptoms such as distention, and the old remedies such as rectal tube, stupes, and enemas are still useful. Prostigmin is often ordered if signs of paralytic ileus appear.

Tuberculosis. Although the total number of active cases of tuberculosis in the United States dropped from 200,000 in 1952 to 120,000 in 1960,[24] there is proportionately more of the disease among the older population than the younger, and this is in direct contrast to the situation twenty-five years ago. The disease is much more common in men than in women when old age has been reached. The incidence of tuberculosis among persons living in homes for the aged and other sheltered care facilities seems high, though it is not known in many instances whether the infection was active on admission. It is known that lesions of tuberculosis can become active after having been inactive for many years.

Many aged persons who have tuberculosis may reveal a history of coughing and expectoration over a period of many years. In the past a chronic cough was accepted as relatively normal in old age. Centuries ago, Hippocrates said, "Old men suffer from difficulty in breathing, catarrh accompanied by coughing."

Many more persons are living to become old, and therefore to spread the disease to those around them if they have it. It may be, though, that tuberculosis is not more common among the aged than it used to be, only that it is now more often diagnosed. The outlook for the future is good as far as the incidence of tuberculosis in age is concerned. Two generations ago, or even one, there was a much higher incidence of primary infection throughout the general population than there is today. In some parts of the world even now, almost 100 percent of the population is exposed to tubercle bacilli in early life. Most of our present aged, however, are products of a time when the nature and control of tuberculosis were not as well understood as they are today, when diagnostic and curative facilities were limited. The future generation of aged persons should have much less tuberculosis, provided that an increasing number of old people do not spread the infection to the young who, if they survive it, will then harbor the infection into their own old age. Developments in use of specific drugs may produce marked changes in present trends.

An older person is most likely to have pulmonary tuberculosis. The lesion is often chronic and accompanied by fibrosis. It may persist for years, with chronic cough and production of sputum. It may progress slowly and may not be accompanied by an elevation of temperature. Night sweats due to weakness are infrequent since diaphoresis is decreased in age, and, except for chronic cough, symptoms may be almost entirely absent. If they are present, weakness and poor appetite are often attributed to old age and other causes and may be ignored as possible signs of tuberculosis.

The nurse has an important function in the control of tuberculosis in the aged. She must do her utmost in the hospital, the clinic, or the home to dispel the often accepted notion that tuberculosis is not a disease of the old. Another belief among certain groups of our population is that if tuberculosis is present in the aged, it is "worn out." Even though the person has been known to have had

Table 4. Mortality from specified chronic respiratory diseases*

By color and sex. United States, 1958-59 and 1949-50

	Average of annual death rates per 100,000									
	Total persons		*White*				*Nonwhite*			
			Males		*Females*		*Males*		*Females*	
Disease	*1958-59*	*1949-50*	*1958-59*	*1949-50*	*1958-59*	*1949-50*	*1958-59*	*1949-50*	*1958-59*	*1949-50*
Total, excluding asthma	9.8	5.1	17.0	8.1	3.8	2.7	9.8	4.2	3.9	2.1
Bronchitis†	1.3‖	1.4	1.9‖	1.8	0.8‖	1.1	1.6‖	1.5	0.9‖	1.3
Pneumoconiosis and other occupational lung diseases	0.8	1.0	1.9	2.1	§	§	0.7	0.5	§	§
Other chronic interstitial pneumonia	2.0	0.6	2.8	0.9	1.2	0.4	3.0	0.6	2.0	0.3
Bronchiectasis	1.3	1.4	1.9	2.1	0.9	1.0	0.9	0.8	0.3	0.4
Emphysema‡	4.2	0.7	7.9	1.3	1.0	0.2	3.5	0.7	0.6	0.1
Asthma	3.7‖	4.5¶	5.2‖	6.2¶	2.3‖	3.0¶	4.7‖	4.2¶	3.0‖	3.3¶

*Courtesy Metropolitan Life Insurance Co.; source of basic data: National Vital Statistics Division, National Center for Health Statistics.

†Chronic and unqualified; includes cases with emphysema.

‡Without mention of bronchitis.

§Less than 20 deaths or rate less than 0.05.

‖1956-1957.

¶1951-1952.

the disease for forty years, he and his family may have come to feel that since it has not killed him in that time it is not dangerous. The elderly patient with a history of "cured" active tuberculosis earlier in his life and a chronic cough may fail to see any relationship between his own history and the death from tuberculosis of some member of his family. Babies are the most susceptible and unfortunately are the ones most frequently exposed to tuberculosis infection by loving grandparents. No one would dispute the right of the elderly to share in the joy of association with the young. Nothing could be further from present concepts of a full and satisfying life for both the oldest and youngest generations. Consequently, safety from the danger of transmitting tuberculosis must lie in regular physical examinations, including x-ray examination of the chest and careful investigation of a chronic cough in older persons. Every older person should be considered a tuberculosis suspect until examination shows him to be free of the disease.

The public health nurse has an excellent opportunity to do case finding and health teaching among the older people in her community. She may have a chance to meet the older relatives when she visits another member of the family. In the prenatal visit, for example, she may inquire about the family circle into which the new member is coming. It is at this time that the confidence of the family should be gained in order that later suggestions may be more readily accepted if a member of the family should have tuberculosis or any other ailment requiring medical investigation.

Skill and tact are required in dealing with persons who have tuberculosis. Sadly enough, in our enlightened age people still fear social ostracism if it is known that a member of the family has contracted tuberculosis. Many people still shun the person who has had the disease even when it is certain that there is no danger of his giving it to others. Recent programs of rehabilitation for patients who have had tuberculosis have emphasized sharply the difficulties of those persons in gaining employment.

The elderly patient may have many emotional problems common to age. These may make it difficult for him to accept a diagnosis of tuberculosis. He may be lonely and insecure. If he lives in a family, he may wonder whether he is really wanted or needed in the family or whether his hospitalization would be a welcome relief to his family. If he has lived alone for years, he may not be able to accept the necessary adjustment of moving to a sanatorium that may be far from friends and familiar surroundings. Furthermore, in his youth he may have learned to look upon consumption as meaning death. For these and many other reasons he may flatly refuse to accept the fact that a cough that he has had for years can possibly be dangerous, either to himself or to others.

The older person who has tuberculosis should sometimes be cared for in a hospital. This should be near enough to his home to allow family and friends to come regularly, so that feelings of rejection and unhappiness will not develop. The trend toward building housing facilities for patients with tuberculosis nearer to the city or as part of the general hospitals may help to eliminate some of the isolation and loneliness that patients with tuberculosis have suffered in the past when they were obliged to go long distances from their homes or families to sanatoriums. Permitting the patient to retain his old-age assistance check while he is in the hospital would encourage elderly patients who live alone to enter the hospital. Often the patient fears and dreads the details involved in reestablishing his right to assistance when he leaves the hospital.

Treatment for the elderly patient with tuberculosis varies with each individual patient, but rest and adequate diet are considered important. The older person may still believe that cold climates and high altitudes are good for tuberculosis. This is no longer considered good therapy for anyone, much less the aged patient who may have cardiac complications.

Drugs now assume a major role in the treatment of tuberculosis. Many patients with active tuberculosis are receiving drugs and being managed completely on an ambulatory basis. This pattern of medical management is particularly fortunate for the aged patient, since it entails very little change from his accustomed mode of living. It is exceedingly important, however, for the nurse to be alert to toxic signs in all patients she sees and that she instruct the patient or the persons responsible for his care so that correct dosages of drugs will be taken, and difficulties will be reported promptly if they occur. The antibiotic streptomycin is now often given in combination with para-aminosalicylic acid. The combination appears to delay development of resistance to streptomycin by the organisms and also allows therapy to be continued for many months without the appearance of toxic signs of streptomycin. Streptomycin is often given intramuscularly twice each week, and para-aminosalicylic acid is given daily by mouth. Toxic signs of streptomycin are disturbance of hearing and of equilibrium, both of which may lead to accidents and may cause the elderly patient who already has defective hearing to take the drug with reluctance. Para-aminosalicylic acid is irritating to the gastrointestinal tract and is usually given after meals with a full glass of water. The tablets are enteric coated and occasionally escape dissolution to be expelled in the stools. If this occurs, it should be reported to the physician at once. Many elderly patients complain of vague gastric disturbances and hesitate to take pills regularly for the year or more that is often necessary. The patient with cardiac disease who is on a low-sodium diet cannot be given the sodium form of the drug, which is less irritating to the stomach.

Another drug, isonicotinic acid hydrazide (INH) or isoniazid, appeared in 1951 and proved to be extremely useful in the treatment of tuberculosis. The drug is given by mouth. The nurse should observe all patients who receive this drug for signs of toxicity to the nervous system. It is now given with para-aminosalicylic acid (PAS) in most cases.

The management of tuberculosis in older people presents some distinct problems. This is true because the traditional plan of care has tended to neglect the needs of the individual personality and to cause feelings of isolation and rejection. The patient in whom the sputum is positive should be treated as one who has an acute communicable disease, and major emphasis should be on teaching the patient how to protect persons about him if he is an active source of infection. The nurse must help in carrying out the isolation regulations in the hospital or agency in which she works. It may be difficult to teach older people measures for control of the spread of infection. The patient may not even believe in the germ theory of disease. In his youth, tuberculosis may have "run in families" or have been "inherited." The older person may not accept some details of general living that are conducive to good hygiene. For instance, some older people refuse to use paper tissues instead of handkerchiefs. Sometimes it is possible to obtain pieces of old muslin that can be used and burned and thus keep the patient happier and the persons around him safer. The nurse must remember that many of the typical changes of age will be present. Patients may not see or hear well and may forget easily. They may have very definite opinions, and sometimes the only way change in conduct can be achieved is to first make the older person feel that the nurse, the doctor, and the hospital are genuinely interested in him and in his welfare.

Some patients are too ill or enfeebled to carry out precautions and will always require strict isolation for the safety of others. It is an impossible task to tell the patient who is terminally ill that he must cover his cough and wear a mask when he is already struggling for existence. Sometimes he may be irrational and cannot be given an explanation.

Many physicians advise a period in a sanatorium or hospital where control of the spread of infection to others can be taught more effectively than is often possible in the home. Many older people, however, cannot or will not go to the hospital. They may particularly dislike the specialized tuberculosis facility that has for decades geared its program to the younger patient. If the patient remains at home, the nurse has the responsibility of teaching him and also the family who may be responsible for his care how he may continue to live in the community and not be dangerous to others. With the aid of the new drugs, the sputum becomes negative in a relatively short time in many of these patients. If this is a probability, it is encouraging to them to know that advised precautions may be only temporary.

The older person with tuberculosis is usually not kept on strict bed rest. He must move about sufficiently to stimulate circulation, and he may be allowed up and about in his room. Exercise must be kept within reasonable limits as prescribed by the physician. Diversion is one of the best forms of therapy for any ill person. Activities in which the patient may keep occupied and produce something useful are beneficial and psychologically uplifting; diversional facilities such as radios, movies, and television help to make the necessary confinement more acceptable and tolerable.

The general condition of many patients may benefit from attention given to bed posture. Lying on a firm bed with a pillow placed against the lower back to produce mild hyperextension for short periods each day aids in more adequate function of lung tissue and prevents further collapse of the rib cage. If the patient is confined to bed, the nurse must see that the range of joint motion is being retained and that no contractures or deformities are developing.

Diet is important for the elderly patient with tuberculosis. Appetite is often poor, and it may be difficult to find nutritious foods that appeal to the patient. As much individual attention as possible should be given to food likes and dislikes.

The nurse should bear in mind that any elderly patient in her care may be an undiagnosed tuberculosis patient. The question has not been settled as to whether the nurse's greatest exposure comes from care of the undiagnosed patient or from her work on the tuberculosis ward. Almost every nurse can name instances from her experience in which she has cared for a patient who was not isolated only to find later that he was suffering from an active tuberculosis lesion and had positive sputum. This points to the need for every nurse to observe the details of preventive hygiene that were impressed upon her early in her nursing preparation. She should wash her hands carefully and often, keep them away from clothing and the face, and wash them most thoroughly before meals.

REFERENCES AND RELATED BIBLIOGRAPHY

1. Baird, K. A.: Chronic respiratory disease in the aged, J. Am. Geriatrics Sec. **10**:1062-1071, 1962.
2. Barach, Alvan L.: The management of respiratory infection in older patients with asthma and pulmonary emphysema, Geriatrics **8**:423-428, 1953.
3. Beeson, Paul R., and McDermott, Walsh (editors): Cecil-Loeb textbook of medicine, ed. 11, Philadelphia, 1963, W. B. Saunders Co.
4. Comstock, George W.: Untreated, inactive pulmonary tuberculosis, Pub. Health Rep. **77**: 461-470, 1962.
5. Davis, Loyal (editor): Christopher's textbook of surgery, ed. 7, Philadelphia, 1960, W. B. Saunders Co.
6. Haas, Albert: Essentials of living with emphysema, Patient publication no. 4, 1963,

The Institute of Physical Medicine and Rehabilitation, New York University Medical Center.

7. Jenney, Florence S., and Cohen, Archibald C.: Changing pattern in causes of death in pulmonary tuberculosis, Dis. Chest **43**:62-67, 1963.
8. Jones, Julia M.: Tuberculosis among the aged, Nurs. Outlook **4**:675-678, 1956.
9. Krug, Elsie E.: Pharmacology in nursing, ed. 9, St. Louis, 1963, The C. V. Mosby Co.
10. Lerner, George C.: Functional treatment of lung disease, J. Am. Geriatrics Soc. **10**:794-799, 1962.
11. Litwack, I. D., and Gardener, John: Reactivation of apparently inactive cases of pulmonary tuberculosis, Pub. Health Rep. **79**:823-828, 1964.
12. McClure, Eugenia J., and Anderson, Leighton L.: Pulmonary emphysema, Amer. J. Nurs. **57**:594-598, 1957.
13. Meyers, J. A.: Chronic disease of the lungs. In Stieglitz, Edward J. (editor): Geriatric medicine, ed. 3, Philadelphia, 1954, J. B. Lippincott Co.
14. Moriyama, Fwao: Chronic respiratory disease mortality in the U. S.: Pub. Health Rep. **78**:743-748, 1963.
15. Murphy, Monica: An emphysema clinic, Amer. J. Nurs. **65**:80-81, 1965.
16. Prindle, Richard A., and Yaffe, Charles D.: Motor vehicles, air pollution and public health, Pub. Health Rep. **77**:955-962, 1962.
17. Proetz, Arthur W.: Disease of the upper respiratory tract. In Stieglitz, Edward J. (editor): Geriatric medicine, ed. 3, Philadelphia, 1954, J. B. Lippincott Co.
18. Reinmann, Hobart A.: Acute disease of the lungs and pleura. In Stieglitz, Edward J. (editor): Geriatric medicine, ed. 3, Philadelphia, 1954, J. B., Lippincott Co.
19. Roberts, Albert: Public Health Service activities in chronic respiratory diseases, Pub. Health Rep. **80**:336-338, 1965.
20. Secor, Jane: The patient with emphysema, Amer. J. Nurs. **65**:75-81, 1965.
21. Shafer, Kathleen Newton, and others: Medical-surgical nursing, ed. 3, St. Louis, 1964, The C. V. Mosby Co.
22. Sieker, H. O.: Pulmonary disease. In Johnson, Wingate M. (editor): The older patient, New York, 1960, Paul B. Hoeber, Inc., Medical Book Department of Harper & Row, Publishers.
23. South, Jean: Expanding objectives for tuberculosis associations, Nurs. Outlook **11**:286-288, 1963.
24. Tuberculosis Branch, U. S. Public Health Service: Cases on current tuberculosis register, Pub. Health Rep. **76**:12, 1963.
25. Welder, Robert J., and Fishbein, Ronald: Thoracic surgery in patients over seventy, Dis. Chest **44**:61-66, 1963.
26. Williams, M. Henry, and Robinson, Faulkner N.: Pulmonary emphysema and nursing care of the patient with pulmonary emphysema, Amer. J. Nurs. **63**:88-96, 1963.
27. Williams, Marjorie J., and Mendel, Julius L.: Pulmonary emphysema, adrenocortical hyperplasia and peptic ulcer, Dis. Chest **44**:303-306, 1963.

Chapter 22

Nursing in diseases of metabolism

DIABETES MELLITUS

Diabetes mellitus, a metabolic disease that involves the use of insulin by the body, is increasingly prevalent with each decade. There are now 2,500,000 persons in this country with known diabetes,[3] and it is a fact that there are many people who have diabetes not yet diagnosed. Recently a survey in a small section of the country indicated that estimates had been too low and that there are at least 4,000,000 persons in the United States who have this disease.[15] Since the highest incidence of diabetes occurs during the fifth and sixth decades of life, it is anticipated that there will be an even greater increase as more and more people live to middle age and beyond.

Several factors may contribute to the statistics that show an increase in diabetes. Extension of life allows more time for persons with predisposing characteristics to develop the disease. Other significant factors may be better diagnostic facilities for early detection of diabetes and the discovery of insulin, which permits a person with diabetes to live longer and to transmit the inherited predisposition to the disease. Before insulin was discovered, a child with diabetes seldom lived more than a few years; now few children die of it. Although it is known that the tendency to develop diabetes is inherited as a Mendelian recessive characteristic, it is thought that additional factors are required to precipitate the disease.

In the United States, the widespread habit of overeating may be a factor contributing to the increased incidence of diabetes. When the disease occurs in persons over 40 years of age it is often accompanied by or follows obesity, and there is some evidence that excessive consumption of carbohydrates can suppress the normal production of insulin. Diabetes is more common in women than in men and often appears after the menopause. Obesity during the childbearing period has been named as one of the most important factors. This would seem to be borne out by a study of a group of married and single women which revealed that the incidence among the married women was almost twice that among the single women. In this study the married women weighed an average of 180 pounds, whereas the single women weighed an average of 160 pounds.

It is yet to be proved, however, that the development of both the obesity and the diabetes is not part of a complex metabolic disturbance aggravated, perhaps, in this instance by the pregnancy.

Diabetes is a very costly disease for our nation. The National Health Survey revealed that only ten diseases were responsible for a greater loss of working days than diabetes with its associated ills. The public expresses little concern over the disease, since diabetes does not have a strong emotional appeal. Voluntary health agencies that give service to patients with diabetes receive only five cents per person per year, whereas only a few years ago more than fifty dollars was given for each person with poliomyelitis. Much of the lack of thought is because the public has not sufficient knowledge of the nature of diabetes and the treatment necessary. Leading public health experts believe that teaching the public about diabetes and initiating programs for detection of the disease are a responsibility of public health agencies dedicated to improving the nation's health.

The American Diabetes Association* publishes literature and promotes case finding, treatment, and research. It makes a simple kit for testing urine to assist in the detection of of the disease. This kit is available free of charge at pharmacies throughout the country. Through recent widespread campaigns for detection of diabetes and education about the disease, the public has become more interested, particularly if diabetes has occurred in some member of a family.

In several parts of the country diabetes detection clinics have discovered the disease in some persons in whom it might otherwise have gone unrecognized for years. Relatives of persons with diabetes have been invited to attend the clinic for diagnostic tests since it is relatively common for diabetes to occur in more than one member of a family. Testing the urine is now such a simple procedure, some physicians are advising the potential diabetic and the close relatives of persons who have known diabetes to test their urine at regular intervals. In the elderly, however, it has been found that sometimes the urine is free of sugar while the blood sugar is elevated markedly. Regular testing of the urine will help to ensure earlier treatment for some persons who develop diabetes although, ideally, much earlier treatment by such measures as weight reduction should be undertaken in an effort to prevent the condition from developing at all.

Routine physical examinations for elderly people by their own physicians should assist in discovering many incipient cases of diabetes before injurious effects have occurred. In the past some promotions aimed at motivating the public to have tests for diabetes overemphasized the "advantages" of a diagnosis of diabetes, with the argument that the continuing medical care the person received might extend his life beyond even that of the person who did not develop diabetes. Although continuous medical supervision of the person with diabetes is indeed important, some of the associated conditions, such as retinal damage, seem to be beyond medical control at the present time; however, other illness, such as a lesion of cancer, vascular changes, or heart disease, may be discovered earlier than when only occasional medical examinations are given.

---

*The American Diabetes Association, 1 East 45th St., New York, N. Y.

Diabetes mellitus develops when a derangement occurs in the secretion or use and distribution of insulin. Insulin normally is secreted by the islands of Langerhans in the pancreas, and its presence makes carbohydrate metabolism possible. When there is insufficient insulin, the liver attempts to use fat in place of carbohydrate in order to produce glycogen, which is essential. The result is that ketone bodies are produced faster than the body is able to dispose of them. What actually causes the islands of Langerhans to cease or alter their function has not as yet been determined. It is now believed that diabetes may be only one manifestation of an extremely complex metabolic disturbance in which several of the endocrine glands and certainly the pituitary are involved. For example, the pancreas may secrete enough insulin, but it may be destroyed by an antagonist. This may occur in acromegaly or when an adrenal tumor develops. It is known that the person who has had the pancreas removed can often maintain a relatively normal blood sugar level if he takes 25 to 30 units of regular insulin per day, yet some young persons with severe diabetes mellitus require 200 or more units per day.

There is still a great deal about the development of diabetes that is not known. For instance, in the young who develop diabetes, there is no relationship whatsoever with obesity. There appears to be no relationship between control of blood sugar at normal levels and the rate of development of retinal changes. It is found that vascular changes develop faster in many persons with diabetes than in nondiabetic persons, even when blood sugar is controlled carefully.

Tumors of the pancreas may interfere with function of the gland and lead to symptoms of diabetes. Cancer of the pancreas is more common in older persons and should be suspected if any symptoms of digestive disturbance or signs of jaundice appear in anyone who has diabetes.

Signs, symptoms, and diagnosis. One of the most characteristic differences between diabetes mellitus in the elderly person and the younger one is that in the elderly, the condition usually is mild. Many aged individuals have diabetes for years without realizing that anything is wrong. Many learn for the first time that they have diabetes when a sudden boil, abscess, toe or foot infection requires medical aid, when failing vision necessitates a visit to the doctor, or when hospitalization for treatment following an accident or other medical problem leads to discovery of the diabetes.

The classic signs—hunger, thirst, frequency of urination, and loss of weight and strength—may be found, though sometimes few of these are present. Drowsiness after meals is common. Patients may recall that they have felt tired a great deal, have had burning on urination, or frequency, which they attributed to "weak kidneys," and have had aching of the legs and feet that they assumed to be part of old age. The aged skin tolerates the high sugar content of the urine poorly, and local pruritus is frequent, sometimes being the first and most distressing symptom. Nonspecific neurologic symptoms and psychic disturbances occasionally occur. Vague pains in the feet and legs are often due to the arteriosclerotic changes that are so characteristically present in chronic diabetes. In this type of arteriosclerosis the intima or inner lining of the arteries is involved and eventually thickens to occlude the free flow of blood. This results in inadequate blood supply to the tissues and causes general pain and discomfort. The patient often attributes his symptoms to advancing years, rheumatism, and like ills and does not report the symptoms until serious damage has occurred. Local gangrene may appear before the person learns that he has diabetes if he has not been under the care of a physician and has not had urinalyses at fairly frequent intervals. Sugar in the urine can occur even in the absence of diabetes, but it points to the need for a thorough and complete investigation as to its cause. It should not be interpreted by the nurse as a sign of diabetes until definite medical diagnosis has been made by the physician.

The diagnosis of diabetes mellitus is made by means of urinalysis and studies of the sugar levels in the blood. Procedures relating to these tests and the nursing care required are no different from those for younger patients and are described fully in current nursing texts.[17] Preparation for tests to be done on the ambulatory patient who is elderly should be written and explained carefully, since he may forget instructions given verbally. Bottles should be labeled clearly with print large enough for ease of reading when urine specimens are to be collected. The time for collecting urine samples, for refraining from meals, and for reporting to the doctor's office or the clinic should be stated definitely.

Medical treatment and general nursing care

Nursing guidance of the aged person with diabetes demands the greatest understanding of the psychology of the individual as well as an ability to reconcile the conflicting opinions of the members of his family in regard to what he should or should not do. Modern treatment of the aged person with diabetes is directed toward removing as far as possible the restrictions that the disease may impose and permitting as normal a life and as many normal experiences as are possible. Some clinics now make special provision for each patient who is diagnosed as having diabetes to have a conference with the nurse after seeing the doctor. Usually, at this time fear is prominent in the patient's mind since he begins immediately to speculate upon how much his life will be limited and if he may become a hopeless invalid. The nurse can contribute substantially to his future adjustment and acceptance of his situation by allaying fear. She should at this time let him talk about his fears, give explanation as needed, emphasize the things that can be done and are not altered by the diagnosis, and make plans with the patient for future visits in which he will learn to care for himself.

Some older people definitely do not wish to accept the limitations that diabetes may impose. They have made their own analysis and planned their own particular solution. In some cases they may have decided to do as they please even though it may mean earlier death, rather than accept any diet change, use of insulin, and possibly other restrictions. Some physicians agree with the patient and feel that such decisions are the privilege of the individual. The nurse must remember that the individual, in the last analysis, must be given the responsibility for his own destiny. She can, however, help to make those necessary restrictions less burdensome and thus more acceptable. She may help the patient to see that by his failure to accept treatment he is affecting others besides himself. By his refusal to take insulin if it is prescribed, the patient may bring added work and unhappiness to members of his family. The aged person with diabetes, as so many other common mortals, may be inclined to say that he wishes to live for today and will let tomorrow take care of itself. When the tomorrow with its irrevocable ills comes, he may regret his decision.

No one can force the patient to take insulin if he is not willing to do so. No one can make him adhere to any prescribed diet. Neither the doctor nor the nurse nor the family can do this if the patient himself does not wish to participate in plans for the treatment of his disease. It should be pointed out to him just what the implications of his actions are to himself and to his family. While leaving personal judgment to the individual, one should be certain that he realizes the significance of the neglect of treatment and the possible aftermath if he ignores the instructions of his physician.

The patient may feel it would be better to die of the disease because he feels he is a burden and thus not welcome in his particular family situation. It is imperative that every effort be made to help him remain as independent and self-sufficient as his age and general physical and mental condition permit. If he is able to do these things safely, the patient should learn the constituents of an adequate diet, administer his insulin, record his weight, and care for his feet.

Some older people welcome diabetes because it brings them solicitous attention from members of the family. To many lonely older people, the trip to the clinic becomes something of a social occasion to which they look forward with pleasure. Some welcome the presence of the visiting nurse in the home because of the break in the monotony of their day, and many appreciate the attention of the nurse more for the companionship she offers than the actual service that is rendered.

Another fear is that if surgery is ever necessary the chances of recovery are lessened by the diabetes. If the condition is known and the patient has followed the regimen prescribed, he faces little more risk than a patient without diabetes.

An obligation of the nurse is to teach the patient or those responsible for him so that the diabetes is treated as prescribed by the doctor, and so that associated conditions that will often develop despite the taking of insulin may not develop into serious complications. To accomplish this, her approach and expectations for both herself and the patient must vary as much as individuals do; the rate at which she achieves her objective will vary also.

Medical treatment. Medical treatment for the patient with diabetes varies with the age of the patient, the severity of the diabetes, the convictions of the physician, and other factors. Some physicians believe that there is insufficient evidence to show the advantage of a regimen that requires keeping blood sugar levels at approximately normal with little or no excretion of sugar in the urine. They point out that arteriosclerosis and retinal changes leading to blindness seem to be much more closely related to the duration of the disease than to the strictness of control of blood sugar level. They believe that treatment should consist primarily of the patient's maintaining his weight at normal, taking insulin or antidiabetic drugs as prescribed without fail, eating normally with avoidance of more than average carbohydrate in the diet, and using a feeling of well-being as an index to the success of treatment. By far the larger number of practicing physicians, however, believe that it is wiser to keep blood sugar levels within normal limits and to avoid the excretion of sugar in the urine. There is general belief that complications may be delayed if the diabetes is "controlled," that is, if the blood sugar level is controlled. It is the nurse's responsibility to maintain the patient's faith in his own physician and to help him follow instructions accurately in the prescribed treatment of his disease. The patient should understand that individuals vary and that what has been recommended for his neighbor is not necessarily good treatment for him.

Diabetes mellitus may be treated by modifying the patient's diet, having him lose weight, and giving insulin or antidiabetic drugs. Diabetes is often less severe in the aged and the development of acidosis is not common. In many instances the disease is relatively well controlled with only minor alterations of diet and without taking insulin. Some patients who have had to take insulin are able to discontinue its use when excess weight is lost and diet has been regulated moderately. All physicians agree that excessive use of carbohydrates is unwise for the person who has diabetes.

Usually treatment also includes teaching the patient so that complications such as infections, signs of limited circulation, and difficulties related to failure in insulin treatment or diet do not occur. Occasionally, the physician feels that the elderly person should spend a period of time in a hospital where he may learn about his diet, how to test his urine if it is necessary, how to give insulin to himself, how to care for his feet, and in general how to live with his disease. Most patients are now learning these things in the clinic or in the doctor's office. Often a public health nurse is called upon to teach the patient in his own home or to follow up after a period of instruction in the hospital.

Diet. Considerable variation in medical thinking exists in regard to diet for the person with diabetes. The trend is toward greater freedom in diet where more liberal use of carbohydrates is permitted. Most geriatricians are agreed that sudden changes in diet are not satisfactory for older people. All are agreed that basic nutritional needs are important for persons with diabetes as for anyone if health is to be maintained. Particular attention should be paid to seeing that the patient receives adequate amounts of the protective foods daily. Older people who are alone are likely to overlook some of these essentials.

It is not sufficient that the diet for the older person with diabetes be adequate for his physical needs. It must also be psychologically acceptable. Modern treatment leans toward liberality in diets for the elderly person, to try to fit the food to the likes, dietary beliefs, and cultural traits of the individual. In order to help the patient adapt dietary restrictions to his particular eating habits, the nurse needs a sound, basic knowledge of caloric, mineral, and vitamin values of common foods and of the normal requirements of these constituents. Furthermore, she must have a generous amount of resourcefulness, plus a genuine interest in her patient's dietary needs, likes, and restrictions. There is little justification for the monotonous diet so often given to a person with diabetes, since imagination and effort will often yield an appetizing meal.

In the older age group food likes and dislikes that are definitely fixed are often encountered. These are so largely a matter of habit and long custom that they are difficult to change. In fact, many physicians experienced in caring for the aged feel that sudden changes in diet are not desirable because some individuals who have sustained a high blood sugar level for years do not respond well to rapid attempts at its reduction. In addition, some of the reactions of the aged to dietary change are unexplained and out of all proportion to the apparent changes being brought about by insulin and diet. When a diet to bring about radical changes in the weight and blood sugar level is ordered, the nurse must watch her patient and report any changes such as disorientation, fatigue, dyspnea, headache, and like symptoms.

The number of calories needed depends upon activity. A liberal amount of protein is generally accepted as good nutritional therapy; at least one to one and one-half grams per kilogram of body weight per day is the amount needed by the aged. Opinions vary regarding the amount of carbohydrate and other dietary essentials that should be given in diabetes. Some physicians still feel that in order to stimulate the islands of Langerhans, liberal amounts of carbohydrate with barely enough insulin to ensure its utilization should be given. Others believe that much of the carbohydrate usually taken in the diet should be replaced by fat in order to decrease the insulin needed.

If the patient is overweight, gradual weight reduction is usually advised. Sometimes there is no longer need for insulin when normal weight has been regained. Food exchange lists prepared by the American Diabetes Association, the United States Public Health Service, and the American Dietetic Association are extremely helpful in assisting the elderly patient to plan satisfactory meals without too many calories These lists (available in booklet form from the American Dietetic Association) give substitutes and equivalent foods and thus enable most people to select foods they can enjoy.

If a weighed diet is ordered by the physician, the patient or persons responsible for his care should receive instruction in the weighing and estimating of food portions. This instruction is usually given by the dietitian or the nurse in the clinic or doctor's office, and frequently by the nurse in the home. A satisfactory method of teaching is to weigh the food and then demonstrate the approximate equivalents since most patients are permitted by their physicians to estimate food amounts. The patient should be instructed to weigh food at weekly or biweekly intervals to be certain that minor errors in the estimation of portions are not becoming habitual.

Insulin. There are now six kinds of insulin—each different in its onset, rate, and duration of action. It is important that the name of the prescribed insulin be written down for the patient. He should be advised to always take the empty bottle to the druggist when he purchases more insulin.

Taking insulin is often a real problem to elderly patients, but it can be made more acceptable when a single daily injection is administered. The patient may associate the use of a syringe and needle with drug addiction or with some chronic disease of a hopeless and disagreeable nature. He may fear what others will think if they discover that he takes insulin. One elderly and seemingly very intelligent woman hid, even from her husband, the fact that she took insulin. Many cannot face the actual details of the procedure of injecting the needle into

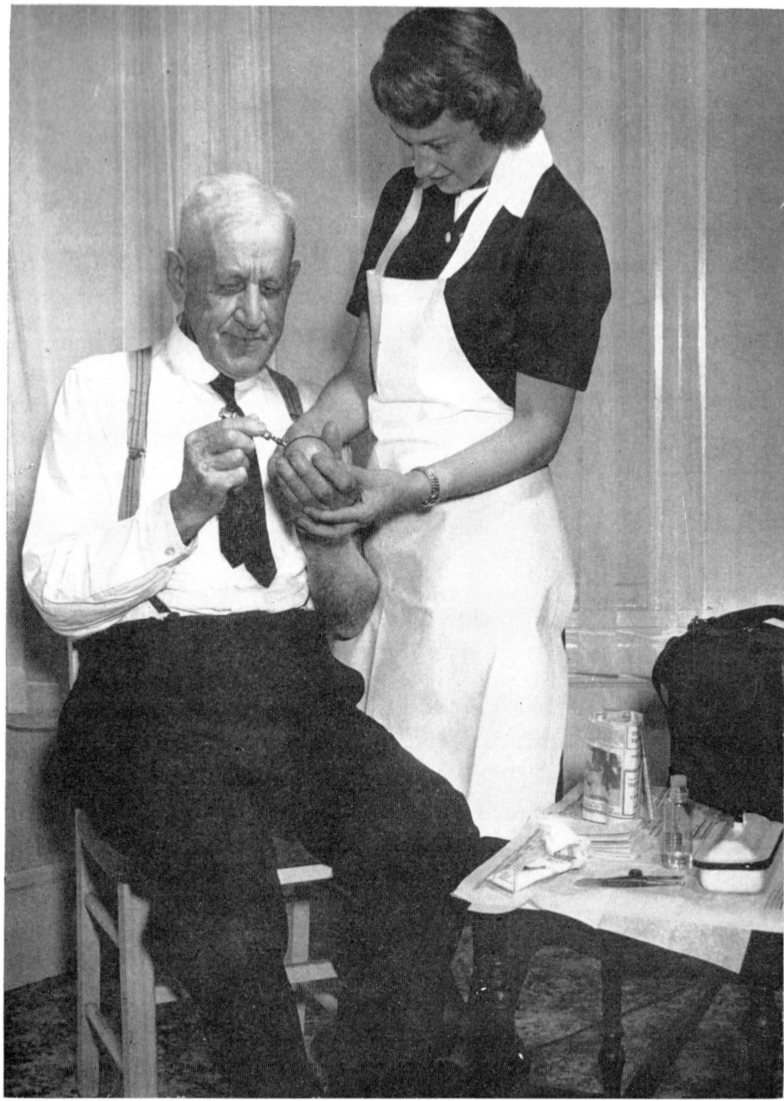

Figure 49. Patience and persistence are needed when the patient learns to give insulin. He may practice on an orange before giving the injection to himself. (Courtesy New York State Health Department; photograph by Freitag.)

themselves, and many resent the time and inconvenience required to prepare the injection and to care for the equipment. Elderly people who are employed fear that the knowledge of their being obliged to take insulin will result in loss of employment and inability to secure another job. Certain forms of insurance are denied the person with diabetes, which may cause the patient to refuse to accept the disease. Some older people interpret the daily need for insulin as a sign of their physical decline and growing helplessness since it gives them a feeling of being tied down and deprived of freedom. Others who have visual disturbance may fear that they will give themselves the incorrect dosage of insulin. For these reasons and many others, the patient may actually reject the fact that insulin is vitally necessary for him. Some believe they cannot afford the insulin. One older lady of limited means chose a biweekly ration of meat for her dog in preference to the purchase of required insulin for herself.

With patience and persistence on the part of the persons who work with them, many elderly people are able to give themselves insulin and are happier for being able to do so. When the patient lives in a family, it is well to instruct another member of the family also. A good deal of supervision is necessary, and it is usually essential that the public health nurse see the patient at home after he leaves the hospital. Questions that need to be answered may arise. Throughout the teaching it is important to stress the need for taking insulin regularly as prescribed. Insulin must never be omitted without medical permission. Aseptic technique must also be carefully supervised, since the patient may often follow procedures quite accurately while he is in the hospital and become careless when he returns home. He also requires supervision in accuracy of insulin dosage. Care must be taken that he understands the strength of the insulin that he is to use and that labels on the bottle are correct and legible. A small magnifying lens is helpful for persons with failing vision. The patient is advised to keep this with his equipment and to use it in reading the label on the bottle and in checking his dosage in the syringe.

Partial or total blindness occurs fairly often among elderly persons with diabetes. Sometimes these patients live alone, and the administration of insulin becomes a real problem. So pressing became this problem that one nurse devised a method of controlling a syringe so that the blinded person could determine the amount of insulin drawn into the syringe. She reported that she had encountered five such patients in her work during one year. A syringe (Cornwall syringe) in which the plunger can be locked at a desired level may be used; in this way the blinded person can be taught to give his own dosage of insulin. The syringe is quite expensive, and the elderly patient, who often has limited financial resources, must sometimes have economic assistance in the purchase of the equipment he needs. It is quite common that older people with diabetes break syringes, since many have somewhat tremulous hands. The cost of the syringe, however, is small in comparison to that of the daily visit of a nurse to administer the insulin. A special stop has been devised that can be fitted to the regular 1 ml. B-D insulin syringe. This can be adjusted by the doctor or nurse and enables many people with limited vision to give their own insulin safely. A magnifying glass with wire attachments. (C-Better) is now available; this can be slipped over the syringe at the place where dosage must be carefully read. Disposable syringes are now available at fairly reasonable cost. It is possible for the patient to have a relative withdraw several doses from the bottle and place them in a safe place in the refrigerator. The small publication *Aids for the Blind,* prepared by the American Foundation for the Blind, Inc.,* lists and describes

*15 West 16th St., New York, N. Y.

many items that would be helpful to the nurse who is assisting an elderly patient adjust to limited vision.

Oral hypoglycemic agents. Several years ago it was noted that certain sulfonilamide drugs produced hypoglycemia, and from this discovery several related drugs have been produced that have proved extremely useful in the treatment of elderly persons who have diabetes in a mild form. The exact mode of action of these drugs is not known, but it is believed that some of them stimulate the secretory action of the cells that produce insulin. They are not effective in treating severe juvenile diabetes, nor in experimental animals when the islands of Langerhans have been removed.

Oral hypoglycemic agents are a boon to the elderly person with failing vision and general difficulty in giving injections. One difficulty encountered, however, is that the patient often fails to realize the seriousness of his condition when he receives treatment by mouth. The ambulatory patient must be reminded of the danger of increasing his dosage to cover dietary indiscretions—a practice that is fairly common among persons who give their own insulin. The patient may also feel that because he can be treated with tablets and does not have to use a needle his condition is not serious, and he may become careless about general health care. He should adhere to the same dietary discretions, must take the same special care if an infection occurs, and must take the same precautions to preserve circulation as the patient who takes insulin by injection.

It has been found that 80 percent of older persons with diabetes mellitus respond to the use of oral hypoglycemic drugs.[3] The oldest and most widely used is tolbutamide (Orinase). The usual dosage is 1 to 2 gm. (15 to 30 gr.) taken daily usually in two doses before breakfast and lunch. The maximum action is reached in four to six hours. Many times the maintenance dose can be reduced to as little as 0.5 gm. (7½ gr.) per day. There are toxic reactions to the drug and these should be watched for and reported at once. They include gastrointestinal disturbances, blood dyscrasia, ringing in the ears, headache, weakness, and paresthesia. Patients taking this drug appear to have a lowered tolerance to alcohol and may develop a typical hypoglycemic reaction if much alcohol is taken. It has been found that medical supervision tends to be less frequent for patients who are receiving drugs orally than for those who take insulin by injection. The nurse must encourage the patient to visit his doctor at regular intervals.

Newer oral hypoglycemic agents include chlorpropamide (Diabinese), which is more potent, destroyed more slowly in the body, and more toxic than tolbutamide. It also acts by stimulating the secretion of insulin, and the toxic reactions are similar to those of tolbutamide.

Another drug that is undergoing extensive clinical study at this time is phenformin hydrochloride (DBI). The action of this drug is not clearly understood but it is believed that it acts by stimulating intracellular glycolysis, or the process by which glucose is broken down into more usable cellular elements.

Testing of urine. The patient may be taught to test his own urine. Benedict's test, the tablet test (Clinitest), the powder test (Galatest), and the paper test (Clinistix) are available. For the older person who lives alone who may have failing vision and uncertain movement, the tablet, powder, and paper tests are simpler and safer although more expensive. These methods require no heat, therefore the older person who lives in a furnished room or a boarding house can do the test inconspicuously in his own room. He is also spared the danger of burning himself as he might do in heating the Benedict's solution over a flame. Some patients are asked to test the urine for acetone. Again, tablets (Acetest Reagent Tablets) that make this simple for the patient are now available.

Complications. Insulin shock and diabetic coma are two complications that can occur. The elderly person seems to possess some resistance to both of these conditions. He goes into shock or coma less easily than the young, active, or growing person. Insulin shock is more dangerous for an elderly person than for a younger person because it may cause myocardial failure, a cerebrovascular accident, or increase in anginal symptoms. Every effort is made to prevent insulin shock from occurring in older patients by impressing upon them the need to take food regularly, even if their appetite is poor. If the patient has digestive difficulty and is unable to eat, he should get in touch with his physician at once. The patient usually is taught that he must never under any circumstances omit insulin without consulting his physician. Some physicians wish to have the patient test his urine regularly to be certain that he has a trace of sugar in the urine so that insulin shock is not apt to develop.

Coma occurs when ketone bodies are produced faster than they can be disposed of and accumulate in the body (ketoacidosis). Signs of coma in the aged are the same as at any age and include headache, flushed dry skin, nausea and vomiting, fruity odor to the breath, air hunger (Kussmaul breathing), and unconsciousness. Patients in coma must be treated immediately by a physician if they are to survive. They must have glycogen, and salt that has been removed must be replaced. Sugar is given to restore glycogen, insulin is given to provide for the utilization of the sugar, and normal saline solution is given to replace fluids and salt lost in the urine. Sugar may be given as glucose intravenously, by gavage in the form of orange juice, or in any other solution containing sugar. Diabetic coma in the aged may be confused with cerebrovascular accident. Some physicians advise their patients with diabetes to carry a small card on their person stating that they have diabetes. In the event of sudden loss of consciousness when they are away from home, this may assist in diagnosis and speed early treatment if the trouble is caused by either diabetic coma or insulin shock.

The best treatment for diabetic coma is prevention. One of the most common causes of coma is the failure of the patient to take the prescribed insulin because he had some ailment and was not eating regularly. It must be emphasized that illness, whether it be a cold, a mild gastrointestinal upset, or something more severe, increases the need for insulin no matter what is eaten.

ASSOCIATED CONDITIONS

Certain abnormal conditions occur often in conjunction with diabetes. They do not seem to be caused by the disease in the strict definition of the term, but they are so often present that some definite relationship may exist. From a nursing standpoint it is not so important just whether diabetes specifically causes or

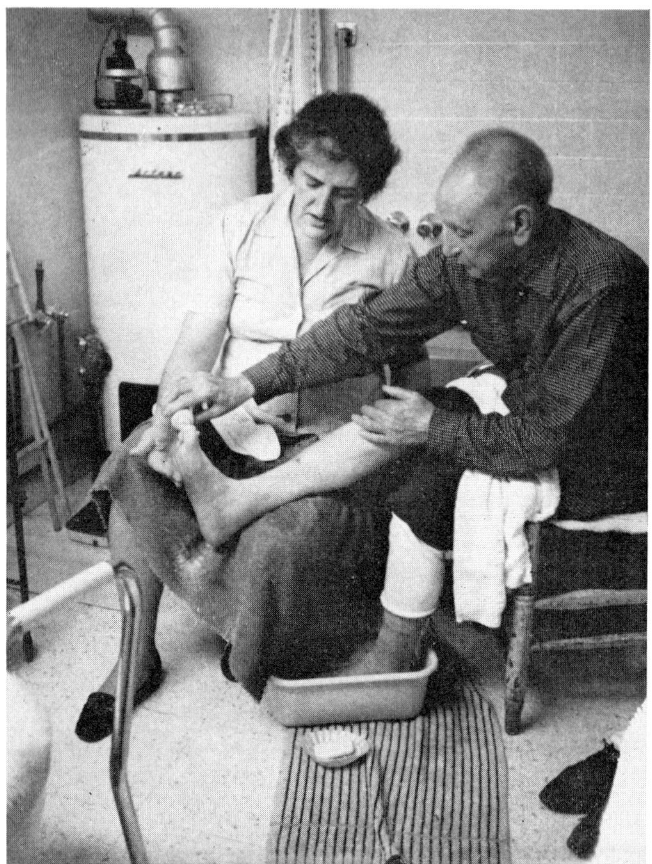

Figure 50. The old person with vascular changes must learn to care for his own feet, but he will need encouragement and help from family members.

does not cause these conditions. It is important that the nurse recognize them. She should know that in their early recognition and management lie much of the hope in protecting the person with diabetes from complete invalidism and dependence upon others.

Arteriosclerosis. Arteriosclerosis is now the most common complication of diabetes mellitus and has far surpassed diabetic coma as a cause of death in those with diabetes. Nothing specific is available at present to prevent the development of atheromatous changes in blood vessels. Much, however, can be done in the care of individuals in whom these changes have taken place in order that crippling complications may not develop. In the diabetic clinic and in her daily contact with patients, the nurse sees a large number of persons with vascular changes of the lower extremities. It is in this area that her responsibility in assisting with the complete teaching and care of these patients is the greatest. Teaching the patient with vascular changes the care of his feet, the choice of shoes, and the avoidance of trauma and infection is an essential part of the nursing care of the aged person since these changes are present in a large number of elderly people who have diabetes. Measures must be taken to preserve what arterial flow still remains. For example, tight garters must be avoided, knees should not be crossed, and special exercises are often prescribed. (For details of care of the patient with arteriovascular changes of the lower extremities, see Chapter 14, Nursing in Cardiac and Renal Disease.)

Albuminuria. Albuminuria occurs fairly often in diabetes and often accompanies arteriosclerosis and hypertension. It does not yield to the administration of insulin. Its damaging effects may be lessened by controlling weight, avoiding infection, and other measures that relieve the work load of the damaged kidneys.

Retinopathy. Diabetic retinopathy occurs quite often in elderly patients, though it seems more closely related to the duration of the diabetes than to the age of the patient. The exact cause is obscure. Diabetic retinopathy often occurs when arteriosclerosis is present, but this is not always the case. The amount of hyperglycemia does not seem to have any direct relationship to the disease process, although it is more frequent and more severe among persons who have gone undiagnosed or failed to limit their diet and to take the prescribed insulin for a long period of time. Unfortunately, this condition does not as yet yield to medical treatment; the main treatment consists of psychologic and physical rehabilitation as the condition progresses.

The nurse caring for the older patient with diabetes should be on the alert for signs of visual impairment. It is important that, as visual difficulties increase, the patient be taught to care for himself in order that maximum self-sufficiency may be preserved. He should be taught some activities that will help to sustain him if he becomes completely blind. He may be taught to read braille, to give his own insulin, and to care for himself in various ways. The patient who realizes that his vision is becoming poor day by day is likely to be discouraged and depressed. He must be kept occupied so that he does not have time to dwell upon his future too much. He needs encouragement. A friendly word about his progress will do much to encourage his efforts toward retaining self-sufficiency.

HYPOGLYCEMIA

Hypoglycemia is a relatively common disorder in which the blood sugar becomes too low. It may drop to abnormally low levels a few hours after a meal or after exercise. The condition is not primarily one occurring in old age, but mild hypoglycemia states may become more pronounced because the patient develops a poor dietary pattern and may eat too much carbohydrate.

Signs and symptoms of hypoglycemia include sudden onset of faintness, headache, feeling of anxiety, and nausea. Pronounced weakness, twitching, convulsions, and complete loss of consciousness can occur, and among the elderly, particularly, these can lead to serious accidents.

Hypoglycemia often is functional with no cause for the condition found. Rarely, it is caused by a tumor of the pancreas, which increases the production of insulin, or by liver disease, which may cause an inability to store glycogen.

Hypoglycemia responds best to a diet high in protein. Excess protein is converted gradually to glycogen while carbohydrate is metabolized more quickly. The elderly person who has symptoms of this condition should have a careful review of his eating practices. Often this will reveal a diet that is deficient in protein. He should eat meals that are spaced regularly and are high in protein. Also, he should carry lump sugar or candy ready for immediate consumption if symptoms appear. Symptoms may be controlled in the elderly patient if he develops the habit of taking a glass of skim or dried milk between meals and before sleep.

OSTEOPOROSIS

Osteoporosis is a condition in which there appears to be a metabolic defect in the relationship of bone formation to bone resorption. There are many secondary causes such as immobilization, but the term usually applies to the demineralization that occurs in later life and is responsible for the fragile bones and the frequency of fracture of the bones among the elderly. It is believed that hormones (notably estrogen) in some way affect the bone metabolism and that their lack permits the resorption of bone at an increased rate.[7] It is known that lack of the anabolic steroids permits a negative nitrogen balance to occur and that this disease is primarily one of protein metabolism and not of use of calcium. The interesting observation has been made that osteoporosis is less common in parts of the country where fluoride occurs naturally in the water supply.[18] It is not known whether a relationship exists between lack of this substance and the disease.

Osteoporosis is much more common in women than in men and occurs frequently following the menopause; 80 percent of clinical cases in geriatric practice occur in women.[16] So frequent is the condition in elderly women that it has been listed as the most commonly seen anomaly in the vertebral column upon roentgenogram examination and exceeds even arthritis in incidence. Actual figures for the incidence of the condition have not been recorded; it is so common that little attention has been paid to it, and it is likely that there is some osteoporotic change in bones of all elderly women. It is estimated that there must be approximately 40 percent demineralization of the bones before roentgenograms show pronounced disease.

Osteoporosis develops most often in the vertebrae and in the long bones. Many times the patient has no knowledge that anything is wrong until a fracture occurs, or until severe symptoms following collapse of a vertebra cause him to seek medical aid. The condition often is discovered when roentgenograms are taken for some other diagnostic purpose. Pain may not be a symptom unless bone changes have altered alignment so much that pressure occurs or strain is placed on nerves and supportive structures. This may be the cause of low back pain in elderly women. Sometimes compression of the vertebral bodies occurs. This decreases the height of the trunk and increases the curve of the thoracic spine. A feeling of lack of stability, noted most when walking on uneven surfaces, and difficulty in maintaining balance may also be noted by the patient. The nurse should urge any elderly person with any of these signs and symptoms to seek medical attention.

Treatment of osteoporosis is not too specific. Effort is directed toward supporting the failing osseous system. Estrogen and androgen therapy has been effective for many patients. Estrogen therapy seems to be most effective for women who have developed the condition quite soon after the menopause. Usually an estrogen preparation such as Premarin is given for one week out of four. A diet high in protein, calcium, and vitamin D usually is ordered. Some studies show that increasing the intake of calcium and vitamin D is of little help unless hormones are given also and may even be harmful.[16] Some physicians feel that sunshine is helpful. If achlorhydria is present, dilute hydrochloric acid may be given.

The patient with osteoporosis must be protected from every possible accident hazard, such as slippery floors, dangling bathrobe cords, and ill-fitting shoes and slippers. If involvement is in the spine, walking on uneven surfaces, such as in the woods, must be done with extreme caution. The patient must be cautioned to take particular care when walking on poorly lighted streets where pavement may be uneven. The patient is advised not to lift any heavy object. He should not, for example, carry a suitcase, and plans must be made for delivery of groceries. Usually the doctor will specify to the patient the number of pounds that can be carried. He may be more comfortable with the weight distributed with part on each arm, but the total weight should not exceed that specified by the doctor. Use of a commode prevents the danger of falling while going to the toilet at night.

The patient must move about since complete immobilization may increase demineralization of the bones. Indeed, many physicians feel that daily exercise is imperative if the condition is to be kept from progressing. If severe pain occurs from further collapse or from injury it is usually treated with the judicious use of muscle relaxants and analgesics, and with rest on a firm bed—but not with complete immobilization.

Most physicians prescribe the continuous use of firm corsets or braces, although some believe that their use may lead to further demineralization from disuse and only encourage their use when the patient is being active. They may be used to enable the patient to be up and about and exercise with a moderate degree of safety and comfort.

The nurse who cares for an aged patient should bear in mind that older persons may have undiagnosed osteoporosis. Since the condition can be made worse by confinement to bed, all elderly patients who have been confined to bed for some time with illness, such as an attack of heart disease, must be mobilized with the greatest of care.

GOUT

Since the treatment and care of gout are discussed in current texts,[17, 20] it will be described only briefly here. The nurse has a responsibility to help correct the many existing misconceptions about the disease.

The classic picture of gout appearing in the great toe of men favored by economic fortune and prone to overindulgence in food is now known to be quite fallacious. Gout is no respecter of class and it is quite common; many of its victims have a high blood level of uric acid (hyperuricemia) and yet no joint pain or other signs.

Gout is a metabolic disorder that is currently undergoing extensive medical and scientific scrutiny. It is primarily a disease of young and middle-aged men, although symptoms may not appear until the patient is elderly. It is caused by a defect in purine metabolism about which much is still unknown. Studies also suggest that faulty excretion may be a contributing factor. The result is accumulation of uric acid in the blood and its ultimate deposit in joints and other locations, such as the tophi under the skin. Women, although having hyperuricemia, seldom develop the joint symptoms. Renal pathology develops in approximately 20 percent of those who develop joint symptoms of gout.

It is important that the patient receive treatment early. In many instances, relatives of persons with known gout have been found to have hyperuricemia. The test for this is not part of the usual physical examination but may become so in the future. The elderly patient should be reminded to tell his physician if he has close relatives with the disease. Typical signs and symptoms of gout are a sudden severe pain in a joint, usually developing during the night and becoming progressively more severe. The great toe, the ankle, or the arch of the foot are most likely to be affected. The joint may be hot and so painful that acute infection is suspected; the patient's temperature, however, usually is normal.

Gout can be treated satisfactorily, and the old standby drug colchicine is still considered the best. Phenylbutazone, probenecid, and adrenocorticosteroid hormones are also used. Other treatment usually includes regular physical checkups with determination of blood level of uric acid, a generous fluid intake, weight reduction if necessary, a normal diet with moderate intake of protein and avoidance of only a few foods that are particularly high in purine, such as liver, kidney, sardines, and anchovy. One of the most common misconceptions about gout is that it cannot occur except following habitual ingestion of large amounts of rich, fatty food. It has been demonstrated that the body manufactures purines far in excess of any amount taken in as food. Because of this conviction on the part of the laity, many persons with symptoms do not seek medical attention as soon as is advisable.

Alcoholic beverages are not contraindicated generally for gout, although occasionally a patient appears to have untoward response to it. For this reason many physicians discourage its use.

REFERENCES AND RELATED BIBLIOGRAPHY

1. Adler, Francis Heed: Textbook of ophthalmology, ed. 7, Philadelphia, 1962, W. B. Saunders Co.
2. Beaser, Samuel B.: A survey of current therapy of diabetes mellitus, Diabetes **13**:472, 478, 1964.
3. Beeson, Paul B., and McDermott, Walsh (editors): Cecil-Loeb textbook of medicine, ed. 11, Philadelphia, 1963, W. B. Saunders Co.
4. Committee of the American Rheumatism Association: Primer on the rheumatic diseases, New York, 1964, The Arthritis Foundation.
5. Couner, J. F., and Miller, B. H.: Clinical experience with oral hypoglycemic agents in an institutionalized group of elderly diabetics, J. Am. Geriatrics Soc. **10**:467-472, 1962.
6. Entmacher, Paul S., Root, Howard F., and Marks, Herbert H.: Longevity of diabetes patients in recent years, Diabetes **13**:373-377, 1964.

7. Frost, H. M.: Postmenopausal osteoporosis; a disturbance of osteoclasia, J. Am. Geriatrics Soc. **9**:1078-1085, 1961.
8. Harrison, T. R., and others (editors): Principles of internal medicine, ed. 4, New York, 1962, McGraw-Hill Book Company.
9. Hatch, F. E., and others: Diabetic glomerulosclerosis, Am. J. Med. **31**:216-230, 1961.
10. Jackson, Helen: Helping a blind diabetic patient become self-dependent, Amer. J. Nurs. **62**:107, 1962.
11. Jay, Arthur N.: Hypoglycemia, Amer. J. Nurs. **62**:77, 1962.
12. Krosnick, Arthur: Diabetic neuropathy, Amer. J. Nurs. **64**:106-108, 1964.
13. Krug, Elsie E.: Pharmacology in Nursing, ed. 9, St. Louis, 1963, The C. V. Mosby Co.
14. Locke, Raymond K.: Foot care for diabetics, Amer. J. Nurs. **63**:107-110, 1963.
15. Public Health Reports: Increase in number of diabetics **79**:878, 1964.
16. Ricitelli, M. L.: The management of osteoporosis in the aged and infirm, J. Am. Geriatrics Soc. **10**:498-504, 1962.
17. Shafer, Kathleen Newton, and others: Medical-surgical nursing, ed. 3, St. Louis, 1964, The C. V. Mosby Co.
18. Stare, Frederick J.: Good nutrition from food not pills, Amer. J. Nurs. **65**:86-89, 1965.
19. Strandness, D. E., Priest, R. E., and Dibbons, G. E.: Combined clinical and pathologic study of diabetic and nondiabetic peripheral arterial disease, Diabetes **13**:366-372, 1964.
20. Talbot, John H.: Gout, ed. 2, New York, 1964, Grune and Stratton, Inc.
21. Yount, Ernest: Metabolic diseases. In Johnson, Wingate M. (editor): The older patient, New York, 1960, Paul B. Hoeber, Inc., Medical Book Department of Harper & Row, Publishers.

Chapter 23

Nursing in diseases of the skin

The skin is a fairly reliable index of age. Probably no parts of the aging process have been more bitterly fought than the wrinkles, sagging, and pigmentation of the skin, baldness, and graying hair. Museums hold many exhibits of materials used by the ancients to prevent, delay, correct, or disguise the skin changes produced by time. Sales of cosmetics in our day indicate that a credulous public still hopes that miracles in rejuvenation of the skin can be achieved by their use.

Much serious scientific thought and study are being given to the skin changes that inevitably occur with age. Aging of the skin begins with birth or before, and unquestionably the process is well under way when complete growth is attained. Rate of change varies greatly, depending upon nutrition, hormone balance, familial tendency, nervous and mental states, and many other inherent factors. The skin loses its pinkish white color and becomes gray or faintly yellow; it becomes thinner, and the blood vessels, though often sclerosed and narrowed in their lumen, become more apparent. Subcutaneous tissues atrophy, elasticity diminishes, and drying of the skin follows. Pigmented areas or freckles (senile lentigines) are common on exposed skin surfaces such as the backs of the hands. These are not treated unless they develop into keratoses.

Skin diseases are somewhat unique in that with the exception of carcinoma, pemphigus, and certain deep mycoses they seldom cause death. They may be annoying out of all proportion to their seriousness, and next to the common cold, skin ailments are the most frequent cause of an older person's visit to the doctor.

There are few skin diseases wholly characteristic of age, except that malignant changes are more common in older people. Individuals, however, who have skin lesions in youth may live to be old; in which case the disease may improve or worsen, depending upon the nature of the lesion. The aged are spared some of the aggravating skin conditions of youth such as acne; psoriasis rarely has its onset after 45 years of age. Certain abnormal skin conditions such as pruritus often become worse as age advances and may be aggravated by lowered resistance to infection, poor circulation, drying of the skin, and other factors.

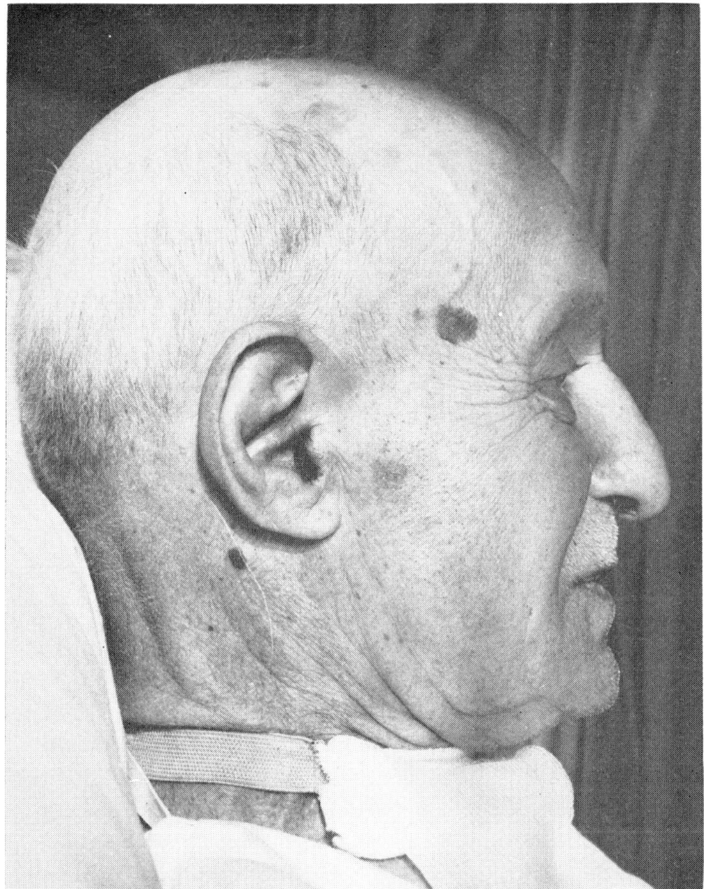

Figure 51. Note the skin changes that are characteristic of age.

PREVENTION OF DISEASE

Prevention of skin disease and control of lesions already present may sometimes be achieved by more adequate diet and fluid intake. Vitamin A and vitamin B are thought to be helpful in preventing skin diseases in the elderly. It may be that these vitamins retard skin changes, but do not prevent them. Diet is important in any skin condition of the aged since poor nutrition makes the skin more susceptible to further damage, and dehydration of the tissues may contribute to pruritus. Special effort should be made to secure the kinds of food that are acceptable to the patient and yet are high in the essential constituents. Elderly people often have a dislike for plain water so that substitutes such as tasty broths, milk, and fruit drinks are used.

Another preventive measure in control of skin disease is the avoidance of local irritation of any kind. Clothing should be clean and free from constricting bands that might cause irritation. Normal perspiration is acid and therefore bactericidal; though when it is allowed to accumulate over too long a period, it becomes neutral in reaction, and its useful properties are negated. Bathing for older people can be overdone, and in many instances it contributes to disease. The details of bathing the normal skin are discussed in Chapter 6, General Hygiene.

Mannerisms or habits of rubbing or scratching the skin (often because of nervousness) may cause irritation and subsequent disease. Alleviation of nervous strain by giving attention to economic and basic sociopsychologic factors will often result in improved skin health. It is useless to repeat to the older person that he should improve his diet and habits of living if the circumstances of his daily living offer no challenge for him to do so. For this reason, the dermatologist in treating his aged patient often leans quite heavily upon the social worker or others in helping him solve the basic issues that may underlie the patient's skin disease.

Teaching patients and their families to consider seriously any skin lesion is important in the field of general health education. Many minor skin ailments progress to a truly troublesome stage because patients attempt self-treatment before seeking medical care.

GENERAL NURSING

The first aim of nursing care for the dermatologic patient of any age is to make the patient feel that he is cosmetically acceptable to those about him. The aged patient may be even more acutely affected by a sense of rejection than the younger one. The deep, unspoken fear of being not accepted, not wanted, and not liked by others is present in each individual and becomes greater for the patient who has unsightly skin lesions on exposed parts of the body such as the face and the hands. The nurse should realize that what may seem a rather trivial ailment to others may be of tremendous importance to the patient, particularly if he is already insecure. One patient who suffered from an incurable and immensely disfiguring skin ailment confidently assured the nurse upon admission that he was able to attend to all of his own needs and would require little care or attention. What must have been the mental anguish that prompted this patient to attempt to forestall any further emotional trauma! Unfortunately, this aspect of nursing is overlooked by some nurses who mistakenly wear gloves, for instance, when the patient's disease is absolutely innocuous and safe to handle, though unsightly.

Skin lesions can be overtreated. An important fact for any conscientious and ambitious nurse to remember is that too much cleansing, treating, and changing of dressings can be more harmful than beneficial. She must be certain that she understands exactly how much treatment the physician wishes carried out.

Every effort should be made to prevent infection and further aggravation of open skin lesions in older people since the blood supply is lessened and healing takes place slowly. Touching, rubbing, scratching, removing dressings, and inspecting the lesion are activities that interfere with healing and yet are a temptation to the patient. Careful aseptic technique on the part of anyone who is dressing skin lesions is important. Hands must be washed thoroughly before applying medications or doing dressings. If the patient is ambulatory, he should be taught to change underwear and bed linen frequently.

Sleep and rest are important. The patient in the hospital is often happier when he is in a ward with other patients since this gives him greater opportunity to talk to others and diverts his attention from himself. The irritations from skin ailments tend to become worse at night when surroundings are quiet and there are few distractions. The patient needs the benefit of nursing measures to induce sleep, such as a warm drink, a back massage, and elimination of light and noise. The aged patient is usually a light sleeper, and when he is suffering from a skin disease, he sleeps even more lightly. If he is sleeping during the day, it is usually best not to disturb him since elderly patients become irritable to distraction from their inability to sleep or from lack of sleep. The room should be kept rather cool since warm air often aggravates skin symptoms and may interfere with rest and sleep. Small doses of phenobarbital are sometimes given to produce mild sedation, but this has the disadvantage of making the patient lethargic and may in itself produce a skin reaction.

Occupational therapy is essential in the complete care of most patients with skin disease, whether they are in the hospital or in the home. Any activity that keeps the patient busy and distracts his attention from his skin ailment or its feared consequences is justified and valuable. Occupational therapy must be carefully prescribed in some instances since the patient may be sensitive or allergic to some of the substances used in a well-equipped occupational therapy department.

The ambulatory patient with a skin lesion and associated pruritus is often advised by his physician to avoid alcoholic beverages, stimulating drinks such as tea and coffee, and occasionally all hot fluids. Since they cause vasodilation, they may increase pruritus.

Bathing. Bathing is done with caution when skin disease is present. Tepid sponges without the use of soap are often ordered instead of baths. The water for bathing may be softened by using a cup of ordinary, uncooked laundry starch or a handful of meal to a tubful of water. In the home, if it is available, rain water is excellent for bathing the delicate skin of the elderly dermatologic patient. While they allay itching in some instances, borax and sodium bicarbonate are not good for old people since they are alkalis and subsequently cause drying of the skin.

An oatmeal or bran bath may be prepared as follows. Add two cupfuls of cereal to two quarts of boiling water and stir the mixture as it boils for five minutes. Pour the mixture into a mesh or gauze bag. Stir the bag about in a tub filled with tepid water for a few minutes. The meal in the bag may be used as a mop to gently pat the skin and remove crusts and debris. Commercial preparations such as Aveeno are now available and their use, although costly, saves time.

A boiled-starch bath is prepared by pouring two quarts of boiling water over a cupful of corn starch moistened with cold water and stirring as it thickens. This may be added directly to the bath without straining through a mesh bag. The patient should stay in the tub for only a short time. Sometimes when itching is particularly severe, he may remain for as long as an hour, but he must be carefully watched for signs of fatigue. After a bath of any kind, the skin should be patted dry with a soft towel. Rubbing should be avoided. Soft, old sheets should be used on the bed, and sometimes "neutral" linen, in which the excess alkali of ordinary laundry soap has been counteracted by rinsing in a mild acid solution, can be used.

The use of water may be contraindicated for patients with skin disease. The physician may approve the use of cold cream as a substitute cleansing agent, and sometimes a cleansing lotion applied with a cotton sponge is refreshing to the patient.

Compresses and dressings. Hot and cold compresses are widely used in the treatment of diseases of the skin. It is often satisfactory for the patient to wash his hands and assist with his own compresses if suitable equipment can be placed at his bedside. However, care must be taken that an older person with impaired vision and uncertain movements does not burn himself if a hot plate is being used. It may take more nursing time to supervise the procedure and assist the patient than to apply the compresses oneself, but the patient is usually happier and is kept moving about in bed if he does this for himself. Both hot and cold or iced compresses should be changed as soon as they reach body temperature. Some elderly patients are annoyed by compresses; they object to what they term the constant fussing in connection with their use, whereas others like the attention they may receive in the frequent changes of compresses.

Hot compresses may be ordered when increased circulation to an affected part is necessary. Cold compresses are used to reduce inflammation and lessen itching. When cold compresses are applied, a piece of ice may be set in a bowl at the bedside, or a basin containing the compresses in solution may be placed in another bowl of crushed ice. If a cake of ice is used, it is obvious that the solution must be changed frequently since it will quickly become diluted by the melting ice. A solution of 3 percent aluminum acetate (Burow's solution) or 5 percent magnesium sulfate is often used for iced compresses.

Wet dressings are used to soften crusts, to promote and remove drainage, to combat infection, and to provide constant protection to healing tissues. A few of the many solutions used for wet dressings are potassium permanganate 1:10,000, hydrogen peroxide and mineral oil in equal parts, thick boiled starch, acetic acid or vinegar, physiologic solution of sodium chloride, and plain sterile water.

Gauze or pieces of old linen are best for the application of wet dressings. Cotton becomes soggy and uncomfortable and tends to hold heat and cause itching. Gauze should be used generously, and the compresses are then covered with waxed paper or oiled silk. An outer wrapping may be used, depending upon the physician's wishes and the purpose of the dressing. If an outer wrapping is needed, old Ace bandages that have lost their usefulness as elastic bandages are convenient for this purpose. An Asepto syringe that is directed carefully to the inner dressing so that contamination is avoided is satisfactory for moistening dressings. Care must be taken to moisten all parts of the inner dressing yet prevent the fluid from running through outer dressings to other parts of the patient's body or onto the bed. The frequency with which complete change of dressings is done depends upon the type of lesion and the amount of drainage. If the skin around the lesion appears macerated, this should be reported; usually wet dressings are alternated with either a dry powder dressing or use of a heat lamp. Certain solutions demand that the entire dressing be changed rather than the inner dressing simply moistened, since frequent moistening may increase the concentration of drug and cause irritation.

Ointments. Ointments with a petrolatum or lanolin base are more often prescribed for older people than pastes, which are more drying. Ointments should be carefully applied in small amounts and removed gently at prescribed intervals, using the solvent ordered. Large amounts of ointment and ointment left on the skin for long periods of time eventually become sticky and uncomfortable. Many healing ointments, such as scarlet red, contain dyes that stain linen; therefore the oldest sheets available should be selected for patients receiving this treatment.

Drugs and other preparations used for skin ailments are often costly. The nurse should know the cost of the preparations used and should direct her patient if he is at home to use enough to be effective yet avoid waste. In the hospital, supplies are often used wastefully.

Patient at home. Many patients with skin diseases are not hospitalized. In the home, the clinic, or the hospital, the nurse must be most specific in her instructions to the patient. Absolute accuracy in carrying out directions is essential because skin conditions often respond to small changes in treatment. For example, a skin ailment may respond to an ointment rubbed on very gently and lightly, whereas the trauma from vigorous rubbing of large amounts of ointment may counteract all the good of the medication and may even make the condition worse. If the skin lesion is an open one, the patient is taught to "butter" the ointment on a piece of gauze and then place this to the lesion. Often pieces of old linen napkin or bed sheeting are preferable to gauze if the patient can be taught to sterilize them by baking or ironing. The nurse must be certain that she herself thoroughly understands the doctor's directions and that she explains them clearly to the patient. The skin may respond to differences in strength of medications; therefore it is important that accurate dilution of medications for soaks, compresses, or dressings be given. Often it is best to write instructions in simple step-by-step form for the elderly patient caring for himself at home.

The older person with a skin disease becomes irritable and discouraged and needs repeated reassurance. Skin conditions are often slow in responding to treatment in persons of any age, and particularly in the very old. The patient and his family need encouragement in returning to the clinic and continuing to carry out instructions upon dismissal from the hospital or the clinic.

DISEASE CONDITIONS

Pruritus. Pruritus is one of the most aggravating conditions of old age and seems in many cases to be caused almost entirely by atrophic changes. It may be furthered by many chronic illnesses that may in themselves cause itching of the skin, such as uremia, jaundice, diabetes, pernicious anemia, and cancer. General hygienic measures already mentioned seem to be the best means of combating pruritus in the elderly. Improvement of chronic systemic disease and emotional health and removal of local irritating factors will often correct symptoms. Massage to improve circulation, use of oil on the skin, and use of superfatted soaps are often helpful. Cod-liver oil taken internally has been found useful for some patients, as has also a diet high in vitamins. Antihistaminic drugs are helpful in some instances. Remarkable improvement often follows the use of hydrocortisone ointment and this preparation, although quite costly, is prescribed widely. It is fortunate that with the exception of fluorohydrocortisone, no systemic effects occur from the topical application of corticosteroid and adrenocorticosteroid preparations, even when treatment is prolonged. Occasionally, when pruritus is severe, these preparations may also be given systemically.

Seborrheic keratoses. Seborrheic keratoses resemble large darkened warts and occur most often in persons who have oily skins. They are often found around the trunk and under the breasts. Although they seldom become malignant, they should be brought to the attention of a doctor. It may be difficult to distinguish them from senile keratoses, which often become malignant.

Senile keratoses. It is important to closely observe senile keratoses because they may undergo malignant change. They consist of small brownish or gray raised areas that appear most often on exposed areas of the body. There seems to be a familial tendency to develop keratotic spots, and exposure to sun and wind appears to hasten their growth. The areas may increase gradually in size and become covered with closely adherent scales, which upon removal leave a bleeding surface. If left undisturbed, they may develop a warty appearance and an inflamed base as the degeneration into epithelioma progresses. In the early stages of growth, keratotic lesions can often be removed by using soap and water, followed by an ointment containing 2 percent salicylic acid. Painting with a destructive acid such as trichloroacetic acid also is effective in many cases. The safest treatment is destruction by means of cautery. The nurse should observe all older patients for lesions of this nature and report their presence to the physician or advise the patient to do so.

Cutaneous horns are excrescences of horny cutaneous cells that project outward and may reach a length of half an inch or more. They may develop from senile keratoses and often have a malignant base. Elderly people who have such skin lesions should be advised to seek treatment also because these lesions are cosmetically so unattractive to those around them. Their treatment usually is the same as that described for malignant lesions.

Moniliasis. Moniliasis, or candidiasis, is a common fungus infection caused by a yeastlike organism *(Candida albicans).* When it occurs at the angles of the mouth, it is called perlèche. It often occurs in this location and is aggravated by sagging of tissues about the mouth, and by poor dental prostheses so that salivation occurs and the creases remain moist. This condition is best treated by improving dental fixtures and by keeping the skin clean and as dry as possible. Ammoniated mercury ointment, 5 percent, may be ordered. Monilial infection can occur in other moist surfaces of the body, such as under the breasts and in the groin.

Epithelioma and carcinoma. The term epithelioma means a tumor of the skin, but has come to be used almost synonymously with malignant lesions of the skin. These growths often follow other skin lesions such as keratoses, some moles, and cysts. They appear most often on the parts of the body exposed to sun and wind, and where prolonged irritation has existed, such as behind the ears and on the bridge of the nose when glasses are worn, on the lips of pipe smokers, and the back of necks of men who wear stiff collars. Some epitheliomas are highly malignant and metastasize early; the squamous cell carcinoma is an example. They do, however, have the positive feature of being where they can be diagnosed early and where they are accessible to treatment. In spite of this, though many older people recognize an irregular lesion on the skin, they neglect it for years before they seek medical advice. The public health nurse often has an opportunity to observe skin lesions early and should urge the elderly person who develops such a lesion to visit his physician at once.

Treatment for any malignant lesion of the skin consists of early and complete removal. This may be done by means of cautery, by surgical excision, by irradiation, or by a combination of these methods. Sometimes the surgical excision must be a radical one, and considerable deformity may result. The problems encountered in nursing care of the elderly following such treatment differs only in degree from that of patients of lesser years. Infection is likely to occur, and skin heals and regenerates slowly in the elderly patient. Meticulous aseptic technique is necessary and much patience is needed. The patient may become discouraged with the length of time required for recovery.

Since malignant skin lesions may recur, the nurse should instruct the patient to report immediately to his physician if any changes occur. Usually the person who has been treated for a malignant lesion of the skin is observed at intervals for many years. The nurse must impress upon him the importance of keeping appointments as directed.

Leukoplakia and kraurosis vulvae. Leukoplakia involving the mucous membrane of the mouth has been considered in Chapter 19, Nursing in Disease of the Gastrointestinal System. Leukoplakia of the vulva and kraurosis vulvae are described in Chapter 26, Nursing in Gynecologic Disorders.

Herpes zoster. Herpes zoster is a rather infrequent but extremely distressing condition caused by virus infection of sensory nerves and nerve ganglia. It causes patches of small blisters along the nerve distribution on one side of the body. Herpes zoster causes a burning pain, redness, and itching that precede the blisters by a few days. When blisters are severe, itching may be severe and persistent. The patient with this condition deserves the most thoughtful and patient nursing care. Prevention of secondary infection is an important nursing responsibility. Like the pruritus of senescence, the condition is aggravating beyond description, and the patient may become exhausted from restlessness and loss of sleep. Soothing local treatment such as application of calamine lotion and use of cotton padding is helpful for the itching. Sedatives and analgesics including codeine, phenobarbital, and aspirin are often ordered for pain and discomfort, and a diet high in vitamins, with additional thiamine chloride, is given. Cortisone and ACTH (adrenocorticotrophic hormone) have been particularly beneficial for some elderly patients. Deep x-ray treatment to the affected spinal ganglia may be resorted to, and occasionally alcohol injection is prescribed.

Allergic disease. Allergic skin conditions do appear in the older person, though less frequently than in the young. The reasons why skin sensitivities have not appeared earlier in life are not always apparent. Sensitivity to environmental factors such as dust or common contactants is more common than sensitivity to food. Persons sometimes develop an allergic reaction to a change of environment or to retirement from work, which thus exposes them more intensively to irritating factors in the home surroundings. Treatment is directed toward finding and removing the irritating substance. Antihistaminic medications have been helpful for many patients.

Stasis dermatitis. Stasis dermatitis is a fairly common skin ailment of the lower extremities of older persons and is usually preceded by varicosities and poor general circulation. Irritation in the tissues is produced by substances normally carried away by the circulation, and it is believed that sometimes autosensitivity or sensitivity to substances in the patient's own tissues develops. Breaks in the skin may be caused by scratching, and infection is added from hands, clothing, and sources elsewhere on the body. For example, chronic vaginitis in elderly women may lead to infection by the same organisms of skin areas on the lower extremities, and these may in turn lead to ulcers, which are resistant to treatment.

The most important part of treatment of stasis dermatitis is prevention by health education in order to eliminate causes of circulatory congestion. People should be taught to avoid obesity, standing for long periods, and the use of tight, rolled garters; they should learn to elevate the lower extremities at regular intervals. Elastic stockings are often helpful in controlling early varicosities and resultant circulatory congestion. The nurse can be most helpful to the patient by helping to plan the day so that rest periods and elevation of the feet can be carried out without too serious interruption of the accustomed mode of living. The nutrition habits of all patients should be carefully reviewed. A high protein diet is usually recommended. Many elderly patients need help in planning their meals so that adequate protein intake is assured.

Dermatophytosis. Dermatophytosis is a fungus infection (athlete's foot). It occurs more commonly in young people with moist skin, but can be troublesome in older people. Older patients with this skin ailment must be reminded of the importance of washing the hands frequently after touching the feet since dermatophytosis spreads easily in the aged. It may spread to the legs and cause an infection and ulcer in tissues where circulation is poor, and it may localize in the genital areas where skin is likely to be moist. Dermatophytosis is commonly treated with undecylenic acid ointment or powder, potassium permanganate soaks, ammoniated mercury ointment, or some combination of these medications.

Corns and calluses. Corns differ from calluses in that they have a center or core which thickens inwardly and causes acute pain upon pressure. The aged patient will avoid serious difficulties with corns and calluses by having his feet cared for regularly by a podiatrist, by consulting an orthopedist, and by being certain that his shoes are correctly fitted. Corns are common in the aged and are often caused by ill-fitting shoes and arthritic changes in the bones of the feet that produce pressure between toes and on the outer surfaces of the toes.

REFERENCES AND RELATED BIBLIOGRAPHY

1. Bozian, Marguerite Wilkenson: Nursing care of patients having dermatologic conditions, Amer. J. Nurs. **52**:873-875, 1952.
2. Carney, Robert G.: The aging skin, Amer. J. Nurs. **63**:110-112, 1963.
3. Davis, Loyal (editor): Christopher's textbook of surgery, ed. 7, Philadelphia, 1960, W. B. Saunders Co.
4. Howell, Charles M.: Common dermatologic problems in geriatrics. In Johnson, Wingate M. (editor): The older patient, New York, 1960, Paul Hoeber, Inc., Medical Book Department of Harper & Row, Publishers.
5. Jeghers, Harold: Herpes zoster, Amer. J. Nurs. **54**:1217-1219, 1954.
6. Ormsby, O. S.: Skin problems of aged (geriatrics), J.A.M.A. **135**:831-835, 1947.
7. Rattner, Herbert: Diseases of the skin. In Stieglitz, Edward J. (editor): Geriatric medicine, ed. 3, Philadelphia, 1954, J. B. Lippincott Co.
8. Sauer, Gordon C.: Manual of skin diseases, Philadelphia, 1959, J. B. Lippincott Co.
9. Shafer, Kathleen Newton, and others: Medical-surgical nursing, ed. 3, St. Louis, 1964, The C. V. Mosby Co.
10. Sulzberger, Marion B., and Wolf, Jack: Dermatology, diagnosis and treatment, ed. 2, Chicago, 1961, Year Book Medical Publishers, Inc.
11. Torrey, Frances: Care of the normal skin, Amer. J. Nurs. **53**:460-463, 1953.
12. Urback, Frederick, and Burgoon, Carroll F., Jr.: Dermatologic aspects. In Cowdry, E. V. (editor): The care of the geriatric patient, ed. 2, St. Louis, 1963, The C. V. Mosby Co.
13. Waisman, M.: Dermatologic problems of elderly persons, Geriatrics **12**:503-514, 1957.
14. Young, A. W., Jr.: Special problems in dermatogeriatrics, New York J. Med. **62**:1407-1412, 1962.

Chapter 24

Nursing in diseases of the eye

Good eyesight that continues throughout active life and into age is a precious asset. As physical capabilities decline, the older person often finds he cannot get about freely, and eventually his social activities are restricted. He may not be able to visit friends, attend ball games, or go for walks. His eyes may become the all-important source of satisfaction and of his contact with the world about him; failing vision, therefore, often leads to severe emotional problems. As the life span of our people extends, the conservation of eyesight becomes more and more imperative.

Many pathologic conditions of the eye occur in age. General slowing of the responses to stimuli tends to make the eyes more liable to injury caused by dust particles and other obstructions. Reduction in secretions and lowered resistance of tissues may predispose to infections. Slower healing may allow infections and other lesions to persist. Visual impairment from vascular degeneration, corneal ulcers, iritis, and detachment of the retina are not unusual. Glaucoma is the eye disease most important from the standpoint of loss of vision, though cataracts are perhaps seen more frequently in hospital patients. The patient may be disturbed by floating spots before the eyes. These are caused by liquefaction of some of the vitreous, with release of the spongy fibrous network of supporting tissue, or to the formation of cholesterol crystals. These spots are annoying but harmless. Changes in the normal function of the ciliary muscle may lessen its efficiency, and this in turn may lessen the accommodation of the eye and may predispose to disease of the ciliary body.

Disease may involve tissues outside the eye itself. Depositions of fat over the cornea from disturbed cholesterol metabolism may appear, as may conjunctivitis. Ectropion and entropion are fairly common in age. They follow loss of muscle tone, laxity of the skin, and loss of fatty deposits under the skin about the eye. Entropion is a rolling inward of the margin of the upper eyelid and may cause damage to the cornea from rubbing of the lashes against its surface. Ectropion is a turning outward of the lower eyelid. In this condition the conjunctival secretions are unable to accumulate, and lubrication of the cornea is impaired. Falling outward of the lower lid often prevents normal drainage into the lachrymal duct. The exposed conjunctiva may become irritated and liable to infection, and the constant tearing of the eye may irritate the skin of the cheek.

The nurse must have more than average knowledge of eye diseases and eye care if she is to be truly helpful to her patients. It is evident that any assumption on her part that certain symptoms may be from a trivial cause may have unfortunate consequences. Only the ophthalmologist should decide the true cause of any eye distress. It is not safe for the nurse ever to reassure confidently the patient who has any symptoms of eye disease unless she has received a report from the ophthalmologist. Patients do need to be encouraged, however, and to be told that something can be done for them, if this is true. For example, the nurse should know that ectropion and entropion can be corrected by relatively simple surgical procedures.

CONSERVATION OF SIGHT

Some conditions that affect the eyes in age, presbyopia or loss of accommodation, for example, cannot be avoided. Many could have been prevented by conservation measures in earlier years. Careless occupational practices and other abuses to the eyes contribute to sightlessness in age. Neglect is most marked during adolescence when physical resources appear unlimited. Prompt treatment when the first symptoms appeared would have arrested the development of some diseases.

Danger signs, neglected in adulthood, later lead to visual loss. Without making persons whom she contacts unduly apprehensive, the nurse should guide them in seeking appropriate treatment if signs of eye disease are present. Frequent headaches, burning sensation in the eyes or the lids, redness of the conjunctiva, and headache associated with reading indicate the need for medical care. Constant dull pain in the eyes, blurring of vision, spots before the eyes, noticed change in visual acuity, and sensation of not having sufficient light for reading are signs that eye function is affected and should be investigated. Frequent changes of glasses and history of repeated visits to optometrists for change of glasses indicate the need for competent medical attention.

Interest in conservation of sight is growing. Conservation of sight and prevention of eye disease present a real challenge to all nurses, particularly to those engaged in community nursing. Industries are becoming vitally aware of the necessity of care of the worker's eyes. More remains to be done in teaching individuals the necessary care of their own eyes during both working and nonworking hours. Sight conservation in schools calls for attention both in teaching students the safe use of their eyes and in the physical construction of the community's schools. Lighting engineers, for example, might well be consulted more widely. In certain outstanding institutions in this country today, students are studying in places not much better lighted than the candle lit monasteries of medieval times. Yet, it is not generally known that a meter to test adequacy of the lighting may be borrowed from almost any electric power company.

Many harmful practices in use of the eyes and their care are typical of man's inconsistent behavior. The human eye was not constructed to do the close reading and other fine work generally imposed upon it. Man was not intended to work in intense heat and light without special protection for his eyes, nor to adjust with rapidity and frequency from bright to dim light and from close to distant vision.

The nurse can be of invaluable help in constantly clarifying unfamiliar terms to the patient and by explaining to him the complexity of the structures of the eye. He should know that conditions of the eyes cannot always be remedied by the prescription of glasses. There is widespread confusion and misunderstanding on the part of the public as to a competent specialist to whom they should turn when having visual difficulty. This is particularly true in the aged, many of whom are from foreign countries and who have trouble keeping up with our changing terminology. One who demands the very best in skilled surgical care when having an abdominal operation may hopefully trust his eyes to a person untrained for the work that he performs. Many people seem to recognize little difference between the *optician* who grinds and fits lenses, the *optometrist* who adjusts lenses to changes in accommodation of the eye, and the *ophthalmologist* who has had intensive training in the diagnosis and treatment of diseases of the eyes. It is surprising to note how many older people purchase their glasses from a store counter and use the glasses of deceased friends and relatives.

Another dangerous belief is that eyedrops that have remained in the family cupboard for twenty years or more can be currently useful in treatment of a new eye ailment. A large proportion of the elder population seems to believe that one kind of eye medication serves many purposes. Much valuable time for treatment can be wasted, and actual harm can be caused to the eyes by the use of old medications. The aged often use old remedies in an attempt to spare the expense of a doctor. The nurse should have at her fingertips the names of doctors and clinics in her local area. She should know the possible sources of financial aid available to her patient. Thus she can help to direct the patient to skilled medical care within his ability to pay.

Another detriment to good eye care is the natural human tendency to put things off, to reject any obvious fact that is unpleasant or disturbing, and to assume that the eye condition will clear up within a few days. This tendency may be coupled with the belief that many conditions are an integral part of old age and must be endured. The nurse in her day-by-day contact with the patient can make him see the ultimate danger of procrastination. Neither the nurse nor the patient can know if an irritation of the eye is a simple conjunctivitis or a beginning of acute glaucoma. The patient must never be permitted to postpone treatment and thus risk further infection or progress of the disease.

No discussion of conservation of the eyes and prevention of eye disease can be complete without a word about the important part that a well-balanced diet plays in eye health. Though it is quite certain that vitamins cannot cure eye disease, it is equally certain that a normal, well-balanced diet and an adequate intake of vitamins may help to delay the aging process, may retard lens opacity, or may deter other degenerative changes. In order to teach the patient effectively, the nurse should know the caloric and vitamin content of the most commonly eaten foods, as well as the approximate amount of protein, carbohydrate, and fat they contain. She should be familiar with the regional eating patterns of her patients and with agencies in her community that give economic aid, since malnutrition may follow poverty.

GENERAL NURSING

A large number of accidents that happen to older people at home are caused by failing vision. Many accidents occur during adjustment to glasses, particularly to the use of bifocal lenses. It is important that furniture be left in the accustomed place, that rugs be anchored carefully, that persons with poor vision avoid the use of gas stoves, and that other potential sources of accidents be considered. The details of accident prevention are discussed more completely in Chapter 6, General Hygiene.

Meeting emotional needs, accuracy in carrying out treatments such as dressings, skill in giving definitive care before and after surgery, and assisting the patient and his family to adjust to the final outcome if some limitation of sight is permanent are important in the nursing of patients with eye disease. Careless though the individual may have been of his eyes, he is much disturbed at the possibility of losing his vision entirely or of having vision markedly impaired. He is fearful of and yet hopeful about the success of any operation or other treatment. Preparation for hospitalization should start as soon as it is known that it will be necessary. Worries over finances should be anticipated, and arrangements with the patient or with agencies who help with finances should be made. Often the doctor will consider it desirable for the medical social case worker to visit the patient in the hospital before the operation to assist in caring for possible problems. By this means the ophthalmologist hopes to eliminate disturbing factors that might affect the patient's recovery after surgery. For example, nervousness might cause a cough, which is harmful in the postoperative period of eye disease. The cough may disappear when its disadvantage is explained to the patient and when the factors contributing to the nervousness have been removed.

Irreparable damage can follow the instilling of unprescribed preparations into the eyes. In the hospital frequent and regular checking of all medication bottles for smearing or obliteration of labels is essential. The patient or persons responsible for his care must guard against the indiscriminate use of incorrect drugs from the family medicine cupboard. Medications for the eyes should be carefully placed in a separate part of the cupboard, and dangerous drugs should be removed if the patient is to select and administer his own medications. The nurse and everyone else who may administer medications must be accurate in the dosage and strength of the medications that they put into the patient's eyes. One ophthalmologist gives this word of warning to all nurses, "If you are unfamiliar with the drug, with the patient, or with eye nursing, question the dosage of any drug of any kind that is over 1 percent in strength."

A large variety of drugs is used for the treatment of eye diseases, and most of them are applied locally as drops, irrigations, or ointments. Mydriatics and cycloplegics such as atropine, 0.5 to 1 percent, homatropine, 2 percent, and Neo-Synephrine Hydrochloride, 10 percent (mydriatic only), are used to dilate the pupil. Miotics such as physostigmine hydrobromide (eserine), 0.25 to 1 percent, and pilocarpine, 1 to 2 percent, are used to contract the pupil. Local anesthetics such as Pontocaine Hydrochloride, 1 percent, or cocaine, 1 percent, are widely employed and are often combined with epinephrine, 1:10,000. Physiologic solution of sodium chloride and mild silver protein (Argyrol) are used as cleansing agents. Antibiotics such as penicillin and neomycin and bacteriostatics such as Gantrisin are used to combat infection. Astringents such as zinc sulfate preparations are often used in the treatment of chronic conjunctivitis. The adrenocorticosteroids are also widely used locally as drops or in ointment.

The techniques of instilling drops, administering ointments, or applying dressings do not differ from those used on any eye patient. The strictest attention is paid to avoid trauma to the eyes and to maintain asepsis. Scrupulous washing of hands before the administration of any medication is absolutely essential. Droppers are held downward to prevent medications from flowing into the bulb. Eye droppers should be separated for washing to remove any medication that may have gotten into the bulb of the dropper. If infection is being treated, a fresh, sterile dropper should be used for each patient.

When the nurse assists with dressings, it is well that she explain the necessary procedure carefully to the patient. It may be difficult to determine whether the patient understands; for example, many patients with impaired hearing depend a good deal upon lipreading and hesitate to admit their hearing or comprehension limitations. It is important that all new experiences be identified for the patient by some means.

Emotional factors in vision loss. The person with marked vision loss often suffers from a sense of isolation. The patient who cannot see depends upon immediate sound and tactile sensation to maintain his feeling of security and of kinship with persons around him. He must be spoken to frequently in a quiet and reassuring voice. Particularly is this true if he is in the strange environment of the hospital awaiting diagnostic procedures and perhaps surgical treatment.

It is upsetting to the patient who cannot see to be touched without first being spoken to; an unfair advantage is taken of his particular situation. This can be irritating and humiliating to the patient, as well as actually dangerous following certain surgical procedures. The nurse must teach all persons who attend the patient and who are under her supervision the importance of making known their nearness to the patient before touching him.

The patient who has marked hearing loss as well as loss of vision presents added difficulties. Tactile contact must then be thoughtfully and quietly made. The nurse must be careful in approaching the patient to touch him very gently at first in order that he may not be suddenly disturbed or frightened. Definite contact must be made, however, and made frequently if the patient is to remain in emotional balance and in harmony with the world around him.

Patient in the hospital. The patient should be helped to feel at home in his new environment. He should be informally introduced to other patients and to nursing personnel. The location of his bed should not be changed about in the pavilion, since moving may cause confusion, particularly when his vision is limited. The location of bedside table, chair, and lamp must be told to him, and they should not be rearranged. If he is to have treatment in which his eyes will be covered, he often feels more secure if he is in a ward with other patients with whom he can talk.

The aged patient with eye difficulty who enters the hospital for treatment must be guarded from accidents and from incurring further eye damage. In acute conditions of the eye and following surgery, the patient must be cautioned not to bend forward and lower his head. If he must stoop, it should always be by bending the knees and hips while holding the head erect. He should be urged not to get up during the night to go to the bathroom, but to use a urinal or bedpan. In many instances side rails are used as a reminder in case he should forget that he is not at home and attempt to step from the high hospital bed.

Preoperative care. Specific routines for preoperative care of patients with eye disease vary somewhat with the part of the country, with the institution, and with the surgeon. The patient usually spends a few days in the hospital while preparation for surgery is made. His general condition and any particular reactions must be closely observed and reported. For instance, signs of upper respiratory disease are contraindications to surgery and must be known.

Sedatives may be given the night before and on the morning of surgery. The nurse must be particularly alert for unusual reactions to sedation. Older people may become restless and confused by sedation, and therefore emphasis should be placed on helping the patient to relax and to feel at home in his new environment and to be less fearful in anticipating his surgery. This is better accomplished by quiet reassurance than by relying upon large doses of sedation.

Enemas are often ordered preoperatively and must be thoroughly expelled. Elderly patients are inclined to retain fluid in the rectum sometimes for several hours; therefore, the enema is usually ordered for the evening before surgery.

Local preparation of the eyes may be started on the pavilion, though some surgeons prefer that a part or all of this preparation be done in the operating room. The eyelids may be gently washed with a very mild soap, the lashes cut, and the eyes irrigated with physiologic solution of sodium chloride at 37° C. (98.6° F.). A topical anesthetic such as tetracaine hydrochloride (Pontocaine Hydrochloride), 1 percent, may be instilled into the eyes at specified times before the patient goes to the operating room.

Procaine hydrochloride (Novocaine), 2 percent, with epinephrine may be injected into the conjunctiva, and tetracaine, or cocaine, 4 percent, may be used to render the site of operation painless. Occasionally a general anesthetic must be used when the patient has severe generalized pain and for certain operations, such as an enucleation. General anesthesia is avoided when possible because of the restlessness which occurs when the patient is reacting. If a general anesthetic is advisable, thiopental sodium (Pentothal Sodium) is the drug most often used at the present time.

Postoperative care. An important postoperative complication of eye surgery in the aged is mental confusion. The patient may move about and impair the result of the operation. He must be observed at very frequent intervals postoperatively. If he moves excessively or shows any inclination to disturb the dressings, he must be watched constantly, and the doctor must be called at once. This situation should be prevented, if possible, by careful observation of the patient for signs of confusion preoperatively and by complete and thoughtful explanation of what he may expect postoperatively. Disorientation is less likely to occur if the unaffected eye is left uncovered; some eye surgeons do cover it, but usually they cover both eyes only when surgery for detachment of the retina or a corneal transplant has been done.

Since the eyes move together, it is important that both eyes be kept as quiet as possible. The nurse can help by explaining the need for quiet to the patient and by anticipating his needs so that it will not be necessary for him to move about and to use the uncovered eye. She should see that the patient's call bell is in place and that he is visited and spoken to frequently. A radio within arm's reach helps to keep him in contact with his environment, and reading to him is also helpful.

Postoperative routines vary with the age of the patient and with the operation. The trend is toward permitting much greater freedom and earlier mobilization than in the past. This, however, depends upon the type of operative procedure. The patient may be permitted out of bed within twenty-four hours. It helps him to accept restrictions if he is told repeatedly that they will be of short duration.

Indications of pain and drainage on dressings must be watched for closely and must be reported since these may be signs of intraocular bleeding or infection. Dressings following eye surgery are always changed by the surgeon.

A soft diet is usually ordered for a few days, though some surgeons feel that a diet that permits moderate chewing will decrease distention and discomfort. If both eyes are covered, the patient should be fed. Otherwise, whether he needs to be fed will depend upon the amount of his eyesight and his general condition. When a person who cannot see is fed, it is important to identify for him the kind of food he is to receive. The nurse must not allow feeding the patient to become a routine procedure.

On about the third day after surgery, mineral oil may be ordered. The patient need not have a bowel movement for four days. This should be explained to him since older people are often unduly concerned with elimination and think that a daily movement is necessary.

The patient should be instructed to follow his doctor's instructions carefully and to keep appointments as specified. Many elderly patients with eye conditions must return to the doctor's office or to a clinic at intervals for a long time—some indefinitely. The nurse caring for the patient in the hospital has a very definite responsibility in teaching this to him, since she deals with the patient when he is most apprehensive and receptive to teaching. The nurse working in the community can be invaluable in arranging for clinic care and in helping the patient and his family to avoid discouragement, teaching them to administer medications as prescribed, and impressing them with the importance of reporting to the doctor regularly.

It is a nursing responsibility to help the patient and his family develop patience and learn not to expect immediate cure from the operation. This demands skill and understanding of the particular patient and of his family. Even though the problem has been explained to him by his physician, the patient often expects that the moment the dressings are removed he will be completely cured. It may take weeks and even months for the patient to become accustomed to the type of glasses he must wear. The sooner during his illness he is acquainted with this fact, the less impatient he will be. The aged patient is often obsessed with the idea that his remaining life may be short, and thus he is more impatient than the younger person. To him time moves faster, and he is anxious to see and do as much as possible in the time left. If he is employed, he may fear that his place in the working world will be taken over by someone else unless he is able to return to work within a short time. If the nurse really understands his problems, she can better help him to adjust to actual circumstances.

DISEASE CONDITIONS

Glaucoma. Glaucoma seldom occurs in persons under 35 years of age, but it is one of the greatest enemies to vision in older people. Twelve percent of all blindness is caused by this disease.[17] Early symptoms of glaucoma most often appear in the late forties. The saving of sight depends upon early diagnosis and continued effective treatment. There are several types of glaucoma, but they all have one common characteristic. Fluid is formed in the eye faster than it can be eliminated so that pressure within the eyeball rises.

Primary glaucoma is of unknown origin. Tendency to inherit a predisposition to the disease is quite certain, and glaucoma occurs most frequently in persons who have a family history of unstable emotional make-up. Increase in the size of the lens may also contribute to the disease in age. Secondary glaucoma follows another disease such as iritis, which may result in interference with the free passage and therefore with the reabsorption of aqueous fluid.

Glaucoma may be acute or chronic; the former is much less common. Acute glaucoma may cause general symptoms, with nausea and vomiting in addition to eye pain and dilation of the pupil. There is edema of the ciliary body and the cornea and an increase of tension within the eyeball (tension of the normal eye is 13 to 29 mm. Hg on the Schiøtz tonometer). Marked increase in tension for over twenty-four to thirty-six hours may cause complete and permanent blindness, hence the urgent necessity for immediate treatment by an ophthalmologist. Morphine may be given for pain, and the miotics may be used to contract the pupil. If symptoms do not subside in a few hours, an emergency operation may be done to permit the escape of aqueous fluid.

Chronic glaucoma may come on slowly, and in the beginning of the disease no symptoms may be manifested. Chronic glaucoma gives one characteristic sign that is tremendously important. The peripheral visual fields are impaired before the central visual fields are affected, so that objects to the side are observed less well. Limitation of vision may not be as apparent as in other eye diseases, and much damage can occur before medical aid is sought. The patient may bump into others in the street or fail to see passing vehicles when he is driving a car; yet he will not realize that the fault lies in his own vision. The community nurse who realizes this may be most helpful in early case finding and prompt referral of patients to the ophthalmologist.

Chronic glaucoma usually begins in a single eye, but, if left untreated, both

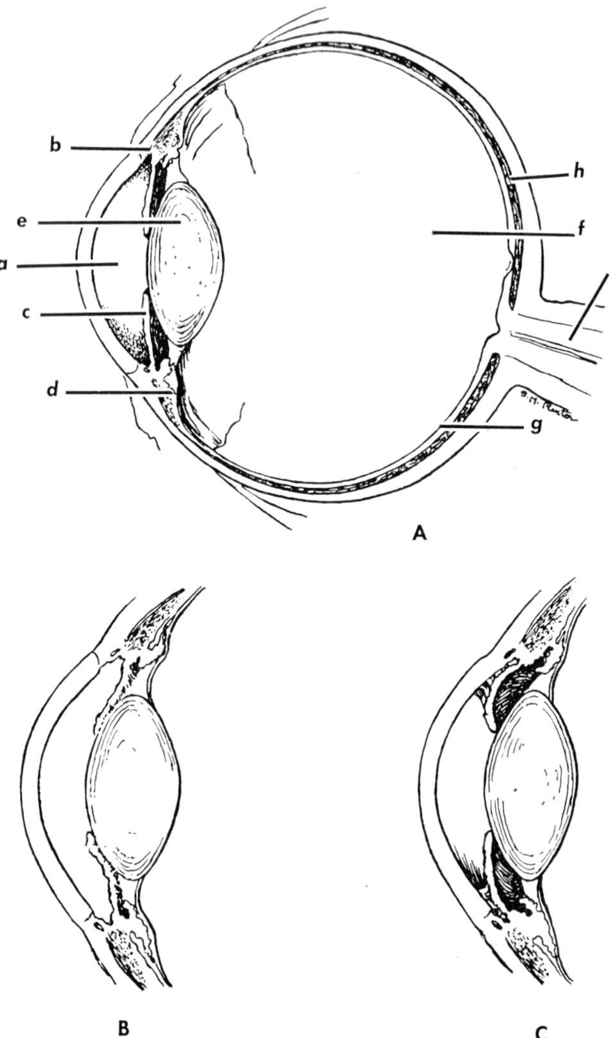

Figure 52. A, Anatomy of the normal eye: **a,** anterior chamber; **b,** Schlemm's canal; **c,** iris; **d,** ciliary body; **e,** lens; **f,** vitreous; **g,** retina; **h,** choroid; **i,** optic nerve. **B,** Adhesion of iris to lens preventing passage of fluid into the anterior chamber—a cause of glaucoma. **C,** Adhesion of iris to the anterior chamber interfering with disposal of aqueous fluid—a cause of glaucoma.

eyes often become affected. Symptoms are most apparent in the morning when a persistent, dull eye pain develops. There may be a steamy appearance to the cornea and a blurring of vision, followed by tearing, misty vision, and a blurred appearance of the iris, which becomes fixed and dilated. Headache, nausea, and vomiting often occur. Halos may be seen about lights, resembling the appearance of lights seen through a steamed windshield, and symptoms may be made more acute by watching movies or television. Early symptoms have been confused with sinus headache. The condition is often precipitated by severe emotional disturbance, worry, or some form of physical ill health.

There is no cure for glaucoma. All treatment is directed toward reducing intraocular tension and keeping it at a safe level. The miotics are widely used, but often surgical measures are necessary. Surgical procedures for the treatment of glaucoma are intended to produce a permanent filtration pathway for aqueous fluid. There are many operations, a few of which are iridectomy, iridencleisis, cyclodialysis, and corneoscleral trephining.

The patient with glaucoma needs assistance in learning to accept his disease. Despite explanation from his physician, he frequently hopes that the operation will immediately end his pain and that the sight he may have lost will be restored. He must realize that the part of the field of vision lost due to glaucoma cannot be restored, but that further loss can usually be prevented. The patient is often advised to avoid stimulants of any kind, including tea, coffee, and certain stimulating soft drinks. He should avoid anything that will increase the blood pressure and in turn the intraocular tension—emotional situations such as arguments, tight-fitting clothing such as constricting collars, constipation with straining at defecation, and heavy lifting. Watching movies and television, driving a vehicle, and work that involves close watching of moving objects must be limited.

The patient with glaucoma must be under medical observation for the rest of his life and receive either drug or surgical therapy or both. Following the operation, he must return regularly to the doctor since one operation does not necessarily mean that drainage will continue. Any obstruction or closing of the artificial pathway will result in reappearance of symptoms and further visual damage.

Cataract. Cataract or clouding of the lens occurs so often in the aged that the term senile cataract is used. At the age of 80 years, about 85 percent of all persons have some lens opacity. Since cataracts may accompany other eye pathology, such as incipient glaucoma, symptoms of other eye disease, such as blurring of vision or pain, must not be overlooked when the patient has been told by his doctor to wait until the cataract is further advanced before it is removed.

The trend is toward earlier removal of cataracts by the intracapsular technic. Any cataract can be removed at any stage by this method. Decision as to when to remove the cataract depends on the patient and the use he makes of his eyes. It is the nurse's responsibility to refer the patient with a cataract to the ophthalmologist and to urge him to accept treatment as recommended. A cataract that is left long past maturity (completely opaque) may be more difficult to extract.

The opaque (aphakic) lens is removed either intracapsularly or extracapsularly. In the intracapsular method the capsule is freed from its supporting structures, and the lens with its capsule is removed. In the extracapsular method an opening is made into the capsule, and the lens is extracted through the opening. The former operation requires a higher degree of surgical skill but yields the best results since the capsule and small particle of lens or desquamation from the lens do not remain to interfere with vision and cause complications. Improvement in surgical techniques appears each year. For example, use of the enzyme alpha-chymotrypsin may soften the ligaments attaching the lens and may facilitate its removal.

Usually only one lens is removed at one operation in case some complications should arise or some unexpected behavior on the part of the patient interfere with good results. If cataracts are present in both lenses, they may both be removed at one hospitalization. This must be explained to the patient's satisfaction, or he may become restless and impatient with the treatment he is receiving.

After cataract extraction, the patient usually lies quietly for twenty-four hours with about 30-degree elevation of the head of the bed. A small pillow may be placed under his head, and another small pillow may be used to support the lumbar spine. On the evening of surgery, the patient is usually permitted to turn toward the unoperated side enough to make good care of the back possible. Patients who have intracapsular cataract extractions are permitted out of bed in one to four days; in about ten days the dressings are completely removed, and temporary glasses may be used.

The elderly patient sometimes finds adjustment following cataract extraction rather difficult. He may be surprised to learn that he needs glasses before he can use the operated eye; that the color of objects seen with the eye in which the lens is removed is slightly different; that, if he has the lens removed from only one eye, he will use one of his eyes, but will not use both together. He needs to be told that it will take some time to learn to judge distance, climb stairs, and the like. The little remaining ability to accommodate the eye is lost when the lens is removed, and the patient must wear glasses. Bifocal lenses are often ordered, and the patient must have perseverance and be given encouragement in becoming accustomed to their use.

Contact lenses are now being used for many elderly patients who have had their own aphakic lenses removed surgically. If contact lenses can be fitted properly and if the patient can adjust to them, they are often most satisfactory because they eliminate the distortion in side vision that occurs when spectacles with thick lenses must be worn.

Detachment of the retina. Detachment of the retina is a forward displacement of the retina from its normal position against the choroid. The amount of visual loss depends upon the location and extent of the area of detachment. Many factors seem to contribute to its cause. Fibers from the vitreous may become adherent and pull the retina forward; extraction of the lens may reduce pressure of the vitreous against the retina sufficiently to allow detachment; a tear in the retina may permit fluid vitreous to seep behind the retina and increase the detachment. A tumor may be the cause. General debility, chronic systemic disease, old age, and trauma seem to predispose to detachment of the retina. Trauma need not be to the eyeball or surrounding structures themselves. For example, a motor accident in which the individual has been severely shaken up but no damage has been done to the head can result in detachment of the retina, if an abnormal and unhealthy condition exists in the retina, the choroid, or the vitreous.

Detachment of the retina is a serious disorder. The amount of permanent visual loss is dependent upon the extent of the detachment and the amount of restoration that can be made. The condition is more serious if it occurs in the upper part of the retina since gravity tends to increase the detachment, and the detached portion may fall downward and obstruct parts of the retina that would otherwise function normally.

The treatment for detachment of the retina is surgical. It consists of attempts to make the retina adhere to its original attachment by the use of penetrating diathermy or by a variety of other surgical means, including "buckling" to reduce the size of the vitreous space. If the condition appears to be the result of a fault of the vitreous with shrinkage and failure to give support to the retina, attempts may be made to compensate for this. Vitreous from the eyes of others can now be desiccated and stored for future use; it is now available from eye banks in some localities.

Before surgery the patient is kept extremely quiet and usually wears pinhole glasses to limit his field of vision. No nursing routines can be established for the patient following surgery. Nursing for the patient with detachment of the retina varies with each patient and must be individual. The patient has both eyes covered and needs constant supportive care. He will usually remain in bed for several days, and attention to his comfort such as that provided by a small pillow to the lumbar spine is important. Whether he is permitted to move from side to side in the bed and to turn depends entirely upon the individual patient and the location and amount of detachment. The nurse must be most careful in checking orders before permitting the patient to turn or sit up in bed following operation for detachment of the retina. Explaining the doctor's wishes to the patient is necessary and helpful. The patient must be cautioned not to sit forward or lift his head from the bed. He is often placed on a soft diet if chewing should be avoided. He is told to avoid sneezing, coughing, or laughing if possible. He must always be spoken to quietly before he is approached since sudden starting or sitting forward may be disastrous.

The patient with detachment of the retina who is placed flat in bed both before and after surgery may complain of abdominal distress. A hot-water bottle may be placed on the abdomen, or a rectal tube may be used. Passive exercises of the arms and legs are necessary, particularly for the patient who is kept extremely quiet for several days. The patient must be instructed to allow the nurse to move his limbs rather than to participate in the exercises himself.

Detachment of the retina may recur. The patient is usually instructed by his physician to avoid bending forward, lifting heavy objects, straining, and vigorous exercise for a period of several months following surgery. General attention to positive health measures such as adequate diet, sufficient rest, and quiet recreation may help to prevent recurrences.

Corneal ulcers. Corneal ulcers may arise from a variety of causes. For instance, they may be caused by viruses and are most common during febrile illness when resistance is lowered. They may follow exposure to irritation, as from the eyelashes in entropion, or they may follow cerebrovascular accident or nutritional deficiencies. Treatment consists of cycloplegics, heat applications, sedatives, and measures to build up general resistance. Infections that are secondary

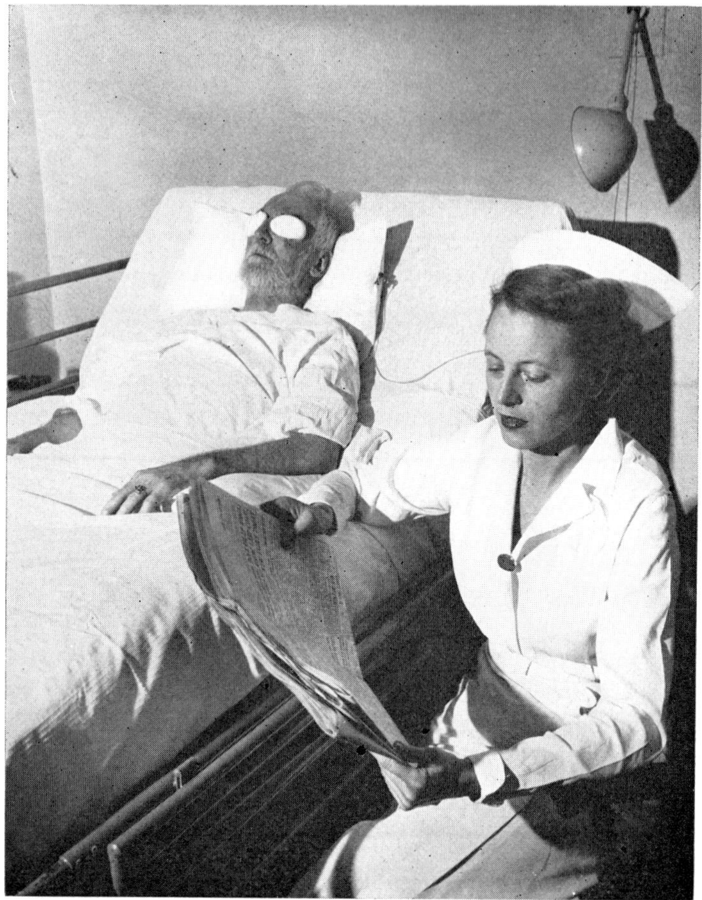

Figure 53. Even the busy nurse should read to the patient who cannot see, to help him maintain contact with the world around him. Note the sideboards that can be turned down during the day.

to the ulcer are treated by use of specific drugs. Sulfonamide preparations and antibiotics may be given both locally and systemically. The greatest care must be taken to prevent additional infection of the ulcer by poor aseptic technique in dressings, and the patient should be instructed not to touch the dressings. Fluorescein may be used to outline the depth and extent of the ulcer. The corticosteroids may be used both locally and systemically. Fever therapy is occasionally used when the ulcer is resistant to other forms of therapy. When this treatment is used, it is important that the nurse observe the patient carefully following the administration of the pyretic agent and take and record his temperature at the requested intervals. Some older people do not tolerate fever therapy as well as younger ones. If the patient is receiving fever therapy, it is important to encourage increase of food and fluid intake. Corneal ulcers are extremely difficult to cure in aged people and may lead to destruction of the cornea and complete loss of vision. Corneal transplants using the cornea of individuals who have recently died may be done; the care of these patients is discussed fully in current nursing texts.[16] Recently, plastic materials have been used to replace a cornea that has been clouded and destroyed by disease.

Eye disease in nutritional deficiency. Much research is being conducted to determine the relationship of nutrition to eye disease. A lack of vitamin A in the diet can cause eye disease marked by changes in the conjunctiva and corneal epithelium. Tears are reduced, and the eyes and lid margins become reddened and inflamed. Sensitiveness to light is often present, and some loss of visual acuity is noticed at night, though this condition must not be confused with true night blindness. This condition responds rapidly to an adequate diet high in vitamin A.

Pathologic changes can occur in the retina as a result of nutritional deficiency, particularly of vitamin B. This condition is found most often in individuals who ingest large amounts of alcohol and pay little attention to their diet. The disease was thought to be due to the alcohol, and the name *tobacco-alcoholic amblyopia* was used. Patients who have suffered optic atrophy as a result of nutritional deficiency will often respond miraculously to a diet high in vitamin B, even though they may continue to take alcohol. Occasionally when damage to the nerve tissue of the retina has been severe and prolonged, a diet high in vitamin B and all other essentials can accomplish only partial recovery.

Eye changes in nephritis and diabetes. Characteristic changes in the retina occur when nephritis with high blood pressure is present. It is often possible for the ophthalmologist to make a diagnosis of nephritis merely by looking into the patient's eyes. No local treatment to the eye is of value, and sometimes the condition causes complete blindness. Treatment is directed toward control of the kidney ailment and reduction of the blood pressure before vision is entirely lost.

Certain pathologic changes occur in the eye of persons with diabetes, but their true cause is obscure and debatable. Corneal ulcers and iritis occur more often in persons with diabetes than in nondiabetic persons, but are thought by some to be the result of a general state of malnutrition and debility that accompanies diabetes before diagnosis is made and insulin is given.

Degeneration of the retina, often called diabetic retinopathy, is caused by increased fragility of blood vessels, allowing many small hemorrhages in the retina that lead to its destruction. It is definitely known that this condition appears in association with diabetes, but it has not been proved that a high blood sugar level is a factor in its development. Diabetic retinopathy is appearing in many young persons who have had diabetes over a period of years. Its development seems to be much more closely related to the length of time the person has diabetes than to whether the blood and urine sugar levels are carefully controlled. Some physicians do believe that the appearance of retinal damage is indication for strict attention to blood sugar levels; they feel that progress of the disease can be partially arrested by adherence to a strict regimen in regard to taking insulin.

Most patients with diabetic retinopathy eventually go on to blindness, if death from some cause does not intervene. Care consists of helping the patient face this reality—helping him to remain independent and self-sufficient.

Degenerative disease of old age. Senile degeneration of the retina is a rather common cause of blindness in very old persons. It is the cause for a proportionately larger number of those blinded each year. There is gradual atrophy of the retina, possibly from impaired nutrition of the retina resulting from arteriosclerosis or atherosclerosis. It may or may not be associated with high blood pressure. There seems to be no real control of this condition at the present time, though attention to adequate diet high in vitamins may assist in retarding the degenerative process.

Night blindness is the result of pigmentary degeneration of the retina and affects the peripheral visual fields first. This condition is fairly common in the elderly and was widely recognized in England during the war when blackouts made it extremely difficult for older people to get about safely. Because of this condition, primarily, it is important that elderly people not move suddenly into an unlighted room and particularly into one with which they are not familiar. Usually they need more light for reading and for carrying on any activity demanding close use of their eyes.

Visual loss may follow vascular accidents to vessels anywhere in the eye or in the main blood vessels outside the eye. A cerebrovascular accident may cause hemianopsia or may cause total blindness, depending upon its location. Thrombosis of the central vein or arteriosclerotic involvement of the central artery of the eye may cause blindness. Generalized arteriosclerosis involving the vessels of both eyes may cause partial or complete loss of vision in both eyes.

REHABILITATION OF THE BLIND

Despite the best efforts of all concerned, some patients will become blind. There are more than one third of a million blind persons in the United States, half of whom are 65 years of age or older. It is the responsibility of the nurse to help the patient achieve a measure of self-sufficiency and satisfaction in living despite his blindness. Persons who are blinded in old age can rarely benefit from state vocational rehabilitation programs, but there are many constructive activities in which they can participate profitably. The most important contribution that the nurse can make to their rehabilitation is in teaching and encouraging them to independence in meeting the functional activities of daily living and in helping family members to see the importance of letting them experience satisfaction in their independence. It is imperative that the patient be given an opportunity to preserve his self-respect and esteem by taking care of his personal needs. He should be urged to feed, clothe, bathe, and otherwise care for himself. The family needs expert counseling and guidance since the natural tendency is to overprotect the patient and thus render him completely helpless. The nurse can make many constructive suggestions in the home that will help with initial adjustment. For example, it is important that accident hazards be removed and that the room be uncluttered so that the blinded person may get about fairly freely without having to request help.

If it appears that blindness may become an actuality, it is usually well while some sight yet remains to direct the patient toward certain activities that it will be possible for him to continue if he does become blind. Occupational therapists are invaluable in helping to meet these needs. If the patient's hearing is good, it may be that he can develop an interest in music. If, without taxing the failing vision, the patient can develop skills that can later be carried on without sight, he might learn such activities as crocheting, carving, pottery-making, and toy-making.

Special provision is made for the blinded under the social security program. There are two national voluntary organizations* devoted to the blind. In addition, some states have their own voluntary or official organizations that are set up primarily to help the person of any age who has partial or complete loss of vision. The nurse should be familiar with resources to help the blinded in her community. The local or state health department or the state department of welfare should be able to give her this information.

---

*The National Society for the Prevention of Blindness, Inc., 16 East 40th St., New York, N. Y., and the American Foundation for the Blind, Inc., 15 West 16th St., New York, N. Y.

REFERENCES AND RELATED BIBLIOGRAPHY

1. Adler, Francis Heed: Textbook of ophthalmology, ed. 7, Philadelphia, 1962, W. B. Saunders Co.
2. Allen, James A.: May's manual of the diseases of the eye, ed. 23, Baltimore, 1963, The Williams & Wilkins Co.
3. Blake, Eugene M.: Glaucoma, Amer. J. Nurs. **52**:451-452, 1952.
4. Blodi, Frederick C.: Glaucoma, Amer. J. Nurs. **63**:78-83, 1963.
5. Brockhurst, Robert J., and O'Donnell, Catherine T.: Detachment of the retina, Amer. J. Nurs. **64**:96-100, 1964.
6. Calhoun, F. P., Kilgoe, Alice P., and Mills, Elizabeth: Detached retina, Amer. J. Nurs. **53**:1316-1321, 1953.
7. Cataract; facts and fancy, New York, 1963, National Society for the Prevention of Blindness, Inc.
8. Clark, Graham, and Shaw, Cora L.: The patient with retinal detachment, Amer. J. Nurs. **57**:868-871, 1957.
9. Eye health, a teaching handbook for nurses, New York, 1946, The National Society for the Prevention of Blindness, Inc.
10. Jones, Ira S., and Bosanko, Lydia: The cataract extraction operation and nursing care of the patient with a cataract extraction, Amer. J. Nurs. **60**:1433-1437, 1960.
11. Kornzweig, A. L.: Eye health needs of persons in an institution for the aged, Sight-sav. Rev. **34**:83-87, 1964.
12. Manhattan Eye, Ear, Nose and Throat Hospital: Nursing in diseases of the eye, ear, nose and throat, ed. 10, Philadelphia, 1958, W. B. Saunders Co.
13. Meyer, William J.: Rural glaucoma screening, Am. J. Pub. Health **52**:75-79, 1962.
14. Pinkerton, Grace: Learning to live with blindness, Nurs. Outlook **3**:432-435, 1955.
15. Rones, Benjamin: The eyes and vitamins, Amer. J. Nurs. **52**:728-729, 1952.
16. Shafer, Kathleen Newton, and others: Medical-surgical nursing, ed. 3, St. Louis, 1964, The C. V. Mosby Co.
17. Sloan, Malachi W., II: Glaucoma control, Am. J. Ophth. **47**:641-649, 1959.
18. Troutman, Richard C., and others (editors): Plastic and reconstructive surgery of the eye and adnexa, Washington, D. C., 1962, Butterworth, Inc.

Chapter 25

Nursing in urologic disease

Urologic disease is common in elderly people. The entire urinary tract, including the kidneys, ureters, bladder, and urethra, changes with age. The renal corpuscles (functioning units or glomeruli) may be reduced in number by damage during life, and remaining glomeruli may be hampered in normal function by vascular changes. Arteriosclerosis in small blood vessels that nourish all of the tract may lessen the resistance of surface tissues to infection and trauma. The muscular portion of the ureters, bladder, and urethra becomes less elastic, and supportive structures may lose tone so that the entire system becomes less efficient.

Every older person should visit his family doctor at the first sign of urinary difficulty since it may be an indication of serious life-endangering disease. An obstruction anywhere along the tract such as caused by the kinking of a ureter or by prostatic enlargement encroaching upon the urethra may cause severe damage to the kidneys if it is left untreated. Carcinoma may reach an inoperable stage if first signs go unheeded. The nurse in her daily work should urge medical care for the person who has any deviation in normal habits of voiding. So often, particularly in rural areas, one encounters families who believe that older people often have such troubles, or that it is part of old age and that little can be done about it. It often requires tact and persistence to get the patient to see the need for medical attention.

Physiologic and pathologic changes follow an obstruction in the urinary tract and inability to excrete urine normally. When urine backs into the ureters and kidney pelves, pressure may damage or destroy the secreting portions of the kidney. Urine retained for a period of time, either in the bladder, the ureters, or the kidney pelves, predisposes to bacterial growth. Cystitis and pyelonephritis may result. These conditions place an added burden on kidneys that may be suffering already from arteriosclerotic changes of the blood vessels to such an extent that they are ill prepared to carry on even normal excretory function. Diverticulosis of the bladder may occur in the aged musculature of a distended bladder. Calculi are frequently associated with infected residual urine, and immobilization increases the chances of this occurring.

There are many geriatric patients in the urologic divisions of the general hospitals. Some are in the hospital because they have failed to understand or neglected to follow medical instructions given them previously. The nurse in the hospital, preoccupied with the immediate needs of the patient, may not stop to consider that she, too, has a responsibility to teach the patient. She should never forget the importance of preventing the complications that follow neglect of the prescribed treatment and care. Some older people with urologic difficulties must visit the doctor's office or the clinic at regular intervals for the rest of their lives. It is the nurse's responsibility to reemphasize this to the patient during the time he is under her care.

GENERAL NURSING

Understanding. Perhaps the most important feature of urologic nursing is the nurse's own attitude toward the urologic patient and his unique problems. It is essential that she understand the patient's personal reactions to his disease and to the changes it may necessitate in his life. Many of the patients on the urologic service are elderly men; therefore the nurse should have a sympathy for and an understanding of male thinking if she is to be happy in this particular kind of nursing.

Emotional reaction is extremely important from the standpoint of case finding and securing early treatment. Many urologic conditions progress to a dangerous state while patients are trying to summon courage to visit the family doctor. Many men fear that their wives will misunderstand their symptoms and react unfavorably to the results of surgery. Many are inclined to misinterpret their wives' reactions because of their own apprehensions and fears. Sometimes the climacteric for either partner adds to the difficulties since both husband and wife may question the behavior of the other. For example, unless the couple is unusually harmonious, doubts may arise as to whether sexual inactivity is the result of aging, illness, or disinterest in the respective mate. Men (and women also) are likely to blame illness on sexual wrongdoing, either real or imaginary. Fears, feelings of guilt, and innumerable conflicts result. The patient may be irritable, apprehensive, and unpredictable with little apparent cause. He may have great difficulty in accepting the surgeon's judgment in regard to treatment.

The ability to function sexually as a normal male is tremendously important to the man, and any threat to this ability is almost intolerable. Even the man of advancing years rebels at circumstances that make sexual activity no longer possible and is unable to accept the thought of himself without it. When symptoms appear that may threaten his procreative activity, a man may refuse to recognize them or to accept their significance as interpreted to him by his doctor. For example, the older man with hypertrophy of the prostate may be cheerful, agreeable, and even manifest considerable interest in diagnostic procedures, only to refuse stoutly to sign a permit for necessary surgery. He may decide that the condition is not serious, and he will not risk being "crippled" by surgery.

Some elderly men who have had no actual sexual activity for years may go into utter depression at the knowledge that removal of the testicles or even ligation of the vas deferens is necessary. If the operation involves ureteral transplants, as well as prostatectomy and orchiectomy, or if amputation of the penis is necessary, the patient may feel that the future is utterly hopeless and that he would rather die than face the operation. It is the surgeon who makes the complete explanation to the patient, but the nurse can be of great assistance by encouraging complete confidence in the surgeon and also by a sympathetic understanding of the patient's emotional conflicts.

A lethargic depression may settle over the older patient who has any urinary tract disease. This must be offset by a cheerful environment and by a kindly interest in each individual patient with thoughtful attention to his personal comfort and to his physical and psychologic welfare. Being assisted out of bed and into a wheelchair where he can be taken to a sun porch or solarium often helps the depressed patient to alter his perspective somewhat and encourages social intercourse.

Observation. All elderly urologic patients and particularly those who have suffered from prolonged retention of urine should be observed carefully for signs of impending uremia. Personality changes, headache, nausea and vomiting, halitosis, and visual disturbances should be reported at once. Many urologists now believe that the patient should have a recording of his blood pressure at least daily, and that tests of kidney function, including blood urea nitrogen determination, phenolsulfonphthalein excretion, and total volume and specific gravity of urine, should be done and recorded at least weekly. The nurse should see that any of these determinations are obtained when requested by the doctor and that their results are recorded, and she should report any difficulties in obtaining them to the doctor.

Care of drainage. Usually a first step in the treatment of urologic disease is to establish adequate drainage of urine. This is to ensure removal from the body of the liberal fluids given as an internal irrigation to remove waste products and combat the infection that so often accompanies urinary tract obstruction. Usually the doctor wishes the patient to get at least 3,000 ml. of fluid per day, although occasionally as much as 5,000 ml. is ordered if not contraindicated by a condition such as cardiac limitation; occasionally smaller amounts are desired in the belief that some concentration of urine may concentrate drugs given and increase their effectiveness. A most important part of nursing care for the urologic patient is attention to urinary drainage. The total intake as well as the total output should be measured carefully and recorded for most urologic patients. Distinction should be made between urinary output and total output if vomiting or diarrhea has occurred, since the urologist will always wish to know what the kidney output for a specified interval of time has been.

A retention catheter usually is ordered when signs of acute obstruction are present. The physician or the specially trained male attendant inserts the catheter for the male patient and anchors it securely. Too much emphasis cannot be placed upon care of the skin. Tincture of benzoin often is used to prevent irritation of the urethral meatus and skin to which adhesive is applied. If any irritation occurs, it should be reported to the doctor promptly. Irritation at the meatus occurs much less frequently when a Foley catheter is used, since this type of catheter is kept in place with a minimum of adhesive. However, when male attendants are responsible for checking the condition of the catheters, they must be reminded by the nurse to watch for signs of irritation. It is important that all drainage tubes be secured to prevent pull on the catheter since this causes discomfort, prevents the patient from moving sufficiently, and may result in the catheter's being pulled out. Tubing can be secured to the bed by means of a large paper clip or by a tape tied about the tubing and pinned to the bed. Neither of these methods causes pressure on the tubing.

When urine must be drained by means of a catheter, either straight or decompression drainage may be used. The method selected will depend upon the patient's difficulty and the physician in charge. In straight drainage, urine simply flows out the tube into a drainage receptacle as it collects in the bladder. This method of drainage is in very wide use today. In decompression drainage, a certain amount of urine accumulates in the bladder, creating a slight pressure that overcomes resistance presented by a Y-tube. The height of the open Y-tube determines the amount of resistance that must be overcome and is ordered specifically by the physician. It is the nurse's responsibility to be certain that the height is maintained as prescribed. Some urologists feel that this second type of drainage has advantages over straight drainage, particularly if infection or bleeding is present since it prevents contact of inflamed bladder surfaces, and the mild pressure produced by the fluid in the bladder gives some hemostasis. If retention has been pronounced and chronic, gradual decompression is often ordered to prevent bladder spasm, hemorrhage, loss of muscle tone, and tubular dysfunction that may lead to loss of too much sodium and to shocklike clinical symptoms.

When retention of urine has been of long duration and renal damage is evident as shown by tests of kidney function, and when the muscle tone of the bladder is poor, a suprapubic cystotomy may be done by the doctor in preference to inserting a catheter into the bladder. This is done because the disadvantages of this type of drainage are few compared with the serious danger of complications following urethral catheterization. These complications include chronic cystitis, epididymitis, prostatitis, and chronic urethritis. A variety of methods of dealing with the urinary drainage from a suprapubic cystotomy and the nursing care involved are described in available nursing texts.[9, 11]

Physiologic solution of sodium chloride is the solution most often used for irrigation. If frequent irrigations are desired, a reservoir for irrigating fluid, tubing, and a Y-tube may be used. If the drainage tube is closed and a prescribed amount of solution is allowed to flow into the bladder, irrigation at regular intervals can be done under aseptic conditions, and the amount used for the irrigation can be accurately measured and controlled. For nearly every patient who has a retention catheter, fluids are forced, and daily irrigation of the catheter is ordered. Retention or indwelling catheters are usually left in place for one to five days or even longer. It is important that the nurse watch for "sanding" or deposit on the inner lining of the catheter, which indicates that there is danger of the lumen becoming clogged and that the catheter should be changed. This sanding, if it appears, should be reported to the doctor since he may wish additional fluids given or a different kind of solution used. This may occur in the

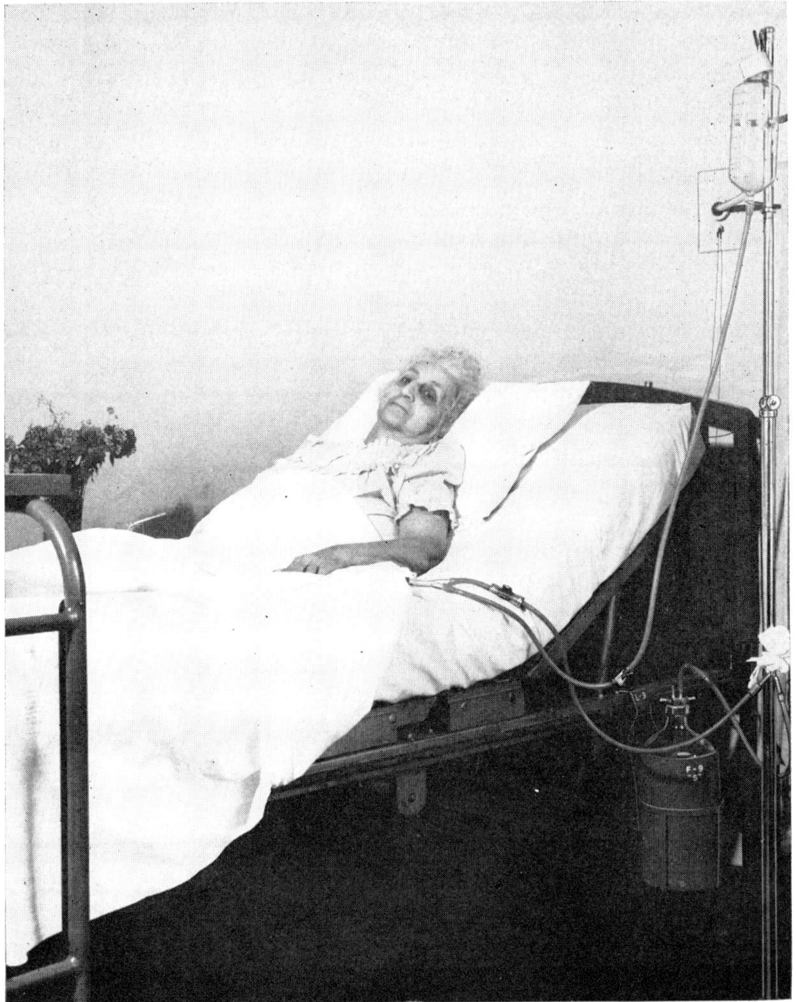

Figure 54. Bladder decompression. The height of the Y-tube attached to the standard determines the amount of resistance that must be overcome before urine drains from the bladder.

older patient who is or has been dehydrated and who may be excreting concentrated urine or residual urine that may contain a large amount of sediment. Urine in the tubing and in the drainage bottles must be watched carefully for any other unusual constituents such as blood.

It is most important that the free flow of urine from the bladder be uninterrupted. Often the patient is allowed out of bed and may sit for hours with the catheter kinked or otherwise obstructed. The nurse should check all retention catheters at least every two hours to be certain that they are draining properly. On some urologic services, emptying drainage bottles and recording output are delegated to an orderly or an attendant. This procedure is safe only if the nurse checks regularly to see that recording is accurate.

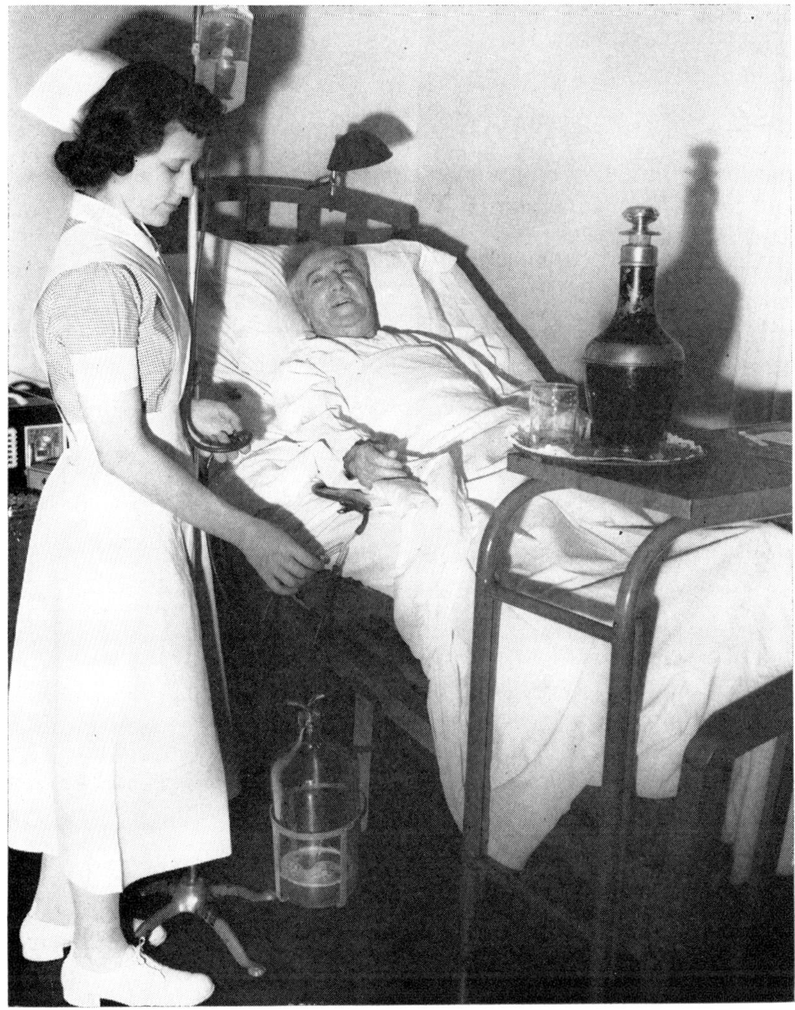

Figure 55. When straight drainage is used, the catheter and tubing are irrigated at regular intervals. The time of irrigation and amount of fluid used can be recorded on a piece of paper kept on the overbed table. Note the large paper clip that anchors the tubing to the bed without causing pressure to obstruct the flow of urine.

The odors that were once taken for granted on the urologic ward are not necessary. Much of this improvement is the result of better surgery and of the use of special equipment. For example, the suction cup that may be applied to any draining sinus has eliminated the need for multiple dressings in many instances, and it has also added greatly to the comfort and emotional well-being of the patient. Modern, efficient methods of intermittent irrigations have helped to decrease odors, as has also the practice of using screw tops for drainage bottles. There is little danger of tubes being pulled from the bottles and of urine being spilled on the floor now that bottles are hung in a rack from the bed. Early ambulation of patients with permission for tub bathing or showers has also been helpful in control of odors on the urologic ward.

Deodorants are often useful in the home if adequate equipment is not available. Oil of pine sprayed on dressings is helpful, and a mild chlorine solution is an excellent deodorant to use in washing equipment, floors, and the like. It is irritating to the skin, however, unless an exceedingly mild solution is used. A few drops of chlorine solution such as common laundry bleach may be used in the home to destroy odors in clothing.

The older person may need assistance and unobtrusive supervision of his personal hygiene. If he is not sufficiently well instructed, he may finger his dressings and may need attention to such details as washing his hands. Many patients who have had surgery such as a cystotomy believe that a bath or a shower is not possible. They must be reassured that a complete bath is a safe procedure. Showers and bathing at odd hours should be discouraged because of the danger of accidents. If the patient is feeble, his need for assistance should be anticipated.

In all urologic wards, there should be an established routine for getting patients out of bed since this helps to prevent pneumonia, emboli, decubitus ulcers, and calculi. This important part of their care should not be overlooked in the busy day. Many times the patient feels so tied down with complicated tubing that getting up does not seem worth the effort. The nurse can and should encourage the patient to be up each day. She must see that the drainage tube is not leaking and that the drainage bottle is convenient. In some urologic divisions, bottles that are easily carried are provided, and patients are taught how to use them when out of bed; 250-ml. intravenous solution bottles or medicine bottles are satisfactory for this purpose. The patient can suspend this small bottle from a belt about his waist or to a binder if he is wearing one, which enables him to move about freely and not feel conspicuous.

Older patients may pull their catheters out of place. They may be confused or may not hear clearly and therefore not realize the importance of leaving drainage equipment undisturbed. It is necessary to explain clearly the temporary nature of catheters and the reasons that they are being used. Hand restraints should not be used unless all other methods of control have failed and then only upon the specific order of the physician.

Occupational therapy is helpful to distract the patient's attention from the annoyance of an indwelling catheter. It is also worthwhile in many instances to place the patient in a ward where he can talk with other patients. Provision should be made for the urologic patient to be out of bed a good deal of the time both preoperatively and postoperatively. A sufficient number of bathrobes should be provided and a supply of warm slippers unless the patients have their own shoes and socks. Shoes give firm support to the feet, and it has been found that older people are less likely to stumble when shoes are worn instead of soft slippers. Consideration must be given to the clothing, heating, and ventilation habits to which the patient has been conditioned throughout life.

In addition to internal irrigation, drugs may be given to combat existing infection and occasionally to prevent infection when a catheter is used. Some of these drugs include methenamine mandelate (Mandelamine) in doses of 1 gm.

four times a day, calcium mandelate, a salt of mandelic acid, in doses of 3 gm. four times a day, and nitrofurantoin (Furadantin) in doses usually of 50 mg. four times a day. Toxic signs of all these drugs are nausea and vomiting. Furadantin should always be given after meals and the fourth dose accompanied by some food to lessen the chances of nausea occurring. Sulfonamide drugs such as sulfisoxazole (Gantrisin) and antibiotic drugs may also be prescribed.

When a catheter has been removed, special attention must be given to voiding. The time and amount for each voiding must be recorded, as well as any discomfort before or during voiding and any abnormality in appearance of the urine. Occasionally a catheter must be reinserted if the patient is not yet able to void normally.

DIAGNOSTIC PROCEDURES

The general condition of most patients is thoroughly appraised before surgery is done. The nurse assists in the diagnostic procedures that are necessary. There are few urologic emergencies if treatment can be started before the symptoms become acute. Such procedures as electrocardiograms, liver function tests, and tests of blood for clotting and bleeding time may be performed, besides the specific tests for condition of the urologic system. Any signs of general weakness or reaction of the patient to diagnostic procedures of any kind or to treatment should be reported at once. Aged patients have become completely exhausted as a result of extensive preparation for procedures such as the taking of intravenous pyelograms. It is necessary to know what procedures the patient is receiving and to be certain that he receives food and fluid as soon as possible. Older people do not tolerate dehydration and starvation as well as young adults.

The nurse should explain diagnostic tests to the patient and should inform him of what his contribution to their success can be. For example, often the hospitalized patient is up and about, which enables him to void in the bathroom when specimens of urine may need to be collected. He may take food in ignorance when he should have nothing by mouth if he has not been instructed carefully so that he understands and remembers the instructions given. He must be told when and why fluids are to be restricted or withheld, and also when they are forced, as for kidney function tests such as urine concentration and dilution tests. One patient believed he was being helpful by refilling his own water pitcher when it had been emptied by the nurse without explanation.

The exact procedure for diagnostic tests varies with the hospital. It is well for the nurse to check instructions carefully before she disposes of any urine and also before food and fluids are served, since these tests may extend over several hours. Spoiling a test entails considerable inconvenience to the patient and, in fact, to all others concerned.

Urography. Intravenous pyelograms, or more correctly, urograms, are often ordered taken for diagnostic purposes. Some urologists depend upon this test for elderly patients instead of ordering a catheterization. Much of the same information—for example, the amount of distention of the bladder—can be determined by this means and it obviates the danger of the serious complications of catheterization.

Usually a cathartic is ordered the night before the test is made; in the x-ray department a radiopaque material (an organic compound containing a relatively large amount of iodine such as Urokon) is given intravenously. It is extremely important that pertinent information about the patient be reported to the physician, particularly if the patient has a history of sensitivity to iodine or has had asthmatic attacks. Sudden fatalities have followed intravenous injections.

Cystoscopy. Cystoscopy examinations are necessary in many urinary tract diseases. This procedure may be particularly exhausting to the aged patient, and he may react to cystoscopy with chills and high temperature, especially if the urinary tract is infected. Cystoscopy reaction may be due in part to apprehension as well as to pain. Much of this can be averted by careful explanation of each step of the procedure by the nurse so that it will not be unfamiliar to the patient. Responsibility for this explanation should be assumed by the nurse on the ward since the patient may be fearful of asking questions of the clinic nurse whom he knows less well, and there is little time for satisfactory explanations in the cystoscopy room. Forcing the necessary fluids before the patient goes to the cystoscopy room will reduce the time required for the procedure. For example, ureteral samples of urine will be obtained much more quickly if adequate fluids have been taken. It is also important that any drug such as morphine be given at the time ordered so that it will have time to take effect before the cystoscopy examination is started.

The cystoscopy table is hard and uncomfortable. A small, soft pillow placed lengthwise under the shoulders may give comfort, and a small pad under the lumbar spine helps to prevent fatigue. The shoulder braces should be well padded since the bony prominences of the older patient are easily traumatized. A warm bath blanket should be spread under the patient as he is placed on the table. Ties and knots should be removed from the back of the gown since these may be uncomfortable. If the patient must remain on the cystoscopy table for an unusually long period, the nurse should remove his legs, one at a time, out of the stirrups for a few moments and straighten them. This will help to prevent discomfort and joint stiffness and improve circulation. Following cystoscopic procedures, fluids are forced, urinary output is checked, and warm tub baths may be given for perineal discomfort. Analgesic medication is rarely necessary.

OPERATIVE CARE

A diet high in protein is usually ordered preoperatively. It is the responsibility of the nurse to note whether the patient can take the diet and to see that meat and other protein foods are in ingestible form if his ability to chew is limited. Blood transfusions and intravenous dextrose or protein solutions may be given preoperatively. When these are given, their purpose should be explained to the patient.

If possible, surgery is not performed until blood protein is approximately normal and/or urinary output has reached around 1,500 ml. per day, with a daily intake of 3,000 to 4,000 ml. of fluid, and/or until existing infection has cleared.

The nurse can be of assistance in preparing the patient emotionally for surgery. She may be able to tell him in more detail than the surgeon's time will permit what he may expect. For example, a preoperative patient may be greatly disturbed to see the drainage from another patient who has recently returned from the operating room. Metal shields or holders may be used to cover the drainage bottles, but even then the ambulatory preoperative patient may encounter some disturbing sights. He may ask if the patient with the bright blood in the drainage bottle had the same operation that he is scheduled to undergo. The nurse could explain that it is usual to have some blood in the drainage and can point out that the drainage is greatly diluted, hence gives the erroneous appearance of containing more blood than is actually there. Many questions that the patient may ask could be safely answered by the nurse, though additional reassurance and specific information about his particular operation must be given by the surgeon, from whom the patient receives his most satisfying encouragement. All questions or misinterpretations relating to potency must be referred to the surgeon at once for further explanation. The patient who is to have a radical operation may benefit from talking to another patient who has adjusted to this operation. In any case the nurse can show him equipment that will be necessary for his rehabilitation and can outline the teaching he will receive.

Postoperatively, the complications that must be watched for in addition to renal failure and poor drainage of urine are hemorrhage, infection, embolism, pneumonia, and mental confusion. Gantrisin is the drug most often ordered to combat infection since it is more soluble and more easily excreted than the other sulfonamides. All complications are described in urologic nursing texts.[9, 11] They are more likely to occur in the aged and are more difficult to deal with than in younger patients. Pneumonia, emboli, and mental confusion are best combated by getting the patient out of bed as soon as possible—often on the day of operation. Some urologists believe that cardiac failure, severe uncontrolled hemorrhage, or shock are the only contraindications to getting the patient up almost immediately.

Hemorrhage may occur following prostatectomy, heminephrectomy, or other urologic operations. Blood pressure should be taken at frequent intervals following surgery since low blood pressure may indicate hemorrhage that is occurring within the body cavity and thus is not apparent. The drainage tubing and drainage bottle must be watched carefully for frank blood. Transfusions are given when necessary. The patient who sees blood in his drainage tube is anxious and needs frequent reassurance from the nurse. If a real hemorrhage is occurring, the patient should not be left alone even for a few minutes. The doctor must be notified at once, and the patient is urged to lie quietly and not watch the drainage tube. Morphine should be given at once if there is an order to cover its use.

Continued suprapubic drainage. Some urologic patients must have suprapubic cystotomies for long periods of time, or even for the rest of their lives. Nursing of the elderly with these urologic problems differs only in that often it is more difficult. The patient may, for example, have visual limitations or poor neuromuscular control that make it difficult for him to change dressings or otherwise care for himself, and he may have no close relatives who are available to help him.

DISEASES OF THE PROSTATE

The most common diseases of the prostate gland are benign hypertrophy and cancer. Occasionally, inflammation of the prostate (prostatitis) accompanies hypertrophy, and this can lead to widespread infection. Occasionally, hemorrhage from varicosities of the large veins of the prostate gland occurs.

Benign hypertrophy. Benign hypertrophy of the prostate is so common that some authorities believe that it is present in about 75 percent of all men over 40 years of age. The cause is unknown although it bears some relationship to the involutional changes of later life. Unfortunately, many men with signs of prostatic enlargement, such as frequency of micturition and difficulty in initiating the urinary stream, put off seeing the doctor until symptoms are severe and damage to the kidneys has occurred. Benign hypertrophy responds poorly to glandular therapy, and the best treatment is surgical removal of a portion of or the entire gland. There was a time when hypertrophy of the prostate presented a threat to the life of an elderly man. Now it is possible to operate with favorable outcome, even upon men who are in their nineties.

Operations for this condition are of four kinds—the suprapubic, retropubic, perineal, and transurethral prostatectomies. The operative procedure is selected for each patient, considering the nature and extent of his lesion, his general condition, and other factors. Although no one type of procedure can be said to be preferable for the aged patient and the perineal route is now widely used, transurethral resection involves no external incision and is sometimes less of a shock to the patient than other procedures. Furthermore, early ambulation is generally feasible and comfortable. However, good supportive treatment has made the other types of operative procedures equally safe for aged patients when they seem most suitable.

Spinal anesthesia is often used for prostatectomy operations. This may be supplemented with thiopental sodium (Pentothal Sodium) or with an inhalation anesthetic. Care is taken to give only enough of the spinal anesthetic to prevent sensation at the operative site, yet not enough to produce blood pressure changes. Many skilled urologists feel that more important than the actual time in surgery is the amount of blood loss, amount of trauma, and other factors. Effort should be made to measure the amount of blood lost during the operation, and, if the amount is excessive, a transfusion should be given either during or immediately after the operation to replace the blood volume lost.

When the patient goes to the recovery room or to his own room, it is important that drainage be connected immediately and that the amount and character of the drainage be recorded. Fluids are forced. When the catheter is removed, the patient is placed on "time and amount" to determine whether urination has been restored to normal.

Cancer of the prostate. Cancer of the prostate has been found in 14.1 percent of a group of males studied at autopsy. It has been found in 21 to 37 percent of a group of males above the age of 65, and its incidence is known to increase with advancing age.[1] In one study 61 percent of prostatic cancer was found to be associated with benign hypertrophy. Cancer of the prostate usually begins in the posterior portion of the gland and consequently may not produce symptoms until the disease is advanced and extension to the paraurethral parts of the glands and elsewhere has occurred. Routine rectal examinations of all men over 40 years of age would reveal some of these lesions long before they are now found. If the disease is diagnosed early, the treatment is complete excision of the gland with its surrounding capsule, the posterior urethra, and the seminal vesicles, through a perineal incision. If the condition is far advanced, the treatment is palliative and consists of a transurethral removal of obstructing tissue and the administration of estrogens, which seem to have an inhibiting effect on malignant cells. The drug most often given is diethylstilbestrol in doses of 5 mg. daily. Orchiectomy is done alone or in conjunction with administration of estrogens in selected cases since this, too, decreases the growth and activity of the malignant cells in most cases. Radiation as a curative measure has not been of much value, but x-ray treatment is used sometimes to produce atrophy of the prostate. Radiation of painful metastatic areas is often good palliation. Cancers of the prostate in the aged are usually slow-growing adenocarcinomas. Even if it is impossible to remove all of the carcinomatous tissue, palliative treatment may give relative comfort for years.

EXTRAPROSTATIC UROLOGIC DISEASES

Cancer of the bladder. Carcinoma of the bladder occurs more often in men than in women and is a fairly common cancer of old age. It usually begins as a lesion on the inner surface of the bladder wall. If it is left untreated, the lesion may develop into a papilloma that may undergo malignant change, developing roots that spread deep into the bladder wall. Often the first sign of the growth is a painless hematuria. The commonly employed treatment when malignant changes have taken place is complete surgical removal of the affected portion of the bladder, with or without transplantation of the ureters, depending upon the location of the lesion. If the lesion has progressed so that complete removal of the bladder is necessary, the ureters may be transplanted either to the abdominal skin or to the colon, provided that the patient has good control of the anal sphincter. Infection and sloughing of the wound or of the ureters from their new attachment are possible; strictures of the transplanted ureters may also occur. The patient needs alert and expert nursing care. More recently a procedure in which a portion of the ileum with its blood supply is resected is sometimes used, and this serves as a new bladder to which the ureters are anastomosed (ileo-bladder). An opening is then made from the new bladder through the abdominal wall to the exterior.

If the ureters are to be transplanted directly into the colon, the patient should have thoughtful explanation of the consequences of the operation to him as an individual. Many patients cannot visualize the rectum being able to accommodate the urine produced. They do not realize that the rectum is capable of distention, and they fear it will require emptying at extremely frequent intervals. If the man hopes to return to work, many uncertainties arise. For example, will the other men with whom he works know that he must sit down to void? Will his company be willing to reemploy him with the inconveniences that may be present? Assistance in meeting such questions may add immeasurably to the ultimate rehabilitation and return of the patient to society as a useful member.

If the patient must go to a hospital for the chronically ill or to an institution for the aged, he still has many questions. Will the institution take him with his irregular new habits? Unfortunately, many homes for the aged and convalescent homes do not admit the patient who requires any special attention such as care of tubing, bottles, or dressings. It is most important that the patient begin to care for his own special needs as soon as he is able. This adds to his feeling of self-sufficiency and makes him a much better candidate for placement in a suitable institution.

There is always the danger of recurrence of malignant growths. The patient must be encouraged regarding his future, yet urged to report to the clinic as directed and to report immediately any further difficulties. The family may be advised by the surgeon not to anticipate too much from the operation in terms of complete and certain cure, depending, of course, upon the findings at the time of operation.

Calculi. The formation of primary or new renal calculi is rare in the aged. Those who have had renal calculi prior to the old-age period may have recurrence in old age, particularly persons who have failed to follow a prescribed medical regimen. Calculi develop sometimes as a result of inactivity. Because of the lessened elasticity and muscle strength of the tissues of the ureters, renal calculi are passed less readily than in younger persons and may become lodged in the ureters. They are dangerous because the obstruction they produce may put too severe a strain upon kidneys already limited in their ability to excrete waste products. The infection so commonly associated with calculi is less readily combated by the older person. Large calculi in the kidney pelves may be removed surgically. If the obstruction is in the ureter, a ureterolithotomy may be done. After the operation the patient usually has a good deal of pain and may believe that he cannot move because of the tube, which is uncomfortable. He must, however, turn or be turned frequently. He can be made more comfortable by the use of rubber-covered pillows to support him toward the operative side to facilitate drainage yet prevent pressure on the tubing. The drainage and the dressings must be carefully watched for the amount of drainage and for the appearance of blood.

Vesical calculi in the bladder are intimately associated with infection and obstruction. They are often found in elderly men who have prostatic enlargement. Fairly large stones may be passed through the normal urethra. Larger stones may sometimes be crushed through the cystoscope in the litholapaxy operation. Very occasionally a suprapubic cystotomy must be done.

Infections. Urinary infections are common in the aged. They are most often associated with or caused by obstruction, calculi, and tumors. Tuberculosis is much less frequent as a cause in the old than in the young. Emphasis in treatment is upon internal irrigation, as described earlier in this chapter, and upon the use of specific antibiotics. Forcing fluids and careful recording of intake and output are important nursing functions in the care of these patients. It is also important that the nurse be on the alert for early signs of overhydration in the event that the cardiovascular system is unable to cope with all the fluids taken.

Stress incontinence. Stress incontinence or the involuntary loss of urine under relatively normal conditions such as coughing, straining, laughing, or distending the bladder is an extremely common urologic condition in elderly women. In fact, it is estimated that 5.5 percent of all adult women have poor urinary control, and almost every elderly woman has stress incontinence to some extent since it is associated with relaxation and poor tone of the related structures.[5]

The elderly woman who has stress incontinence should be urged to seek medical attention since improvement in the condition can sometimes be achieved and thus enable her to live a happier and more normal life. The urologist first attempts to distinguish true stress incontinence from incontinence from other causes such as neurologic disease or upper urinary tract involvement.

Stress incontinence is sometimes treated surgically by various operations intended to restore relaxed structures to their normal position; the results from these operations are varied. Quite remarkable improvement has been reported from the use of exercises that were first identified and prescribed by Kegel and are therefore known as Kegel exercises. The patient is taught to consciously contract the muscles involved and by so doing strengthen them. Occasionally, exercise against resistance by using a resistometer is also prescribed. The patient needs encouragement since the exercise regimen is a tiresome one that must be conscientiously adhered to for a long period of time. If treatment is not successful, the patient can often be helped to care for herself so that she can mingle with others and lead a fairly normal life. Details of care are described in basic nursing texts.[11]

REFERENCES AND RELATED BIBLIOGRAPHY

1. Campbell, Meredith F.: Urology, vols. I, II, and III, ed. 2, Philadelphia, 1963, W. B. Saunders Co.
2. Ceccarelli, Frank E., and Smith, Perry C.: Studies on fluid and electrolyte alterations during transurethral prostatectomy, J. Urol. **86**:434-441, 1961.
3. Chute, Richard: Preoperative and postoperative care of aged patients undergoing urological surgery, J.A.M.A. **148**:184-187, 1952.
4. Heckel, Norris J.: Diseases of the bladder, the prostate and the urethra. In Stieglitz, Edward J. (editor): Geriatric medicine, ed. 3, Philadelphia, 1954, J. B. Lippincott Co.
5. Kegel, Arnold H.: Physiologic therapy for urinary stress incontinence, J.A.M.A. **146**:915-917, 1951.
6. Mossholder, Irene B.: When the patient has a radical retropubic prostatectomy, Amer. J. Nurs. **62**:101-104, 1962.
7. Krug, Elsie E.: Pharmacology in nursing, ed. 9, St. Louis, 1963, The C. V. Mosby Co.
8. Murphy, John J., and Schoenberg, Harry W.: Urologic aspects. In Cowdry, E. V. (editor): The care of the geriatric patient, ed. 2, St. Louis, 1963, The C. V. Mosby Co.
9. Sawyer, Janet R.: Nursing care of patients with urologic diseases, St. Louis, 1963, The C. V. Mosby Co.
10. Scott, Roger B.: Common problems in geriatric gynecology, Amer. J. Nurs. **58**:1275-1277, 1958.
11. Shafer, Kathleen Newton, and others: Medical-surgical nursing, ed. 3, St. Louis, 1964, The C. V. Mosby Co.
12. Walsh, Michael Adrian, Ebner, Marion, and Casey, Joseph William: Neobladder, Amer. J. Nurs. **62**:107-110, 1963.
13. Wasmuth, Carl E., and Higgins, Charles C.: Anaesthesia for the aged and poor-risk candidates for genito-urinary surgery, Geriatrics **10**:100-104, 1955.

Chapter 26

Nursing in gynecologic disorders

In gynecologic nursing, more than in any other part of geriatrics, the nurse is needed in case finding and intelligent referral of patients. The nurse is frequently consulted about some problem of a gynecologic nature that the patient may be reluctant to discuss with her family or her physician. Years of discomfort from chronic ailments could be prevented in many instances by medical intervention. Many deaths from cancer might be avoided if all women over 35 years of age had regular, complete pelvic examinations including cytological smears (Papanicolaou, or pap smear). Yet physicians are often confronted with elderly women suffering from malignant disease conditions that have spread widely.

There are several reasons why gynecologic disease may go untreated. Fear of cancer is one of them. The fear of cancer, even more pronounced in the elderly than the young, makes the individual put off seeking what may be bad news, makes her shut her eyes to obvious physical findings rather than face whatever eventuality may be in store. Some elderly women hesitate to submit to pelvic examination because of embarrassment at the thought of having the genital area exposed. Another reason for failure to seek medical aid is that many women accept discomfort dating from obstetrical trauma as a natural aftermath of having children. With age and relaxation of tissues, the condition becomes worse; yet they assume that added discomfort is part of growing old and must be endured. Some believe that they are too old to have an operation. They have no conception of the surgical skill now developed, of surgery that can be done under local anesthesia, or of the supportive measures available. The nurse by her understanding, her knowledge, and her optimism can encourage patients to seek treatment that may add to their enjoyment in living.

In addition to the effect of decreased hormonal influence on tissues, the older woman is affected by atrophic changes in the genital system that are part of general aging. Although hormones may stimulate growth in youth, there is no evidence that their use retards senescence. Neither can hormones provided artificially compensate for the gradual loss of the body's own resources. The rate of physical change from these causes varies considerably with individuals and usually is gradual. Reabsorption of subcutaneous fat and general atrophy of the external genitalia occurs. The labia lose tone and become smaller, pubic hair becomes scanty, and mucous membranes may become pale, thin, and dry. The vaginal wall becomes shrunken, particularly at the introitus; the rugae become flattened, and sometimes adhesions form within the vaginal canal. A smaller amount of vaginal secretion is produced and this becomes less acid and therefore less effective in inhibiting bacterial growth. The cervix becomes more fibrous, and the uterus may revert to adolescent size and become firm and fibrous. Ligaments and other supportive tissues may lose tone so that good support for structures sometimes is lacking.

The cessation of menstruation and beginning of slow atrophy of structures do not mean that sexual activity must cease. Gonadotrophic hormones from the pituitary gland that stimulate follicular activity at puberty continue to produce estrogenic hormones in small amounts after ovarian output of hormone ceases. This production accounts in part at least for the very gradual progress of the physical changes. For many women, normal libido and participation in sexual activity persists beyond 65 years of age. There is a very wide variation in sexual interest and activity in both men and women in the older age group. It is probable that this is affected by hormonal influences, psychological reactions, relationship to spouse, and other factors.

Some conditions related to menstruation and to its cessation occur in elderly women. Although it is estimated that only 10 percent of women have true menopausal syndrome, a large percentage have some marked emotional response to the climacteric, and for a few this may persist into the time of late maturity. Acute menstrual disorders no longer occur, but vaginal bleeding is seen occasionally following administration of estrogens, which may be prescribed for a number of difficulties such as severe depression, vaginitis, and osteoporosis. The patient receiving estrogens usually is warned by the doctor that vaginal bleeding may occur lest she fear cancer, which, however, is not ruled out by the fact that the patient is receiving estrogens.

Gynecologic conditions occurring quite often in elderly women include disorders of the vulva, vaginitis and dyspareunia, perineal herniation including rectocele, cystocele, and partial or complete prolapse of the uterus, carcinoma anywhere in the genital system, and benign fibroids in the uterus. A few general aspects of the nursing care of these conditions will be considered before a brief description of the diseases and their treatment and care are discussed.

GENERAL NURSING

Appreciation of the emotional problems of the gynecologic patient is important for nurses. Normal women (and men) derive satisfaction from the features, qualities, and characteristics that make them distinctly feminine (or masculine). Experts in the study of emotional adjustment in age point out that the longer that aging people can retain these distinctive features, the more satisfactions will be had, and the happier they will be. Many women who value their femininity sharply resent the withering changes that come with age. Even after the childbearing period is over, they are reluctant to permit operations entailing the removal of the uterus or ovaries. When a mutilating operation such as an amputation of the vulva appears necessary, the psychic reaction may be severe. Understanding care with this in mind may help to prevent postoperative emotional disturbances.

Fear of cancer haunts a large percentage of older women, particularly those who are being treated for some gynecologic ailment. Without giving direct information, the nurse should give reassurance if this is possible. She should report the marked fears and apprehensions of the patient to the doctor so that his reassurance may be given.

It must be remembered that many elderly women are quite unfamiliar with hospitals and their routines. Many had their children at home and have never been subjected to questionings in large and open wards. Provision should be made for histories to be taken in private, even if this means placing the patient in her bed in another room for the time of the history taking. The patient should be carefully draped, and the doctor should be ready to do the pelvic examination as soon as she is prepared since the position on the examining table is particularly uncomfortable for the older person. Complete, kindly, and matter-of-fact explanations should precede each step of the preparation for any treatment and the care following any treatment.

Preoperative care. It is important that the patient void immediately prior to surgery. For certain operations catheterization and the instillation of methylene blue into the bladder are necessary before surgery. Many operations are performed under local anesthesia. The preparations used for anesthesia are described in Chapter 13, Anesthesia and Operative Care. It is most important that the patient who is placed in Trendelenburg position for gynecologic surgery have a small pillow under the lumbar region. The patient in the lithotomy position should be so placed that the pull on the legs is not excessive and back strain is prevented. Leg holders should turn upward and outward, and the patient's hips should never be lifted off the table by the pull on her feet in the stirrups.

Postoperative care. Unless special precautions are taken, emboli may occur after pelvic surgery. Surgeons differ in their orders for mobilization, but the nurse may expect the patient to be out of bed in one or two days following major surgery. Before she is permitted up, the patient must be urged to take deep breaths at regular intervals, to cough, and to move about while in bed. Unless cardiac complications are present, the nurse should encourage the patient to move herself since active exercise is much more beneficial than passive exercise. The prognosis is poor if embolism occurs. Nursing emphasis should be on the prevention of phlebothrombosis and hence of pulmonary embolism. All elderly patients should be observed closely for pain in the leg or thigh that might indicate the development of phlebothrombosis. If the patient has pronounced varicosities of the lower extremities the doctor may order that Ace bandages be applied before she gets out of bed. Some surgeons advocate that the limbs be raised at intervals postoperatively to drain the blood from the leg veins. If symptoms of thrombosis do occur, the patient should be urged not to exercise or rub the limb, and the doctor should be notified at once. The nurse should never minimize any complaints of pain on walking. Thrombosis may not be apparent until the patient walks for the first time after the operation.

It is imperative that distention of the bladder be prevented postoperatively, and often a catheter (Foley catheter) is inserted and left in the bladder for a few days. When it is removed the time and amount of voiding is recorded carefully. No patient should be permitted to go over eight hours without catheterization if normal voiding is impossible. Some surgeons order catheterization every four to six hours, depending upon obvious distention of the bladder and complaints of discomfort by the patient. The patient should void within four to six hours after surgery and every four hours thereafter. This is especially important in the care of patients who have had perineal repairs of any kind.

Following most pelvic surgery, no effort is made to have the patient have a bowel movement for three to seven days. Mineral oil may be given each night, starting on about the third day postoperatively. If no bowel movement occurs in three to five days, an oil retention enema usually is ordered.

NONMALIGNANT DISEASES

Pruritus vulvae and vulvitis. Pruritus of the vulva is a relatively common and extremely troublesome condition. There are many causes, including atrophy of tissues, sugar in the urine, uncleanliness, vaginal, rectal, or urethral infection, allergy, trauma, and psychogenic factors. Vulvitis is believed to be primarily the result of atrophic changes in the tissues that lead to inflammation. Irritation from this, often aggravated by scratching and subsequent contamination from a variety of organisms, can lead to pronounced infection that is difficult to cure.

Treatment of pruritus vulvae is directed toward removal of the cause if it can be determined. Hydrocortisone ointment, 1 percent, has been found extremely useful and is prescribed widely for both pruritus and vulvitis. Systemic estrogen therapy and local irradiation are of little or no value. If itching continues to be severe and other treatment fails, the pudendal nerve may be resected. Occasionally alcohol, 95 percent, is injected subcutaneously at numerous points over the perineum, and this treatment may give relief for several months.

Conservative treatment of pruritus vulvae and vulvitis often produces surprising improvement. This includes the administration of small doses of sedatives such as phenobarbital or chloral hydrate or one of the ataractic drugs, sitz baths, and the careful avoidance of trauma. The patient should be instructed to wear the softest of undergarments with no constriction on the perineum. Frequent bathing is advised, but soap should be avoided and the area should be patted dry and not rubbed. Some physicians advise the use of mineral oil for cleansing.

Kraurosis vulvae. Kraurosis vulvae is shrinkage of the skin and subcutaneous tissues more than is consistent with normal physiologic atrophy. It rarely leads to cancer. The labia and clitoris may almost disappear, and shrinking of tissues may interfere with urination and with sexual function. Estrogen therapy may be helpful, but does not cause return of tissues to normal. Hydrocortisone ointment is often used. Irradiation is of no value. Treatment is surgical excision of troublesome strictures and vulvectomy in severe cases that do not respond to treatment with hydrocortisone.

Vaginitis. Following the menopause the walls of the vagina atrophy somewhat, Döderlein's bacilli, which are found in the vagina in large numbers during the reproductive years, may disappear, and the vaginal secretions are no longer acid in reaction. These circumstances appear to encourage mild vaginal infections that may become chronic and difficult to cure. Vaginitis may cause bleeding and the formation of adhesions in the vagina and may produce a discharge that is irritating to the mucous membrane and to the outer surrounding skin. Adhesions may also form about the urinary meatus and the introitus.

Vaginitis often responds well to estrogen therapy. Diethylstilbestrol (usually 0.1 mg. daily) in a vaginal suppository may be ordered, or an estrogen such as Premarin may be ordered to be taken by mouth. Improvement of symptoms is often reported within a few days, although treatment usually is continued for several months or indefinitely. It is important to instruct the patient with vaginitis to avoid douching unless she is ordered to specifically, since douching may dilute the already limited natural secretions. Douches with mild acid solutions such as vinegar, however, are often ordered by the doctor and in some cases may be the only treatment that is required. Fungus infections may complicate the problem if a low bacterial count in vaginal secretions has followed administration of antibacterial drugs. Careful cleansing of the perineal area with water and a very mild soap after excretory function will help to prevent irritation and further infection. Sitz baths are also often ordered.

Dyspareunia. Dyspareunia or painful intercourse is fairly common in elderly women. Usually it is associated with vulvitis, kraurosis vulvae, or chronic vaginitis. It occurs most often in women who have not borne children. The elderly woman who mentions this problem to the nurse should be encouraged to seek medical care, since response to treatment is often excellent. The condition is treated by giving small doses of estrogens such as diethylstilbestrol or Premarin. Estrogens may be given locally as suppositories or systemically by mouth. Occasionally, surgical excision of adhesions is necessary.

Tissue changes after complicated surgery or radiation treatment for a malignant lesion of the vagina, vulva, or adjacent tissues may cause dyspareunia. In such cases estrogen treatment is of little value.

Perineal herniation. Perineal herniation may include rectocele, cystocele, and partial or complete prolapse of the uterus. The term *procidentia* is used when prolapse of the uterus is complete. Perineal herniation is common in elderly women, usually when the patient has had children; but occasionally prolapse occurs in the nullipara. The condition is often the result of stretching and tearing of structures at the time of delivery, though symptoms may not appear until the involutional changes of age take place, and supportive structures are less effective. Symptoms are a dragging, pulling sensation in the lower abdomen and low back, incontinence, frequency or incomplete emptying of the bladder, and feeling of a mass in the vagina. Pain in the low back is frequently named as a symptom of a gynecologic condition when in reality it may often be from faulty posture and body mechanics.

Treatment depends a great deal upon the extent of the herniation and upon the age and general health of the patient. Rectoceles have little tendency to become worse with age, and often their repair can be done surgically under local anesthesia. Cystoceles are more difficult in that they tend to increase with age, and often urinary involvement occurs. Surgical repair is often relatively simple and is usually the best treatment for the older woman. Treatment for prolapse of the uterus is usually a vaginal plastic operation in which the cervix and fundus of the uterus may or may not be removed.

Postoperative care and treatment vary with the surgery and with the individual patient. Often the patient may be permitted out of bed immediately, and tub baths may be ordered. If the patient remains in bed, she may be instructed to lie with the legs somewhat abducted in order that free circulation of air may have access to the perineum. External perineal care may be ordered once or twice each day, and a light and cradle may be used if any tendency to sloughing of sutures is apparent. Extreme caution must be exercised not to burn the patient if a light is used. The bulb should never be more than 25 watts and should be placed at least 12 inches from any skin surfaces. If the patient cannot be relied upon to lie quietly while the light is being used, she must be attended constantly.

A retention catheter that may be drained at regular intervals to stimulate normal bladder filling and emptying may be left in place for several days. Intermittent bladder irrigation is sometimes ordered, and about 200 ml. of physiologic saline solution is used every four hours, and fluids by mouth are forced.

The use of pessaries dates back to pre-Christian times. With the improvement in operating techniques and in preparation for surgery, usually they are now resorted to only if the patient refuses surgery. Plastic material usually is used. The Gellhorn pessary is by far the most widely prescribed for the elderly patient. If the pessary cannot be removed by the patient, she must report to the doctor regularly for careful examination to detect pressure or irritation to the supported tissues. If the pessary is to be removed by the patient, she must have careful instruction in douching if it is ordered and in removal and care of the pessary.

Tampons are extremely unsatisfactory supports for uterine prolapse and are used only for extremely old and debilitated patients who cannot tolerate surgery and who are unable to wear a pessary. Tampons must be changed at least twice each day, and vaginal douches are usually ordered when they must be used.

MALIGNANT DISEASES

Leukoplakia. Since at least 50 percent of cancer of the vulva is accompanied by leukoplakia, it is usually considered a precancerous condition. Leukoplakia is characterized by shiny, thickened, white patches on the labia, clitoris, and fourchette. Extreme pruritus often accompanies leukoplakia, and estrogenic therapy yields no benefit. Because of the tendency of leukoplakia to become cancerous, complete vulvectomy is usually performed. Operation may be done under local anesthesia in extremely old and debilitated patients. Leukoplakia is an extremely difficult condition to treat and may recur along the margin of the surgical excision. Dilute hydrochloric acid is often given since many persons with leukoplakia have achlorhydria. Large doses of vitamin A are given. Cod-liver oil may be given by mouth and applied locally as an ointment, and ointments containing vitamin A and vitamin B are also used. Pyribenzamine ointment and hydrocortisone ointment have given quite remarkable relief in some instances. Radiation therapy is occasionally employed, but is generally considered to be unsatisfactory.

Carcinoma. Any vaginal bleeding after the menopause should be considered as caused by cancer until proved otherwise. The nurse cannot emphasize too greatly the necessity for investigation of any bleeding no matter how slight it may be. No further signs may appear until the lesion is far advanced and perhaps inoperable. Increase in vaginal discharge or leukorrhea is also significant and indicates the need for thorough medical examination. One study[11] showed that approximately 60 percent of a group of women past the menopause who had vaginal bleeding were suffering from cancer somewhere in the genital tract.

Carcinoma of the vulva is fairly common in older women and should be suspected when any lesion on the external genitalia occurs. The treatment is radical vulvectomy, with excision of the inguinal nodes. Carcinoma of the vagina is extremely rare.

Carcinoma of the cervix occurs most often around the time of the climacteric, but many cases are reported in the age interval after 60 years. Prevention by routine physical examination and treatment of conditions that may predispose to the development of cancer are important. Trauma to the cervix at childbirth may predispose to the development of cancer; therefore either cauterization, excision, or other treatment of lacerations and erosions of the cervix is performed.

There is no unanimity of opinion as to the ideal treatment of cancer of the cervix. Treatment varies with the extent of the lesion, the general condition of the patient, and the preference of the surgeon. Radiation therapy is used widely in some centers, while others tend to use extensive surgical procedures more often. Surgery may be followed by radiation therapy.

The incidence of cancer of the endometrium is highest in the sixth decade of life. The disease may occur in the absence of fibroids or may, occasionally, develop from fibroids that have persisted for years. Most gynecologists believe that every woman with postmenopausal bleeding should have a curettage, that smears (Papanicolaou) should be studied, and that a biopsy of any suspicious lesion should be obtained. Benign fibroids of the uterus tend to diminish in size after the menopause; if they do not do this, it is believed generally that a hysterectomy is advisable. This is because malignant changes may be occurring even though the endometrium has not yet been invaded so that the results of examination by smears (Papanicolaou) and curettage would be negative.

Treatment for malignancy of the uterus consists of total hysterectomy and bilateral salpingo-oophorectomy. This may be preceded by radiation therapy. Occasionally, when it is not given preoperatively, radiation may be used postoperatively. Radiation alone may be used, and in this case curettage is done first, and then the radioactive substance in a tandem and colpostat such as shown in Figure 56, or needles containing a radioactive substance such as radium or irradiated cobalt, is inserted into the uterus and left a specified time, depending upon the dosage ordered and the material used. The care of patients receiving this treatment is described in basic nursing texts.[9]

Carcinoma of the ovary is fairly common in older women. The only hope for control is early diagnosis, every woman having yearly or six-month pelvic examinations during which palpation of the ovaries is done. In most instances, metastasis has occurred before diagnosis is made. Malignant changes in the ovaries

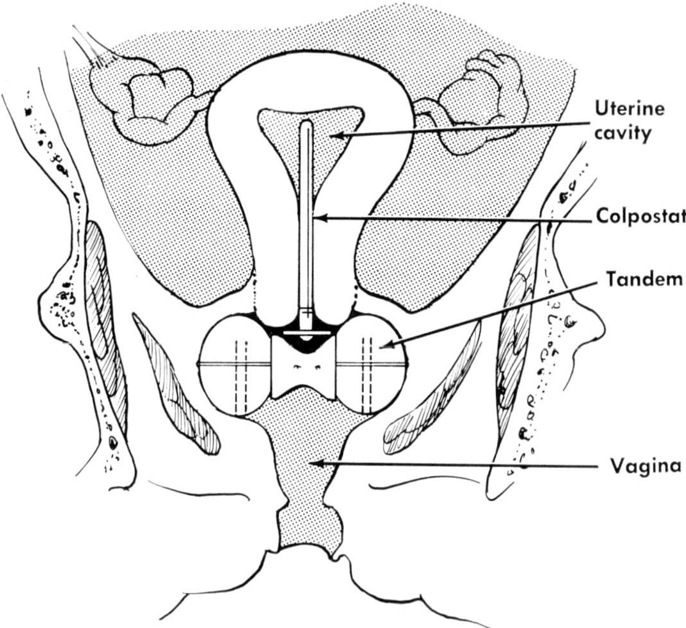

Figure 56. Schematic drawing showing a tandem and colpostat being used in radiation treatment of the cervix and body of the uterus. (From Schafer, K. N., and others: Medical-surgical nursing, ed. 3, The C. V. Mosby Co.)

may cause uterine bleeding and other irregularities. Cancer of the ovary is often suspected if vaginal bleeding occurs when there is no other known cause, such as the administration of estrogens, when no cervical lesion is found, and when curettage fails to reveal any abnormality in the uterus. Unfortunately, unexplained enlargement of the abdomen due to ascites in far advanced disease may be the first sign of trouble.

Treatment of cancer of the ovary consists of radiation or surgery or a combination of these. If metastasis has occurred, the patient usually has to return to the hospital outpatient department or to the doctor's office at intervals for paracentesis to remove fluid accumulated in the abdominal cavity. Radioactive gold (Au^{198}) may be instilled into the abdominal cavity.

Nursing care when radiation treatment is used. When radiation material has been placed in the uterus, cervix, or vagina, the elderly patient must be watched very carefully. She may become confused and may attempt to alter the position or remove the radioactive material and she may not understand or remember the instructions to lie quietly for the time that it is being used. There is danger of severe injury to surrounding structures if rays are permitted to focus on normal tissues. A mild laxative followed by cleansing enemas may be ordered to ensure the bowel being empty when treatment is started. Usually a catheter is inserted into the bladder, the vagina is packed with gauze, and the patient is instructed to lie very quietly. The amount of activity is determined by the doctor and depends upon the material being used and its stability in its location. In some cases the patient may be out of bed, while in others even spreading the legs wide apart in bed would be contraindicated. Any special problems the patient has, such as back stiffness, and the nursing measures that are helpful should be recorded on the nursing care plan or other equivalent place to aid all who give nursing care to the patient.

Transportation may be a real problem for patients who must come to the hospital for radiation treatment or for dressings. Social services should be called upon to assist patients who cannot afford suitable transportation. A public health nurse in the community may help the patient to plan for assistance so that she does not travel to or from the treatment center alone, and she may assist her to care for herself in many other ways. Careful scheduling of treatment so that patients will not be fatigued by long waiting helps to ensure continuance of treatment.

Radiation therapy may cause adhesions that interfere with the patency of the cervical opening; infection in the fundus of the uterus (pyometra) may follow. Adhesions may also form at the urinary meatus. Women who have had treatment, particularly of the vulva, should be instructed to report any difficulty in voiding in order that retention of urine with its attendant complications of infection, kidney destruction, and formation of vesical calculi will not occur.

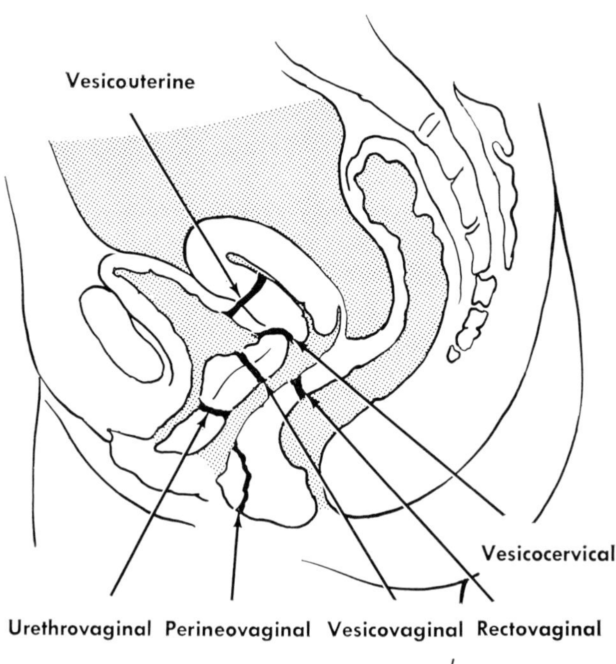

Figure 57. Types of fistulas that may develop in the uterus and vagina. (From Shafer, K. N., and others: Medical-surgical nursing, ed. 3, The C. V. Mosby Co.)

The patient usually is instructed by the doctor to report at regular intervals following treatment and to report any signs of infection or of abnormality in voiding.

A variety of fistulas, including vesico-vaginal and rectovaginal fistulas, may occur in advanced malignancies of the uterus and related structures (see Figure 57). They may also be quite rare but extremely distressing complications of radiation treatment. These conditions are often difficult to treat and can be of long duration in elderly women. The complicated nursing care involved is described in current nursing texts and periodicals.[9, 10]

Certain patients with cancer of the cervix or the uterus that has eroded to the bladder may be treated by means of radical excision of the uterus, the tubes and ovaries, the cervix, the bladder, and surrounding tissues. The ureters are transplanted to the rectum if the rectal sphincter is good. If the rectum is pathologically involved, a resection of the bowel may also be done with a permanent colostomy, and the ureters may then be transplanted to the abdominal wall, with an external opening through which the urine drains. Some patients get along very well with ureteral transplants to the rectum, provided that the malignant lesion has been completely excised and controlled. The rectum is able to distend sufficiently to accommodate urinary secretions with relatively little difficulty, though it first may be necessary for the patient to empty the rectum at frequent intervals. If a permanent colostomy has been necessary and the ureters are transplanted to the abdominal wall, the patient faces a tremendous adjustment. The nurse can be most helpful in this period by her prompt attention to change of dressings and to frequent change of drainage tubes or bottles. It is imperative that the patient be kept as clean and odorless as possible in the early period when emotional adjustment is most difficult.

Odors present a nursing problem in caring for the patient with advanced carcinoma of the genital tract. Frequent perineal or vaginal douches are helpful if the lesion is of the vulva or if much vaginal discharge is present. Potassium permanganate is useful as a douche and "phenol and menthol compound," containing phenol, menthol, boric acid, and alum, is also helpful. Oil of pine needles is useful, and trade preparations containing chlorophyll (Air-Wick) are acceptable to some patients as room deodorants. Sodium hypochlorite, one tablespoon to a pint of water, is a good disinfectant and a valuable deodorant. Chlorine solutions such as common laundry bleaches are useful in washing solutions to destroy odors on equipment. Thorough rinsing should follow their use, and they should not be put directly on the skin.

Pain may be severe and prolonged in carcinoma of the genital tract. Some physicians fear the miseries of drug addiction in addition to pain of the disease and therefore restrict narcotic drugs. Others believe that narcotic drugs should be given freely in increasing doses, as needed. Alcohol injections are sometimes effective in controlling pain for days and even weeks. Endocrine treatment has been found to be of little value. Rhizotomy and cordotomy procedures are often helpful in alleviating pain in uncontrolled malignancy (Chapter 16, Nursing in Neurologic Disorders). The nurse can help alleviate pain suffered by the terminally ill patient by her cheerfulness and by her genuine, kindly interest and willingness to do seemingly simple things that help make the patient attractive and comfortable. Such details as combing the hair attractively, using gay hair ribbons, giving a manicure, a careful bath, and the like, help to make the pain and discomfort of advanced malignancy more endurable.

REFERENCES AND RELATED BIBLIOGRAPHY

1. Bieren, Roland: Vaginitis in older women, Geriatrics **8**:429-433, 1953.
2. Brewer, John I.: Textbook of gynecology, ed. 3, Baltimore, 1961, The Williams & Wilkins Co.
3. Cinberg, Bernard L.: Management of descensus uteri in the aged, Geriatrics **3**:151-156, 1948.
4. Crossen, Robert James, and Campbell, Ann Jones: Gynecologic nursing, ed. 5, St. Louis, 1956, The C. V. Mosby Co.
5. Davis, M. Edward: Gynecology of senescence and senility. In Stieglitz, Edward J. (editor): Geriatric medicine, ed. 3, Philadelphia, 1954, J. B. Lippincott Co.
6. Grollman, Arthur: Disorders of the endocrine system. In Johnson, Wingate M. (editor): The older patient, New York, 1960, Paul Hoeber, Inc., Medical Book Department of Harper & Row, Publishers.
7. Hofmeister, Frederick J., Reik, Robert P., and Anderson, Nancy Jane: Vulvectomy; surgical treatment and nursing care, Amer. J. Nurs. **60**:666-668, 1960.
8. Scott, Roger B.: Common problems in geriatric gynecology, Amer. J. Nurs. **58**:1275-1277, 1958.
9. Shafer, Kathleen Newton, and others: Medical-surgical nursing, ed. 3, St. Louis, 1964, The C. V. Mosby Co.
10. Volk, William L., and Foret, John D.: The problem of vesicovaginal and ureterovaginal fistulas, Med. Clin. N. Amer. **43**:1769-1777, 1959.
11. Zeman, Frederic D., and Davids, Arthur M.: Gynecologic surgery in the elderly patient with special reference to risks and results, Am. J. Obst. & Gynec. **56**:440-446, 1948.

Index

D